Essentials of Medicine and Surgery for Dental Students

CHURCHILL LIVINGSTONE DENTAL SERIES

A Manual of Paedodontics
Second edition
R. J. Andlaw and W. P. Rock

Aids to Oral Pathology and Diagnosis
Second edition
R. A. Cawson

Clinical Pharmacology in Dentistry
Fifth edition
R. A. Cawson and R. G. Spector

Essentials of Dental Surgery and Pathology
Fourth edition
R. A. Cawson

Notes on Dental Materials
Fifth edition
E. C. Combe

Anatomy for Students of Dentistry
Fifth edition
A. D. Dixon

An Introduction to Removable Denture Prosthetics
A. A. Grant and W. Johnson

Occlusion in Restorative Dentistry
Technique and theory
M. D. Gross and J. Dewe-Mathews

Essentials of Pathology for Dental Students
W. Lawler, A. Ahmed and W. J. Hulme

Clinical Anatomy for Dentistry
R. B. Longmore and D. A. McRae

Dental and Maxillofacial Radiology
J. McIvor

Principles and Practice of Orthodontics
Second edition
J. R. E. Mills

Introduction to Dental Anatomy
Ninth edition
J. H. Scott and N. B. B. Symons

Principles of Pathology for Dental Students
Fourth edition
J. B. Walter, M. C. Hamilton and M. S. Israel

Basic and Applied Dental Biochemistry
Second edition
R. A. D. Williams and J. C. Elliott

Essentials of Medicine and Surgery for Dental Students

A. C. Kennedy
MD, FRCP (Lond., Edin. and Glasg.), FACP (Hon.), FRACP (Hon.), FRSE
Muirhead Professor of Medicine,
University Department of Medicine,
The Royal Infirmary, Glasgow

L. H. Blumgart
BDS, MD, FRCS (Eng., Edin. and Glasg.)
Professor of Surgery and Director,
The University Clinic for Visceral and Transplantation Surgery,
Inselspital, Bern, Switzerland

G. D. O. Lowe
MD, FRCP (Edin. and Glasg.)
Senior Lecturer,
University Department of Medicine,
The Royal Infirmary, Glasgow;
Director, West of Scotland Haemophilia Unit, Glasgow

J. R. Anderson
MB, FRCS (Edin.)
Senior Lecturer,
University Department of Surgery,
The Royal Infirmary, Glasgow

FIFTH EDITION

CHURCHILL LIVINGSTONE
EDINBURGH LONDON MELBOURNE AND NEW YORK 1989

CHURCHILL LIVINGSTONE
Medical Division of Longman Group UK Limited

Distributed in the United States of America by Churchill
Livingstone Inc., 1560 Broadway, New York, N.Y. 10036,
and by associated companies, branches and representatives
throughout the world.

Third edition 1977
Fourth edition 1982
Fifth edition 1989
  Reprinted 1992
First two editions published under the title *Essentials of
Medicine for Dental Students* by A. C. Kennedy

ISBN 0-443-04087-7

British Library Cataloguing in Publication Data
Kennedy, A. C. (Arthur Colville)
  Essentials of medicine and surgery for dental students.
  1. Man. Diseases & injuries
  I. Title
  616

Library of Congress Cataloging-in-Publication Data
Essentials of medicine and surgery for dental students/A.C. Kennedy
  . . . [et al.]. — 5th ed.
    p. cm. — (Churchill Livingstone dental series)
    Rev. ed. of: Essentials of medicine and surgery for dental
  students/A.C. Kennedy, L.H. Blumgart. 4th ed. 1982.
    Includes index.
    1. Internal medicine.   2. Surgery.   3. Dental students.
  I. Kennedy, A. C. (Arthur Colville)   II. Series.
    [DNLM: 1. Dentistry.   2. Medicine.   3. Surgery.   WB 100
E785]
  RC46.K53   1989
  616'.00246176 — dc19
  DNLM/DLC
  for Library of Congress   88-30256
                                                            CIP

The
publisher's
policy is to use
**paper manufactured
from sustainable forests**

Produced by Longman Singapore Publishers (Pte) Ltd
Printed in Singapore

Preface

In 1960 one of the authors (A.C.K.) published the first edition of *Essentials of Medicine for Dental Students*. The reception accorded to the book indicated that it was of value to dental students in Glasgow and throughout the country and it became quite widely used.

When faced with the question of producing a third edition in 1977 a decision was made to incorporate the elements of surgery, and in that year a volume combining the essentials of medicine and surgery for dental students was written by two of us, A.C.K. and L.H.B. It is relevant to note that L.H.B., in addition to being a practising surgeon, is also qualified in dentistry. In that edition we expressed our hope that the work would prove acceptable to dental students and would provide them with the essentials of medicine and surgery necessary for their studies. The sales of the book indicated that it clearly met a need and a reprint was required in 1979/1980, and a fourth edition in 1982.

The fifth edition has been thoroughly revised and updated by G.D.O.L. and J.R.A., who currently teach dental students in Glasgow. A new chapter on hepatitis B and immunodeficiency viruses and the control of cross-infection in dentistry has been added, in view of the major importance of these infections in recent years.

The original intention to present a simplified account of the various medical and surgical disorders has been maintained. Many of the details which are required by the doctor for the actual practice of medicine or surgery are omitted and in particular details of management which are firmly within the realm of medical, as opposed to dental, practice. The description of many of the diseases is, of necessity, incomplete but as before we have tried to avoid statements which are incorrect. Disorders such as facial pain, haemophilia, swellings about the face, and surgical conditions related to the mouth are dealt with at rather greater length since the dentist should have a full knowledge of such matters.

The majority of the chapters and sections open with a brief description of the relevant anatomy and physiology, as we have found, in the course of teaching, that most students welcome a brief refresher in these pre-clinical subjects. Line drawings, tables, and illustrative clinical photographs and X-rays are included throughout the text. It is our belief that these will be of considerable value and interest to the student.

Lastly, it is a pleasure to record the help given to us by the publishers.

Glasgow and Bern, 1989
A.C.K.
L.H.B.
G.D.O.L.
J.R.A.

Contents

1

Diseases due to infection — medical aspects

GENERAL CONSIDERATIONS

Infection of man with pathogenic microorganisms has been an extremely important cause of disease since antiquity but it is only within the last hundred years that we have gained precise knowledge regarding the causal agents. Bacteriological knowledge has been followed by truly remarkable advances in the prevention and treatment of the infectious disorders and, in consequence, several diseases, which were previously widespread, have been almost eliminated from many countries, e.g. diphtheria, or even more remarkably, as in the case of smallpox, eliminated throughout the world. Despite such striking achievements there is still much to be done; this is especially so in the tropical and semitropical areas of the world but it is also true in the temperate zones. Indeed, having regard to the laws of nature, it is almost certain that man will never be free from the risk of infection with pathogenic organisms, although he may possess increasingly effective remedies. This is illustrated by the recent epidemics of hepatitis B virus and human immunodeficiency virus (HIV) in western countries (see Ch. 2).

In this chapter a brief account will first be given of some general principles applicable to all the infectious diseases and this will be followed by a description of several of the commoner diseases grouped according to the causal organism. Those infectious diseases which produce effects predominantly on one organ or system of the body are dealt with under that system.

Pathogens and commensals

According to their ability to produce disease in the human, the microorganisms may be grouped as follows:

1. Active pathogens which almost invariably cause disease when they gain access to the body in sufficient numbers unless the individual has a high degree of natural or acquired immunity.

2. Commensals which multiply on the skin and mucous membrane surfaces of the body, and within the body (e.g. in the intestines), without causing damage.

The division into these two groups is, however, not a rigid one and many commensals are capable of causing disease under certain circumstances. Thus the pneumococcus, which is usually present in the normal flora of the mouth and throat, may cause bronchopneumonia if the resistance is lowered by diseases such as measles or influenza. Another example of a potential pathogen is the production of subacute bacterial endocarditis by the usually harmless *Streptococcus viridans*.

Results of infection

Infection of the tissues of the body with pathogenic organisms is not necessarily followed by recognizable disease. The outcome depends on the balance between the resistance of the individual and the intensity of the infection. Factors favourably influencing resistance are natural immunity from previous contact with the organism, artificial immunity as a result of prophylactic vaccination, etc., and a satisfactory state of the general health and nutrition. Factors influencing the intensity of the infection are the number of organisms concerned, their virulence which is not a constant for any given species, and the portal of entry. Depending on the resultant of these various factors there may be produced:

1. A subclinical infection.
2. A clinical infection, of varying severity, but with recovery.
3. A clinical infection which proves fatal.

Sources of infection

The infection may be derived from the excreta of cases or carriers of the disease, both human and animal.

An important factor favouring the spread of infection from cases is the high infectivity of many of these diseases in the earliest stages, often before a diagnosis has been reached and preventive measures and treatment instituted. Spread of the upper respiratory tract infections, such as the common cold, is facilitated by the widespread custom of continuing one's ordinary activities during the illness.

A *carrier* is an apparently healthy individual who harbours a pathogenic organism. In some instances this follows a clinical attack of the disease, but in others this is not so. One example is the typhoid carrier who may excrete pathogenic organisms in the faeces and urine for several years and be responsible for many cases of typhoid particularly if engaged in the preparation or handling of food. Hepatitis B and HIV infection are usually transmitted by the blood of asymptomatic carriers, or from mother to baby, before they develop symptoms (see Ch. 2).

Modes of transmission

A healthy individual may become infected with pathogenic organisms in the following ways:

1. By *direct contact* with someone suffering from the disease, e.g. the venereal diseases, impetigo.

2. By *contact with some intermediate object* such as improperly sterilized syringes, needles, and other instruments, and common articles of cutlery and crockery.

3. By *airborne transmission* of the organisms. Many organisms are sprayed into the atmosphere during speaking, coughing and sneezing, and they may remain airborne, in fine droplet form, for considerable periods and thus be inhaled by several individuals. Even after the droplets have dried the risk is not over, for the fine particles of dust which are formed may contain resistant organisms such as the tubercle bacilli. Airborne transmission is the principal mode of spread in many of the common infectious diseases of childhood, e.g. measles, whooping cough.

4. By *ingestion* of infected food and water. This may be responsible for large-scale outbreaks of typhoid fever, bacillary dysentery, and cholera.

5. By *vectors* including the house fly, which is responsible for the mechanical transmission of many organisms, the body louse (epidemic typhus) and the mosquito (malaria).

Prevention and control

The principal measures employed to prevent and control the infectious diseases may be grouped as follows:

1. *Isolation of cases* is vitally important in the highly infectious disorders such as cholera and dysentery. Isolation used to be standard practice in Britain for the majority of children suffering from the common infectious diseases such as measles, scarlet fever, etc., and many special hospitals were built for this purpose. Due to the wide-scale use of immunization, the reduced virulence of some of the organisms, the improvement in living standards, and the introduction of the antibiotics, these diseases are now much less frequent and less dangerous. Isolation is still carried out in the occasional cases of diphtheria which occur but otherwise hospital admission is usually necessary only when the home circumstances are very unsatisfactory, or the attack is particularly severe.

2. Detection and treatment of *carriers*.

3. Maintenance of a *clean water and food* supply, and control of sewage.

4. Control of *vectors* such as flies, lice, and mosquitoes.

5. The production of *active immunity* in vulnerable individuals by the use of vaccines and toxoids. A vaccine is a preparation of killed or attenuated bacteria or viruses which retain their antigenic properties, i.e. stimulate the production of antibodies, but are no longer capable of producing disease. A toxoid is a toxin artificially modified so that it is no longer poisonous but remains antigenic.

Prophylactic immunization is now widely practised and in Britain it is usual to advise immunization of young children in the first year of life against diphtheria, tetanus, pertussis (with the so-called triple vaccine), and poliomyelitis. Immunization against measles, mumps and rubella is now offered at age 1–2 years, and rubella immunization is offered to girls aged 11–13 years not previously immunized. Live vaccines should not be given without expert advice to patients with immune deficiency, i.e. HIV infection (see Ch. 2), or during treatment with immunodepressant drugs. Under such circumstances the organism may cause widespread disease. Immunization against many other diseases is also available and may be required in the special circumstances of war or in the tropics — e.g. against typhoid and paratyphoid fever, cholera, and yellow fever.

6. *Passive immunity*, which is short-lived, may be conferred on susceptible individuals before or just after infection has taken place, by the injection of gamma globulin containing antibodies to the organism concerned. Examples are hepatitis A and B, tetanus, rabies, and antivaricella zoster which is offered to immunodeficient persons exposed to varicella zoster virus.

It may be noted in passing that the infant has a natural passive immunity, of some months' duration, to many infectious diseases, derived from the transplacental passage of antibodies from the mother during intrauterine life.

Clinical features

Many of the infectious diseases have clinical features in common. The onset is usually sudden after an incubation period ranging from a day or two to several weeks, but which is relatively constant for a given organism. In general, the patient feels unwell, has a poor appetite, may vomit, has a coated tongue, a rapid pulse, and an elevated temperature. A lesion may be present at the portal of entry of the organism. In several instances, skin rashes occur and these may be sufficiently distinctive to be of diagnostic value. Symptoms otherwise largely depend on the localization of the organism, e.g. in the liver in cases of infective hepatitis, or in the lung in lobar pneumonia.

A leucocytosis develops due to a polymorpho-nuclear increase in the bacterial infections and there is an increase in lymphocytes in viral infections.

VIRAL INFECTIONS

Viruses are the smallest microorganisms known to cause disease. Electron microscopy is necessary for their visualization. As far as is known, they multiply only within living cells. Certain viral infections such as poliomyelitis and chickenpox produce a long-lasting immunity whereas in others such as the common cold and influenza, the immunity is, unfortunately, short-lived since new strains develop.

Among the more important viral diseases are the common cold, influenza, poliomyelitis, hepatitis, infectious mononucleoses, measles, German measles, mumps, chickenpox, herpes zoster, and HIV infection.

Measles (*morbilli*)

The incubation period of measles is 10 days to the onset of the first symptoms, and 14 days to the development of the rash. It is spread by droplet infection.

The illness starts with an upper respiratory tract infection and, during this stage, the child appears as if he has an extremely severe head cold. In addition, the conjunctivae are usually infected ('pink eye'), while examination of the buccal mucosa at this stage will reveal the presence of Koplik's spots which are small, whitish-grey spots set on an erythematous base. They are most often seen along the line of closure of the molar teeth. After three or four days a blotchy, purplish rash develops particularly on the face and trunk; it is often first apparent behind the ears. In most cases fever lessens and the rash begins to fade in a further three or four days.

The main complications are secondary bacterial infection spreading to the middle ear (otitis media), and bronchopneumonia, both of which are less frequent and serious since the introduction of antibiotics. Encephalitis may also occur.

Gamma globulin derived from the plasma of individuals who have had measles may be used to give passive immunity to exposed, immunodeficient persons for whom an attack of measles might be particularly dangerous. Vaccination with an attenuated virus is offered to children age 1–2 years.

German measles (*rubella*)

The incubation period is two to three weeks after droplet infection.

It is usually a relatively mild febrile illness associated with rhinitis, tender enlargement of the cervical lymph glands, and a transient rash which is often maximal behind the ears. Koplik's spots do not occur.

The condition is of little importance except in pregnant women. If infection occurs in the first four months of pregnancy, it may cause congenital heart disease and other defects in the offspring. Hence immunization is offered to children in the second year of life; to nonimmunized girls aged 11–13 years; and also to women found to have no antibodies to rubella during pregnancy, who are offered vaccination *after* delivery to protect them in further pregnancies.

Mumps (*epidemic parotitis*)

The incubation period of mumps is two to three weeks, after droplet infection.

The characteristic feature is tender swelling of the parotid glands with inflammation of the orifice of the duct. Occasionally the other salivary glands are also involved.

The main complications of mumps are inflammation of the pancreas (pancreatitis) and the testes (orchitis). These are more liable to occur in adults. Meningitis and encephalitis may occur.

There is no specific treatment for mumps. A fluid diet is usually required until the acute parotid swelling subsides. Oral hygiene is important. Vaccination with an attenuated virus is now offered to children aged 1–2 years.

Chickenpox (*varicella*)

This is caused by a herpes virus (varicella zoster virus, VZV) which has an incubation period of two to three weeks. It is spread by droplet infection or by skin contact with the blisters.

The infection usually causes relatively little general upset. The characteristic feature is the occurrence of many small blisters, or vesicles, filled with a clear fluid, on the skin, particularly of the trunk, and on the mucous membranes. The lesions are superficial, intensely itchy, and they occur in successive crops. Secondary infection of the vesicles may occur due to scratching and may cause small permanent scars. Encephalitis is a rare complication.

The principal object of treatment is to prevent scratching and secondary infection of the vesicles. A vaccine is available in the USA but is not yet licensed in Britain.

Herpes zoster (*shingles*)

The virus of herpes zoster is identical to that of chickenpox and the illness may occur in those in contact with chickenpox, and vice versa. It has a predilection for the posterior nerve roots particularly those of the trunk and for the fifth cranial nerve. The condition is always unilateral.

The infection starts with three or four days during which the individual feels unwell, has mild fever, and experiences pain, which is often severe, in the sensory area of the affected posterior nerve root. A red rash then develops along the sensory distribution of the affected nerve followed by the occurrence of small vesicles filled with a clear fluid. These vesicles usually last for about one week and if secondarily infected they may leave a permanent scar. The discomfort and pain produced by the vesicles is often extreme. If the ophthalmic division

Fig. 1.1 Herpes zoster of the ophthalmic divison of the fifth cranial (trigeminal) nerve.

of the fifth cranial nerve is involved (Fig. 1.1) the lesions may occur on the eye causing corneal scarring with resultant impairment of vision. After the condition has cleared there may be persistent pain in the affected area. Postherpetic neuralgia is more common in the elderly (see also Ch. 18).

The vesicles should be kept dry and free from infection and analgesics are given to relieve pain. If immunodeficient patients are exposed to VZV, they should be offered passive immunization with human VZV immunoglobulin. When the infection develops in such patients, antiviral drugs are given — acyclovir or vidarabine, by intravenous infusion. Antiviral drugs may also be given for zoster infections in normal people; they may shorten the duration of symptoms if started as early as possible, but are expensive. Oral acyclovir or topical idoxuridine may be used.

Herpes simplex

This is another herpes virus which causes painful ulcers on the lips (see Ch. 9), genitals or cornea. Encephalitis is a serious complication, and generalized infection occurs in the immunosuppressed. Such persons are treated with intravenous acyclovir. Acyclovir cream or tablets may be prescribed by dentists for oral herpes of the lips and mouth respectively, and should be started as early as possible. Clinical dental staff have transmitted herpes simplex to patients.

Smallpox (*variola*)

This is due to a herpes virus with an incubation period of about 12 days. Smallpox used to be common in Britain and in the Middle Ages it is said that a woman could lay some claims to beauty if she possessed a skin unblemished by its ravages. The prefix 'small' was used to distinguish it from the 'great' pox, syphilis.

There is a short prodromal stage of malaise and fever followed by an extensive rash which is at first papular, then vesicular, and then pustular. The great majority of the lesions occur at the one time and not in successive crops as in chickenpox. They are maximal on the peripheral parts of the body, e.g. the face and the distal parts of the limbs. The pustules rupture, or dry up, with the formation of scabs; when

these separate they may leave very disfiguring scars. The mortality rate is considerable in severe infections.

In the late eighteenth century Jenner, an English country doctor, noted that persons who had been infected with a rather similar illness affecting cows (cowpox) either did not develop smallpox, or at least got it in a mild form. This inspired clinical observation led to vaccination (inoculation of the skin with the cowpox virus, vaccinia) and a subsequent marked reduction of smallpox in countries where vaccination was widely practised.

This dangerous infection was eradicated from its only host, man, in the late 1970s.

The infectious mononucleoses

The infectious mononucleoses are caused by a group of three agents which may each produce a 'glandular fever' illness, usually in adolescents and young adults. During the acute infection, transformed 'atypical' lymphocytes appear in the peripheral blood, hence the name mononucleosis. All three agents usually cause a subclinical illness, especially in young children. Chronic latent infection may result, which may be reactivated or transmitted to others, usually by close contact (e.g. kissing) or occasionally by blood transfusion. Case-to-case clinical spread is uncommon. Patients with immunosuppression (e.g. HIV infection, see Ch. 2) may develop severe, generalized and fatal infections. In pregnant women, two of the three agents can cause fetal infection and disease.

Infectious mononucleosis

The Epstein—Barr virus (EBV) is a herpes virus. Clinical symptoms of this type of mononucleosis, which is the commonest, include fever, sore throat (often with a white exudate on the tonsils and small petechial haemorrhages on the palate), lymphadenopathy (especially the posterior cervical nodes), splenomegaly, skin rashes, and viral hepatitis (see Ch. 10).

The diagnosis is confirmed by presence of atypical lymphocytes on a blood film, and a characteristic heterophil antibody in serum, which agglutinates red blood cells of other species. The specificity of this antibody is shown by the Paul—Bunnell or Monospot tests.

Treatment is symptomatic, e.g. gargles and aspirin. If antibiotics are given for suspected streptococcal pharyngitis (see later), ampicillin and similar drugs should be avoided as there is a high risk of an allergic skin rash. A short course of corticosteroids may be given for severe pharyngeal oedema. Intrauterine infection and congenital disease do not occur.

Cytomegalovirus (CMV)

This is another herpes virus which can cause a similar glandular fever illness to EBV. Patients tend to be older (25–35 years), and viral hepatitis is more common. The Paul–Bunnell and Monospot tests are negative; there is a rise in antibodies to CMV in the serum. Treatment is again symptomatic.

Toxoplasmosis

This is due not to a virus but to an intracellular protozoon, *Toxoplasma gondii*, which is found in all mammals. Infection can occur by eating undercooked meat, or by contact with cat faeces (1% of cats excrete the cysts), either directly or from infected soil. Lymphadenopathy, fever and malaise are the main symptoms. The Paul–Bunnell and Monospot tests are again negative; there is a rise in Toxoplasma antibodies in the serum. Treatment is with the antibiotics spiramycin or co-trimoxazole for severe or protracted illness.

Infectious mononucleoses in pregnancy

In pregnant women, CMV and *T. gondii* can cause intrauterine infection and fetal abnormalities. No pregnant women should be exposed to patients with infectious mononucleosis-type illnesses, hepatitis, or HIV infection (see Ch. 2) in which generalized subclinical or clinical CMV infection is common. This applies to dentists and clinical dental assistants.

RICKETTSIAL, MYCOPLASMAL AND CHLAMYDIAL INFECTIONS

The *rickettsiae* are microorganisms which are intermediate between viruses and bacteria. They occur naturally in various arthropods, which act as vectors of infection.

Rickettsial infections are still widespread in many parts of the North American continent and in the Pacific area although their incidence has been much reduced by the use of insecticides to control the vectors. Examples are scrub typhus and Rocky Mountain spotted fever.

Epidemic typhus (gaol fever or camp fever). This is the most serious of the rickettsial infections. The vector is the human body louse, *Pediculus corporis*. Typhus was common in Europe until the end of the nineteenth century and was again a scourge in Russia and Eastern Europe during and shortly after the First World War. An outbreak in Naples during the Second World War was prevented from spreading by prompt application of strict hygienic measures. Chloramphenicol and tetracycline are effective remedies for rickettsial infections.

Mycoplasmas which may cause pneumonia (see Ch. 8) and *chlamydiae* which cause nongonococcal urethritis are similar to rickettsiae in that they are intermediate between viruses and bacteria, and are sensitive to tetracycline.

BACTERIAL INFECTIONS

The number of bacteria which are actively or potentially pathogenic to man is very large. They are usually grouped according to their reaction to Gram staining.

1. Gram-positive bacteria—streptococci, staphylococci, pneumococci, diphtheria bacilli, tubercle bacilli, tetanus bacilli, and gas gangrene bacilli (*Clostridium welchii*).

2. Gram-negative bacteria — gonococci, meningococci, *Bordetella pertussis*, *Escherichia coli*, members of the typhoid and dysentery group, *Vibrio cholerae*, and the plague bacilli (*Pasteurella pestis*).

Streptococcal infections

The haemolytic streptococci are very important pathogens responsible for several infectious diseases. In addition, an immunological reaction to streptococcal infection is generally considered to be the cause of rheumatic fever, chorea, and some cases of acute glomerulonephritis.

Penicillin has greatly facilitated the treatment of streptococcal infections.

Streptococcal sore throat. Infection of the throat (pharyngitis) with the haemolytic streptococcus is a common ailment. The infectivity is high and the incubation period short. It occurs more frequently in the autumn and winter months and affects particularly children of school age and young adults. Small epidemics may occur. Cross-infection may occur in the dental surgery.

The throat shows evidence of acute inflammation and is fiery red on inspection. The tonsils, if present, are enlarged and points of pus may be visible on the surface; in some cases a thin, yellowish membrane, which is easily removed, covers the tonsillar area. The cervical lymph glands are enlarged and tender. Constitutional upset shown by fever, tachycardia, malaise and leucocytosis is usually associated and, in severe infections, may be marked. Swallowing may be painful and difficult (dysphagia).

A throat swab should be sent to the bacteriology department to establish whether the infection is streptococcal or viral. Most cases of pharyngitis are viral (e.g. adenovirus, Coxsackie, Epstein–Barr virus) and cannot be distinguished from streptococcal infections clinically. Treatment of viral infections with antibiotics is wasteful and may have adverse effects (e.g. skin rashes). Confirmed streptococcal infection is treated with penicillin (or erythromycin in penicillin-allergic patients), which is effective in prevention of the complications (otitis media, rheumatic fever, chorea, glomerulonephritis).

The infection may cause an abscess in the tonsillar area (quinsy throat) requiring incision to permit drainage; this complication is now infrequent.

Scarlet fever (scarlatina). This is due to infection of the throat with strains of haemolytic streptococci which possess a toxin capable of producing a red rash in susceptible individuals. The disease is now much milder than it used to be and cases occur where the rash is slight or absent. The incubation period is a few days.

The essential clinical feature is acute inflammation of the throat as described under streptococcal tonsillitis. When present, the red rash is widespread but it does not involve the area around the lips which appears pale relative to the rest of the face (circumoral pallor). The tongue is thickly coated with a white fur in the early stages. Later this peels off leaving a red tongue with engorged papillae,

sometimes referred to as a strawberry tongue. Complications and treatment are as for streptococcal sore throat.

Erysipelas. This is a local infection of the skin with haemolytic streptococci. The incubation period is a few days.

The affected area is red, oedematous, has a raised border, and spreads rapidly. The face and legs are the commonest sites. *Cellulitis* is a similar spreading infection in the subcutaneous tissues (see Ch. 3). Treatment of erysipelas or cellulitis is with penicillin or erythromycin.

Impetigo. This is due to infection of the superficial layer of the skin with streptococci alone or in combination with staphylococci. It is most often seen on the faces of poorly cared for children who may also harbour head lice and have scabies.

The lesions commence as small vesicles filled with yellow pus which forms honey-coloured crusts or scabs. Impetigo is highly contagious.

The principal aspects of treatment are initial cleansing to remove the crusts, application of a topical antibiotic ointment which does not cause allergic reactions (e.g. fusidic acid) as indicated by a skin swab culture, and attention to the general health and hygiene.

Puerperal fever. Childbed fever, due to streptococcal infection of the raw lining of the uterus, used to be a dreaded complication in maternity hospitals and was responsible for many maternal deaths. Fortunately, it is now very rare.

Staphylococcal infections

Many of the infections due to staphylococci are essentially surgical problems and are dealt with in Chapter 3. Cross-infection may occur in the dental surgery.

Sycosis barbae (barber's rash). This is a staphylococcal infection of the hair follicles in the beard area in men. Numerous small yellow pustules develop and close inspection reveals that each is centred by a hair. The condition is very contagious but fortunately it usually responds to local antibiotic applications. The patient may have to stop shaving for a few days.

Diphtheria

This is another bacterial pharyngitis due to infection

with the *Corynebacterium diphtheriae*. The incubation period is short (two to seven days). Fortunately, the incidence of diphtheria has been greatly reduced following the widespread adoption of immunization of children with the toxoid in the first year of life. Despite the small number of cases now occurring, it is important that the immunization programme is maintained.

The child with diphtheria is usually extremely ill and toxic. Examination of the throat shows a grey-yellowish membrane covering the tonsillar area; the membrane is very adherent and, if it is forcibly removed, small bleeding points are left. The throat is not fiery red as in streptococcal infections. Enlargement of the cervical lymph glands is present.

Diphtheria is an extremely serious illness as the toxin produced by the organism may produce myocarditis and various forms of paralysis, the commonest being paralysis of the soft palate. Furthermore, the membrane in the throat may be so extensive as to obstruct the airway necessitating tracheotomy to prevent asphyxiation (see Ch. 3).

Suspected cases are hospitalized and given penicillin and diphtheria antitoxin as soon as possible.

Whooping cough (*pertussis*)

This is caused by the organism *Bordetella pertussis*. The incubation period varies from one to almost three weeks. It is spread by droplet infection and usually affects children under 5 years old.

The illness starts with what appears to be a severe upper respiratory tract infection, associated often with conjunctivitis. After a short period it is noted that the child is having paroxysms of severe cough with an inspiratory whoop at the end of each paroxysm. The whoop is due to forced inspiration through a glottis which is in spasm. Vomiting frequently occurs at the end of each severe paroxysm and, if this is prolonged, it may lead to serious malnutrition. The paroxysms of coughing may cause ulceration of the fraenum of the tongue.

Whooping cough may be complicated by bronchopneumonia and, in some instances, there is collapse of small portions of lung tissue with danger in the future of bronchiectasis.

Antibiotics are required if any of these respiratory complications occurs, but their efficacy is debated. Vaccination in the first year of life is valuable in prevention. Unfortunately, over-concern about its very rare association with encephalitis has decreased public acceptance of vaccination, and hence increased the incidence and fatality of this preventable disease.

Bacillary dysentery

This bowel infection is caused by a group of bacilli (*Shigellae*) which bear the names of some of the most distinguished bacteriologists (Sonne, Flexner, and Shiga). The incubation period is short. The usual mode of infection is by contamination of food and drink. Cases occur mainly in the tropics but it is also common in Britain. Serious epidemics were a scourge of many military campaigns in the past and there is an old reference to the disease as 'the bloody flux which decimated armies'.

The main features of the illness are colicky, abdominal pains associated with intense diarrhoea with blood and mucus in the stools, and a high fever. The condition is extremely infective. In severe cases there may be serious dehydration and shock.

Treatment involves rehydration with oral or intravenous fluids, and careful hygiene to avoid faecal−oral transmission. Antibiotics are usually not indicated unless septicaemia occurs, when intravenous antibiotics are given.

Typhoid and paratyphoid fever

Typhoid and paratyphoid fever, or the enteric fevers, are caused by bacteria of the Salmonella group which produce acute inflammation of the small intestine. The infection is transmitted in a similar way to bacillary dysentery, but in the first few days the microbes enter the bloodstream, from which they may be isolated.

There is a prodromal period of toxaemia and pyrexia before severe diarrhoea develops. At this stage rose-coloured spots occur on the trunk and the spleen becomes enlarged. After several days of extreme illness the temperature gradually falls. The main complications are perforation of the gut and intestinal haemorrhage.

Chloramphenicol has greatly improved the prognosis and ampicillin is also of value. Vaccination is recommended for visitors to high-risk areas.

SPIROCHAETAL INFECTIONS

The spirochaetes are elongated, spiral organisms which, although motile, do not possess flagella. The major systemic spirochaetal diseases are syphilis (p. 16), Weil's disease, yaws, and relapsing fever. Vincent's infection of the buccal cavity is due to the combined effects of fusiform bacilli and a spirochaete (see Ch. 9).

Weil's disease (*Leptospirosis icterohaemorrhagica*)

The usual mode of infection is contamination of minor skin abrasions with water to which rats, which are carriers of the spirochaete, have had access. Sewage workers are mainly affected. The disease is a serious one and is characterized by severe liver damage with jaundice and a tendency to haemorrhage. Cases of moderate severity usually respond to penicillin, but acute liver failure or acute renal failure may occur in severe cases.

FUNGAL INFECTIONS

The fungi are multicellular microorganisms often forming long branching filaments. Localized infections of the skin, such as athlete's foot, are quite common. Systemic fungal infections are rare in Britain but frequent in North America. However they are increasing in frequency with the spread of HIV infection (see Ch. 2).

Ringworm (*tinea*)

This is a general term which includes several varieties of localized infection of the skin and adnexae caused by closely related fungi.

One of the commonest sites is between the toes (athlete's foot) where the skin becomes thickened and sodden, small blisters develop, and an offensive odour results. This infection may secondarily involve the fingers and other parts of the body such as the groin.

Other varieties include ringworm of the scalp (tinea capitis) which causes scaly areas on the scalp associated with a patchy loss of hair, and tinea circinata characterized by reddish, ring-shaped lesions on the skin.

Actinomycosis

This is dealt with in Chapter 3.

YEAST INFECTIONS

The commonest yeast infection is with *Candida albicans*, which causes painful inflammation with white exudates (thrush) in the mouth (see Ch. 9), the vagina and urethra, or under the breasts in obese people. It is common after antibiotic therapy, in diabetes mellitus (see Ch. 15) or in the immunosuppressed. The antibiotic nystatin is effective.

PROTOZOAL INFECTIONS

Protozoa are unicellular parasites which are extremely important causes of disease in tropical and semitropical countries. The most important protozoal infections of man are malaria, amoebiasis, trypanosomiasis or sleeping sickness, and leishmaniasis or kala-azar. In western countries, *Trichomonas* is a common cause of vaginitis; and *Giardia lamblia* a common cause of gastroenteritis. Both respond to treatment with metronidazole. Recently *Pneumocystis carinii* has become the major cause of death in HIV infection, by producing a diffuse pneumonia (see Ch. 2). Cryptosporidiosis and toxoplasmosis are also common in such patients.

Malaria

This is caused by a protozoal parasite of the genus Plasmodium. The parasite has two stages in its lifecycle, one being passed in the mosquito and the other in the red blood cells and reticuloendothelial system of man.

The classical feature in benign tertian malaria, which is one of the common forms, is recurring bouts of fever occurring every 48 hours. At the start of each bout the individual feels intensely cold, has a rigor, and experiences aching in the muscles; he then becomes extremely hot and the temperature rises quickly; the third stage is that of profuse sweating with fall of temperature; thereafter he usually falls into a sleep. Enlargement of the spleen is a characteristic finding. In chronic cases anaemia develops.

The traditional drug used in the treatment of malaria is quinine, but there are now also many synthetic preparations, such as primaquine and chloroquine available both for the treatment and prophylaxis of malaria. The main step in the eradication of the disease is control of the mosquito and, in particular, destruction of its breeding grounds.

Amoebic dysentery

This is caused by a protozoan parasite known as the *Entamoeba histolytica*. The illness is usually less acute than bacillary dysentery. Diarrhoea, weight loss, and pyrexia occur. There is a tendency for chronic infection to be established in the bowel and for spread to occur to the liver, producing amoebic hepatitis or amoebic abscess.

The main therapeutic agents are metronidazole and chloroquine.

METAZOAL INFECTIONS

The metazoa are multicellular, invertebrate animals, several of which are parasitic to man.

Examples which may be seen in western countries are threadworms and tapeworms. Other parasitic worms of great importance include schistosomal infection of the intestine and bladder which is common in the Middle East, fluke infection of the liver and lungs seen especially in the Far East, and hydatid disease caused by the larval stage of the tapeworm *Echinococcus granulosus* which is encountered particularly in Australia.

Threadworms

Infection of the gut with threadworms is quite common in western countries especially in children. The adult worms measure about 1 cm in length and are actively motile.

No symptoms are produced by the presence of the worms in the gut, but the female worm emerges from the bowel at night to lay eggs in the perianal region and this causes intense local itching. The fingers of the individual commonly become infected with the eggs due to scratching and subsequent reinfection through the mouth is common. Threadworms are popularly believed to cause children to grind their teeth at nights but it is doubtful if this is so.

The main steps in treatment are improved hygiene to prevent reinfection and the use of a drug which has a lethal action on the worms.

Tapeworms

The beef tapeworm, *Taenia saginata*, is a more common intestinal parasite than the pork tapeworm, *Taenia solium*. Infestation arises from eating undercooked meat or pork which contains the worms in cyst form. The worms lodge in the small intestine, being attached to the mucosa by a row of suckers on the head, and may grow to many feet in length. Ripe segments, which contain eggs, become detached from the terminal portion of the parasite and are passed with the faeces. Treatment consists in the administration of drugs which have a toxic action on the worm.

THE ARTHROPODS

The arthropods are a special group of metazoa including flies, fleas, lice, the parasite of scabies, spiders, and scorpions. They may cause disease in man by transmitting infection, by parasitic infestation, or by injection of poisons.

Lice

Only the head louse, *Pediculus capitis*, and the body louse, *Pediculus corporis*, will be described.

The head louse is most likely to be seen in the hair of ill-cared for children and adults. The ova, or nits, are small white oval objects firmly attached to the hairs by a special cement. The adult lice are larger, flat, and mobile. The ova hatch within one week and mature in two weeks so multiplication takes place at a great rate. Head lice produce considerable irritation of the scalp, and secondary infection of the resultant scratch marks is common; chronically infested individuals, however, appear able to harbour vast numbers of lice without discomfort.

The body louse, which is rather larger than the head louse, lives on non-hairy skin and usually chooses the seams of clothes as a site for depositing the ova. Irritation of the skin leads to scratching, excoriation, and secondary infection. The body louse is of great importance in the transmission of typhus.

Proper hygiene is the main factor in the prevention of louse infestation. Ova may be removed from the hair by the use of a fine comb dipped repeatedly in weak acetic acid which loosens the cement. Malathion, applied locally, is an effective insecticide for the adult lice.

Scabies

Scabies, which is caused by a parasite known as the *Acarus scabiei*, is spread by close contact. The female acarus burrows under the horny layer of the skin to lay its eggs. The small tell-tale burrows are seen especially around skin folds such as between the fingers, at the wrists and the axillae and groin. Scabies causes intense itching, especially at night, and scratch marks and secondary infection are commonly present. Benzyl benzoate ointment, applied liberally to the whole body after hot baths, is a common remedy. Clean clothes and improved hygiene are indicated.

TUBERCULOSIS

Incidence

Tuberculosis has been known since the earliest days of medicine and has been variously termed the 'captain of the men of death', consumption and phthisis; these latter terms were descriptive of the wasting which is a striking feature of the advanced forms of the disease.

The incidence of tuberculosis was very high in Britain in the nineteenth century when it was a major cause of death. The poor social conditions which were commonplace during the Industrial Revolution were largely responsible for the prevalence of the infection. The marked improvement in living standards which has occurred since the nineteenth century contributed greatly to the decline in the incidence of tuberculosis and the advent of antituberculosis drugs accelerated the fall. Fig. 1.2 shows the striking fall in the mortality figures in the present century; these contrast markedly with the increasing mortality rate for bronchogenic carcinoma.

Tuberculosis is still far from being a rare disease, however, and there is no room for complacency. Many thousands of new cases of respiratory tuberculosis are detected annually in Britain. The

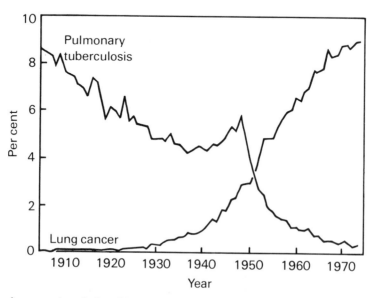

Fig. 1.2 Deaths from pulmonary tuberculosis and lung cancer in men in Scotland as a percentage of deaths from all causes (prepared by Professor A. J. Haddow from material derived from the Registrar General's returns).

incidence is higher where social conditions are poor and in the coloured immigrant population. There is also an increased risk in diabetes mellitus, patients on immunosuppressive drugs, and HIV infection (see Ch. 2). All ages are at risk.

Bacteriology

The tubercle bacillus (*Mycobacterium tuberculosis*) was discovered by Koch in 1882. It is a rod-shaped organism with certain individual staining characteristics which are of great importance in its recognition; with the Ziehl–Nielsen technique the bacillus is stained red and this colour is not removed by acid, hence the term acid-fast bacillus. The tubercle bacillus has a high resistance, and will live for weeks outside the body under certain conditions, e.g. in dust. It is, however, killed by exposure to strong daylight, by boiling for at least two minutes, and by autoclaving.

There are two types of tubercle bacillus of importance to man. The human variety, which is endemic in man, causes pulmonary tuberculosis and most cases of bone and joint tuberculosis, genitourinary tuberculosis, and meningeal tuberculosis. The bovine variety, which is endemic in cattle in some countries, causes most cases of alimentary and lymph gland tuberculosis.

Mode of spread

The majority of cases due to the human strain of the organism are spread by droplet spray from the lungs of patients with 'open' pulmonary tuberculosis. The dentist is, by nature of his work, particularly prone to this form of infection.

The bovine variety of the organism is spread to man by ingestion of milk from an infected cow unless the tubercle bacilli have been killed by pasteurization or boiling.

Pathology of pulmonary tuberculosis

The tubercle bacilli are inhaled, settle in the lungs and cause a small local reaction known as the primary focus, or Ghon's focus. The main histological features of the 'tubercle' are a central area of coagulative necrosis, termed caseation, and a cellular section in which epithelioid and giant cells are characteristic. The lymph glands at the hilum also become infected. The term primary complex is used to describe the lung lesion plus the associated lymph gland lesion.

1. In most cases firm healing of both the lung and the gland components takes place, at first by fibrous tissue and later by the deposition of calcium salts. Small healed, calcified areas are quite commonly seen in the chest X-ray of adults who give no past history of pulmonary tuberculosis. The individual is now sensitized to tuberculin (see below) and has acquired a partial immunity.

2. In some individuals the infection persists and spreads in the lungs to produce either local, or diffuse, tuberculosis of all degrees of severity. The lesions may vary from a single small area of caseation to multiple lesions, with large cavity formation, throughout both lungs. The disease may manifest itself soon, or many years after the primary infection has taken place.

3. In a minority of cases blood spread occurs to the bones and joints, the kidneys, the nervous system, and throughout the lungs themselves.

4. There may be recrudescence of activity from an apparently healed primary focus under conditions of impaired resistance or following prolonged steroid therapy.

Tuberculin sensitivity

Within a few weeks of a person becoming infected with tubercle bacilli he develops a sensitivity to tuberculin which may be revealed by a positive reaction to the intradermal inoculation of a very small amount of the diluted substance, as in the Mantoux technique. Tuberculin sensitivity is an extremely valuable phenomenon as it enables us to separate those who have been infected with tubercle bacilli from those who have not. A positive Mantoux reaction is not to be taken as an indication that someone is suffering from tuberculosis but only that at some time in the past he has been infected with tubercle bacilli.

Clinical features of tuberculosis

Active tuberculous infection is associated with lassitude, malaise, loss of appetite, and loss of weight. The pulse is rapid, there is a tendency to evening pyrexia associated with night sweats, and the erythrocyte sedimentation rate is elevated. In addition there may be local features depending on the organ involved.

Pulmonary tuberculosis

Pulmonary tuberculosis may take several forms (Figs 1.3–1.6).

1. *The primary complex.* The individual may be quite unaware of the primary infection, there may be a vague illness which passes undiagnosed, or there may be evidence of 'tuberculous toxaemia' as described in the preceding section.

2. Occasionally the primary infection causes a brisk pleural reaction with the formation of a straw-coloured effusion containing lymphocytes.

3. *Acute spread* through the lungs. In some unfortunate individuals the tubercle bacilli spread rapidly through the lungs producing a very active, extensive, lesion almost like a pneumonia in its rate of spread. This is the variety which used to be termed 'galloping consumption'.

Fig. 1.3 Calcified pulmonary and glandular component of primary tuberculous complex.

Fig. 1.4 Snowstorm appearance in miliary tuberculosis.

Fig. 1.5 Bilateral active tuberculosis.

Fig. 1.6 Tuberculous cavity at left apex.

4. *Fibrocaseous pulmonary tuberculosis*. This is the commonest form of tuberculosis of the lungs. The lesions are most often at the apices and in the absence of treatment progressive caseation causes much tissue destruction and cavities develop. Cough and spit, haemoptysis, breathlessness and discomfort in the chest may all be present in addition to the features of toxaemia described above. A chest X-ray is an essential step in diagnosis. Finger clubbing occurs in chronic cases where there is much suppuration.

5. *Miliary tuberculosis*. This is caused by the haematogenous spread of the organism, and in the lungs it is represented by the presence of literally thousands of small tubercles which, on chest X-ray, give the appearance of a 'snowstorm' lung.

Alimentary tuberculosis

This may be a primary infection due to ingestion of milk infected with bovine tubercle bacilli or it may result from swallowing infected sputum in chronic pulmonary cases.

1. Lesions of the buccal cavity are uncommon. Superficial painful ulceration of the tongue may occur in chronic pulmonary cases with infected sputum.

2. The ileocaecal region is the part of the alimentary tract most frequently affected as the temporary hold-up in intestinal contents at this site gives the tubercle bacilli a greater opportunity to invade the lymphatic tissue in the wall of the gut. Diarrhoea is the principal symptom.

3. The infection may spread from the gut to the abdominal lymph nodes and peritoneum causing ascites. The swollen abdomen contrasts with the general wasting which occurs.

Tuberculous lymphadenitis

The two main sites for tuberculous lymphadenitis are the neck and abdomen. The latter has already been described. Disease in the neck is usually fairly well localized and is more common in the upper cervical region where it is the result of tonsillar infection reaching the jugulodigastric node but later extending to other nodes. The lesion is a primary focus and not secondary to tuberculosis elsewhere. However, infection of the lower cervical glands can occur, and this is always secondary to disease elsewhere, usually the apex of the lung. Very rarely there is a diffuse enlargement of the cervical nodes related to blood spread of tuberculosis. Following the initial reaction resolution may occur or the lesion proceed to caseation, the necrotic tissue extending towards the surface and perforating the ensheathing layer of deep cervical fascia and then later the skin (collar stud abscess).

Bone and joint tuberculosis

The main sites of skeletal involvement are the vertebrae, the hip joints, and the knee joints. Local bone destruction occurs producing pain, deformity and impaired joint function. Severe hunchback deformity can result from involvement of the spine and there may be cold abscess formation with pressure on adjacent structures, e.g. the spinal cord.

Genitourinary tuberculosis

Involvement of the kidneys and bladder is always secondary to tuberculosis in some other site. Frequency of micturition is a common symptom. Microscopic examination of the urine commonly reveals pus and blood.

Tuberculous meningitis

Involvement of the covering membranes of the brain and spinal cord is seen especially in children. It is due to blood-spread from the primary site of infection. The child becomes drowsy, irritable and obviously ill. Evidence of meningeal irritation is shown by stiffness of the neck. Examination of the cerebrospinal fluid, obtained by means of lumbar puncture, is the main diagnostic step.

Diagnosis

From the *clinical* point of view the main points to be considered are the family history, the individual's personal history regarding any of the symptoms mentioned in the preceding sections, physical examination, and the result of the Mantoux reaction.

Radiological examination of the lungs, bones and joints, of the kidneys etc., is essential if tuberculosis of these sites is suspected.

The *bacteriological* demonstration of the organism is the final proof of diagnosis. It may be found in the sputum, the urine, the faeces, the cerebrospinal fluid, and in pus or scrapings direct from lesions. It should be looked for in direct smears after staining by the Ziehl–Nielsen technique, by culture, and, if these measures are negative, by guinea pig inoculation. The bacteriologist can also give very valuable information regarding the sensitivity of the organism to the antituberculous drugs. However culture and sensitivity testing take several weeks.

Prophylaxis

The main aspects of prophylaxis are:

1. The eradication of undesirable *social factors* such as poor housing, overcrowding, and faulty nutrition.

2. The *early diagnosis and treatment* of active tuberculosis. If cases can be detected early, and treated effectively, then the reservoir of infection will obviously be steadily reduced. All contacts of active cases (including dentists) should be traced and investigated.

3. *Elimination of tuberculous milk* may be achieved by the buildup of herds of cattle which are free from infection and, secondly, by the pasteurization of milk so that if any tubercle bacilli should be present they are rendered harmless.

4. The *protection of uninfected individuals* who are particularly at risk by a vaccine prepared from an attenuated, avirulent strain of tubercle bacilli such as the bacillus Calmette Guérin (BCG). This is offered to children aged 10–13 years in high-risk areas, and to nurses, medical students, and dental students. Only those who are 'Mantoux negative' should be vaccinated, i.e. those who have not been infected. BCG vaccination does not give complete protection but there is now ample statistical evidence as to its worth in reducing the incidence of the disease in vulnerable groups of the population.

Treatment

Treatment of tuberculosis may be considered briefly under three aspects:

1. *Isolation* of patients while infectious, i.e. coughing up infected sputum. Chemotherapy usually renders patients non-infective within a few days.

2. *Chemotherapy* is with a combination of drugs specially reserved for treatment of tuberculosis, in order to prevent drug resistance occurring in the organism. Treatment should be given for several months, to prevent relapse. Rifampicin and isoniazid are commonly used; a third drug such as ethambutol, pyrazinamide or streptomycin can be added.

3. *Other measures.* The patient's resistance should be built up by rest and adequate nutrition. In bone and joint disease, prolonged immobilization in plaster casts may be needed. Surgical removal of the lobe of a lung (lobectomy) or a kidney (nephrectomy) is sometimes required.

Dental considerations

From the immediate practical point of view the dentist should remember the following important points:

1. The possibility of encountering tuberculous lesions of the buccal cavity.

2. The personal risk to himself should he undertake treatment in someone who has active pulmonary tuberculosis. Facial protection should be worn.

3. The necessity for proper sterilization of instruments after dealing with anyone suspected to have tuberculosis.

THE VENEREAL DISEASES

In the great majority of cases venereal diseases are spread by sexual intercourse. It is important to realize that, in many instances, the persons suffering from the disorder may be unaware that they are a source of infection.

There is a risk that the dentist, doctor, or nurse may accidentally acquire the infection through examination of the mouth of a patient who is suffering from the secondary stage of syphilis. Syphilis may be transmitted from the mother in utero. Gonococcal infection of the eyes of the newborn child may occur at the time of birth if the mother is suffering from an active stage of gonorrhoea.

The venereal diseases represent a considerable social problem in practically all countries both in times of peace and, even more, in times of war when promiscuous sexual activity tends to increase. Syphilis is now uncommon, but increased promiscuity in recent decades, as well as the use of oral contraceptives rather than condoms, has caused epidemics of all other venereal diseases in western countries. HIV infection (see Ch. 2) has reminded everyone that the use of condoms and limitation of sexual partners, preferably to one, are essential measures in prevention of venereal disease.

Syphilis

Historical aspects

There is some doubt about the precise origin of syphilis, or lues, but it is generally believed that the infection was carried back by the sailors of Columbus from the New World since when it has been an unwelcome feature of civilization. It is likely, however, that the infection was present many hundreds of years before this time, and certain Biblical references to illnesses associated with extensive skin rashes may refer to what we now know as syphilis.

The causal organism was detected in 1905 and three years later an extremely valuable serological test was introduced by Wassermann.

Bacteriology

Syphilis is caused by a sphirochaete, the *Treponema pallidum*. It is a delicate organism with a corkscrew shape, slightly greater in length than the diameter of a red blood corpuscle. It is able to penetrate the intact skin. It may be seen readily by dark-ground illumination after staining with a silver impregnation method but it does not stain with ordinary dyes. It has a low resistance outside the body and is relatively readily killed by antiseptics.

Natural history of the infection

On an average, some three to four weeks elapse from the time of acquiring the infection to the first sign of disease in the absence of treatment. The effects of the infection can most readily be understood if the disease is considered in three stages — primary, secondary, and tertiary — although it should be appreciated that the process is a continuous one and that the rate of progress from one stage to the other may show considerable individual variation.

Primary syphilis

The characteristic lesion of primary syphilis is termed the primary chancre, or hard sore. It is highly infectious. It develops some three to four weeks after infection and is usually situated on the genitalia. The lesion starts as a small, firm, raised swelling which breaks down in the centre to form an indurated ulcer which has a firm, rubbery feel. It is not painful unless secondary infection occurs. The lymph nodes in the area of drainage (usually the groin) become firm, and slightly enlarged. In the absence of treatment the primary chancre will gradually heal and may or may not leave a fine scar. By this time, however, the spirochaetes have invaded the rest of the body.

Extragenital chancres may develop on the lips, or other anterior parts of the buccal cavity, from kissing a person suffering from the secondary stage of the disorder, or on the fingers of dentists, etc., who inadvertently examine the buccal cavity of an individual with secondary syphilis. Anorectal lesions also occur, from anal intercourse.

Secondary syphilis

The manifestations of secondary syphilis usually appear a few months after the primary stage. In the absence of treatment they may last from one to two years. The individual shows evidence of a general constitutional upset, the main features being irregular pyrexia, anorexia, headache, and limb pains. Skin rashes are common on the trunk and limbs and may be very varied in type; perhaps the most characteristic rashes are a coppery, macular eruption, and a deep red, papular eruption. Lesions of the buccal cavity are of considerable dental importance. They may take the form of mucous patches of sodden, greyish epithelium or superficial 'snail-track' ulcers. Both are extremely infective. Infective lesions also occur in the perineum (condylomata lata). The hair tends to fall out (alopecia), usually in a patchy distribution. Slight enlargement of the superficial lymph glands is commonly present.

Tertiary syphilis

The tertiary manifestations of syphilis may develop as early as 2 and as late as 25 or more years after the primary infection. The characteristic feature of this stage is a proliferative endarteritis of the small arteries resulting in their partial obliteration. This causes diminished blood supply to the affected organ, tissue destruction, and replacement fibrosis.

The two main *cardiovascular lesions* of tertiary syphilis are aneurysms of the aorta and incompetence of the aortic valve. In both instances the basic change is fibrous tissue replacement of the middle coat of the aorta so that stretching of the wall of the aorta occurs. Aortic aneurysms, which are now rarely seen, may be considerable in size and cause pressure on adjacent structures such as the bronchi, the left recurrent laryngeal nerve, and the oesophagus. The valve lesion, which is less uncommon, produces the same effects on the heart as aortic incompetence of rheumatic origin (see Ch. 7).

The major *central nervous system lesions* of tertiary syphilis are tabes dorsalis and general paralysis of the insane. Tabes dorsalis, which is also known as locomotor ataxia, is due to involvement of the posterior nerve roots of the spinal cord. It is characterized by difficulty in walking, loss of tendon reflexes, shooting or lightning pains in the limbs and trunk, loss of sensation in the deep structures of the legs, a painless arthritis (Charcot's joints), and loss of bladder control. The pupils are smaller than normal, irregular, and do not contract when stimulated by light (Argyll Robertson pupils). General paralysis of the insane is characterized pathologically by extensive invasion of the cerebral hemispheres by the spirochaete with subsequent death of brain tissue and fibrous tissue replacement. Delusions of grandeur are followed by progressive dementia and paralysis.

A *gumma* is the term given to the mass of granulation tissue which is produced as a reaction to the localization, in the tertiary stage of the disease, of spirochaetes in various tissues. Clinically the lesion usually takes the form of a hard, painless lump. Gummata may occur anywhere in the body but the more common sites are in the skin and subcutaneous tissues, bone, palate, nasal septum, liver, and brain. Gummata situated in a superficial site tend to break down with the formation of indurated ulcers with 'punched-out' edges and a yellow, 'wash-leather' slough on the floor.

Latent syphilis

The term latent syphilis is used where there is no obvious clinical lesion to be found in the individual but the Wassermann reaction is positive. This type of case is seen frequently after treatment with antisyphilitic remedies.

Congenital syphilis

Congenital syphilis is due to infection passed from the mother to the fetus in utero via the placental circulation. It is much less common nowadays because a high proportion of pregnant women attend antenatal clinics where serological tests are routinely determined; patients with a positive reaction receive immediate treatment.

If the infection of the fetus is very severe, death in utero will occur; if the infection is less pronounced a live, but infected, child will be born.

The syphilitic lesions which are commonest in the early months of life are inflammation of the mucous membranes of the nose producing 'snuffles', destruction of the nasal cartilages leading in later years to a saddle-nose deformity, moist papules at the angles of the mouth which heal leaving fine radiating scars known as rhagades, a papular rash especially over the buttocks, poor general health, anaemia, and enlargement of the liver and spleen.

In later childhood characteristic changes occur in the permanent teeth. The incisors become widely spaced, taper from the base to the cutting edge, and frequently show a notch on the margin (Hutchinson's teeth). The first molar teeth tend to show rounding or doming (Moon's molars). Involvement of the corneal tissues of the eyes (interstitial keratitis) produces a ground glass appearance of the cornea with visual deterioration and possibly blindness. Other lesions that may occur include involvement of the eighth nerve producing deafness, painless joint effusions (Clutton's joints), and periostitis of the tibia leading to a sabre deformity.

Diagnosis

A history of exposure to infection is very helpful in

suspected cases of syphilis but there may be reluctance to inquire, and the patient may attempt to conceal his or her indiscretion.

Regarding the clinical aspects of individual lesions one should remember that syphilis has been termed 'the great imitator', as it may produce a very wide variety of lesions which may mimic many other diseases. Suspicion should always be raised in the presence of painless firm ulcers, superficial ulcerated lesions in the mouth not apparently due to Vincent's infection, and in skin rashes which do not readily fit the pattern of the common skin disorders.

All suspected cases should be referred to a venereologist. The serological reactions for syphilis may be negative very early in the infection and in a proportion of later cases but, in general, they are positive in the majority of cases. If syphilitic disease of the nervous system is suspected the cerebrospinal fluid should be examined.

The spirochaete may be demonstrated in scrappings from ulcerated lesions such as the primary chancre, or the secondary lesions of the buccal cavity. Since the organism is readily killed by antiseptics these must not be applied to the lesion prior to the samples being taken.

Prognosis

The prognosis in syphilis has been much improved since the introduction of penicillin. It is still essential, nevertheless, to make the diagnosis as early as possible because, once extensive tissue involvement has taken place, e.g. of the brain, complete cure cannot occur.

Treatment

Penicillin is given by daily injections for 14 days. Careful follow-up and tracing of contacts by the venereologists is essential.

Gonorrhoea

Gonorrhoea is caused by the gonococcus (*Neisseria gonorrhoeae*), a Gram-negative diplococcus which is mainly intracellular. The incubation period is usually about four to five days.

Clinical features

The main feature of the illness in the male is acute inflammation of the anterior urinary passages causing a purulent discharge and considerable discomfort and frequency of micturition. In chronic cases the infection may become established in the prostate gland, or cause a urethral stricture. Gonococcal arthritis, which is usually monoarticular, is a relatively uncommon complication due to blood-spread. The temporomandibular joint may be affected. In the female there is a purulent vaginal and urethral discharge, often of relatively slight degree. Infection may spread to the fallopian tubes causing lower abdominal pain, fever, and later sterility.

Diagnosis and treatment

The diagnosis is established by the demonstration of the organism in stained smears of the discharge.

Acute cases usually respond well to prompt treatment with penicillin. If the organism is resistant to penicillin, either co-trimoxazole or spectinomycin hydrochloride may be used. The latter drug does not mask incubating syphilis and may be useful in cases where both diseases are suspected.

Other venereal diseases

Chlamydiae are the common cause of non-gonococcal urethritis. Tetracycline is effective.

Candida albicans and *Trichomonas vaginalis* cause vaginitis and urethritis. Treatment is with nystatin and metronidazole respectively.

Herpes simplex causes painful, recurrent ulcers, often resistant to treatment (acyclovir cream or tablets).

Papilloma viruses cause genital warts, and possibly cancer of the cervix uteri (neck of the womb).

Hepatitis B virus and HIV are considered in the next chapter.

2

Infections due to bloodborne viruses (hepatitis B and immunodeficiency) and the control of cross-infection in dentistry

CROSS-INFECTION

Cross-infection may occur in the dentist's surgery in three ways:

1. *Infection of the dentist or clinical dental health care workers by the patient*. Examples include tuberculosis (infected sputum) and syphilis (contact with infectious oral lesions).

2. *Infection of the patient by the dentist or clinical dental health care workers*. For example, outbreaks of hepatitis B and of herpes simplex have occurred in patients of infected dentists or dental health care workers (CDC 1986a).

3. Theoretically, *cross-infection between patients* may occur if there is re-use of instruments contaminated with blood or saliva by the dentist or clinical dental health care worker; however documentation of such transmission is currently lacking (CDC 1986a).

In Chapter 1, infections with several organisms which may cause such cross-infection were noted: herpes simplex, cytomegalovirus, staphylococci, streptococci, tuberculosis, and syphilis. A large number of upper respiratory tract viruses (see Ch. 8) are also transmissible.

Historically, dentists and dental health care workers have been unique amongst surgeons in not routinely using such precautions against cross-infection as gloves, masks, and gowns. In recent years, concern has arisen about cross-infection during surgery in general, with three bloodborne viruses, hepatitis B and D viruses, and human immunodeficiency virus (HIV), which has prompted reassessment of infection-control practices for dentistry and the issue of guidelines in the United States (CDC 1986a) and in Britain (BDA 1986).

Hepatitis B virus (HBV). This virus is fairly infectious, and frequently causes serious disease (acute and chronic hepatitis, hepatic cirrhosis, and hepatocellular carcinoma). Its prevalence is increasing in western countries. Increases in serological markers of HBV in recent years amongst dentists suggest that previous infection-control practices were inadequate (BDA 1986, CDC 1986a). Safe and effective vaccines have recently been developed which are recommended for all clinical dental personnel, to protect both themselves and their patients against HBV (BMA 1987).

Hepatitis D virus (HDV, delta antigen). This is a recently discovered virus which occurs only as a co-infection with HBV, and which greatly increases its severity and associated mortality. It is also increasing in prevalence, and is prevented by measures that prevent HBV infection.

Human immunodeficiency virus (HIV). This is another recently discovered virus which causes the acquired immunodeficiency syndrome (AIDS) and other severe and fatal diseases. It is spreading epidemically worldwide. HIV-related disease is largely untreatable and appears uniformly fatal. No vaccine is currently available. However HIV is much less infectious than HBV, and preventive measures against HBV should also prevent infection with HIV.

At present, there is no documented case of HIV transmission by dental surgery. However there are several cases of other health care workers who have acquired HIV from infected patients, through needle-stick injury or at operation; one surgeon has died from such infection. These cases, and the epidemic spread of HIV infection, reinforce the need for good routine infection-control practice in dentistry, and in particular the need for great care to avoid needle-stick injuries and other injuries with blood-contaminated instruments.

These three viral infections are reviewed in turn, before summarizing current recommendations for infection control in dentistry. Further information is available from the guidelines (BDA 1986, CDC 1986a) and from recent reviews (CDC 1986b, Greenspan et al 1986, Pinching 1986, BMA 1987).

HEPATITIS B

Epidemiology

Hepatitis B was originally defined epidemiologically as hepatitis that occurred six weeks to six months after injection of blood or blood products, or after use of inadequately sterilized syringes or needles (hence the old names of serum or syringe hepatitis). These features contrast with hepatitis A (see Ch. 10) which has a shorter incubation period (two to six weeks) and which is usually spread by the faecal—oral route (hence its old name of infectious hepatitis).

Since specific laboratory tests for hepatitis A and B (antigens and antibodies) were developed in the 1970s, it has become apparent that some cases of hepatitis are due to other agents (non-A, non-B hepatitis, see Ch. 10), which are probably also bloodborne viruses since this is now the commonest type of post-transfusion hepatitis. Study of non-A, non-B hepatitis is hindered by the lack of laboratory markers.

Hepatitis B tests have shown that there are a huge number of asymptomatic carriers, estimated as 280 million worldwide (over 5% of the world's population). HBV infection is the World Health Organization's primary target for eradication of an infectious disease. The prevalence of previous HBV infection (defined as presence of serum antibody to the viral surface antigen, HBsAb) and of the HBV carrier state (defined as presence of serum surface antigen, HBsAg) varies markedly worldwide:

1. *China, South-East Asia, Tropical Africa* — 70–95% of the population have antibody and 8–20% are carriers.
2. *Eastern Europe, the Mediterranean, USSR, Central and South America* — 20–55% of the population have antibody and 2–7% are carriers.
3. *Northern, western and central Europe, North America* — 2–6% of the population have antibody and 0.1–0.5% are carriers.

Even with the low prevalence of carriage in Britain, it is estimated that general dental practitioners could be treating up to 400 undiagnosed carriers of HBV every day. The prevalence of the carrier state is increasing. It is associated with living in towns and with poor socioeconomic conditions. Groups at increased risk include: immigrants and visitors from, and returned visitors to, high-risk areas; the mentally handicapped living in institutions, especially patients with Down's syndrome (see Ch. 19) and staff in close contact with such patients; persons with multiple sexual partners, including prostitutes, and homosexual or bisexual men; intravenous or percutaneous drug abusers; those living or working in institutions (e.g. prisons, drug and alcohol rehabilitation centres) which have a high prevalence of high-risk persons; haemophiliacs and other persons who have received regular transfusions of blood or blood products (e.g. renal dialysis, oncology and immunocompromised patients); dentists and other clinical dental staff (four times increased risk compared with the general population in Britain); doctors and other hospital staff, especially surgeons, accident and emergency unit personnel, and those working in drug dependency units, renal dialysis units, liver units, and with haemophiliacs or other multitransfused patients; laboratory staff, especially those working in blood-banks and pathology laboratories; partners and close relatives of the above groups, not necessarily with sexual contact; and children of infected mothers.

Virology

The hepatitis B virus (HBV) is a DNA virus which differs strikingly from other DNA viruses in that it uses an RNA copy of the genome to integrate itself within the host's chromosomes. It infects hepatocytes causing acute hepatitis which is often asymptomatic, and which may become chronic resulting in hepatic cirrhosis. Hepatocellular carcinoma may also occur in chronic infection. The virus is also found in leucocytes in all body secretions (blood, saliva, semen, vaginal and menstrual secretions, breast milk, tears, vomit, faeces, sweat, and urine). The concentration of infective virus particles in blood can be very high (up to 10 trillion/ml during acute infection).

Electron microscopy of blood shows several viral forms: intact virus containing the DNA core (42 nm diameter), and tubular and spherical forms of the surface antigen (22 nm diameter). HBV is a very sturdy virus which can remain viable in the environment for weeks. It is resistant to boiling for less than 30 minutes and to common antiseptics such as chlorhexidine. It can be destroyed only by steam-heating under pressure (autoclaving) or in hot-air ovens, sodium hypochlorite (household bleach), iodine, or glutaraldehyde.

Transmission

The high resistance of HBV to inactivation and its high concentration in blood and other body fluids account for its high infectivity by inoculation with blood or body fluids. Only traces of blood are required, especially if the e antigen from the virus core is present in serum. Following needlestick injury from an HBeAg-positive person, the risk of HBV transmission is 40%. Three main routes of transmission are recognized:

1. Transmission from carrier mothers to their babies (vertical transmission) occurs during the perinatal period, especially if the mother has a high titre of HBsAg or contracts acute hepatitis B during or shortly after pregnancy. Most children infected perinatally become chronic carriers of HBV, but this can be reduced by immunization (see later). Vertical transmission is a major factor determining the high prevalence of HBV in eastern and tropical countries.

2. Sexual intercourse, heterosexual or homosexual, is also an important method of transmission, especially if unprotected by condoms. Thus, HBV can be a venereal disease.

3. Inoculation of blood or other body fluids through the skin or mucous membranes may explain cases of non-sexual transmission, and is of most concern to health care workers, especially those involved in invasive procedures. Inoculation can occur in several ways:

a. Transfusion of blood or blood products. This is largely, but not completely, preventable by asking at-risk persons not to donate blood, and by routine testing for HBV. Similar considerations apply to organ transplantation and donation of sperm or breast milk.

b. Dental, surgical and medical procedures, especially:

(i) Injury of health care workers by contaminated needles or other sharp objects (e.g. scalpels, bone fragments during surgery).

(ii) Contamination of broken skin (e.g. cuts, abrasions, dermatitis of the hands).

(iii) Inadequate sterilization of dental and surgical instruments prior to re-use, or inappropriate re-use of disposable needles, syringes or other invasive apparatus.

(iv) Aerosol spread of infected blood or saliva, e.g. that produced by modern dental equipment, which may infect clinical dental workers through the conjunctivae, mucous membranes or broken skin.

c. Laboratory accidents.

d. Intravenous or percutaneous drug abuse.

e. Tattooing, ear and nose piercing, acupuncture, bloodletting, circumcision.

f. Sharing of razors and toothbrushes.

g. Biting and spitting.

h. Theoretically, by bloodsucking insects.

Clinical spectrum and diagnosis

Acute hepatitis (see also Ch. 10). Symptomatic infection occurs in only 20–30% of cases. After an incubation period of six weeks to six months, a prodromal influenza-like illness is followed by jaundice (yellow colour of the skin and sclera of the eyes) which may be mild or severe, dark urine, and pale stools. The liver may be slightly enlarged and tender. About 5% of cases are complicated by acute glomerulonephritis (see Ch. 11), and about 1% by hepatic failure (see Ch. 10) with coma and bleeding. Most patients make a clinical recovery within six months, but often feel generally unwell and depressed during this time.

The diagnosis is established by high serum levels of bilirubin and transaminases (see Ch. 10) and the presence of HBV surface antigen (HBsAg), core antigen (HBcAg) and e antigen (HBeAg). The e antigen correlates with the number of intact viruses in serum and the infectivity of the blood. These antigens disappear from the serum during convalescence in most persons, but persist in some who become chronic carriers. Antibodies to c, e, and s antigens appear in that order during convalescence. The presence of HBsAb indicates immunity and lack of infectivity.

It should be noted that blood samples from all persons with suspected or known HBV infection should be taken with great care, and sent to laboratories properly packaged to prevent spillage and labelled to indicate high risk of infectivity.

Acute subclinical infection. In most persons acute HBV infection is subclinical, i.e. there are no symptoms or perhaps only nonspecific tiredness or malaise. Diagnosis is retrospective, by discovery of the presence of HBV antigens or antibodies in serum.

Chronic infection. About 3–10% of healthy heterosexual adults retain the virus for more than six months after clinical or subclinical infection: most of these remain seropositive for HBsAg. A higher percentage of the young, old, and certain risk groups, become carriers. Impaired immune response may partly account for persistent carriage: recent studies have shown that treatment with human interferon by injection for several months may produce clearance of the virus.

Diagnosis of carriage may be by follow-up of acute hepatitis, or by discovery when investigating chronic liver disease or performing liver function tests or HBV tests for other reasons. Carriers are usually infectious. The presence of HBeAg (18%) is associated with high infectivity; HBeAb indicates low infectivity in western countries, but not in endemic areas. Liver biopsy may show normal histology, but usually shows chronic hepatitis.

Chronic persistent hepatitis has a better prognosis than chronic active hepatitis, which more commonly progresses to hepatic cirrhosis and/or hepatocellular carcinoma (hepatoma, see Ch. 10); 80% of hepatomas are caused by HBV. Most carriers are asymptomatic and unaware of their condition, so their contacts cannot be warned of their infectivity.

Management and prevention of HBV infection

Treatment of acute hepatitis, chronic hepatitis, cir-

rhosis, or hepatoma is symptomatic (see Ch. 10). No treatment is effective. While recent studies suggest that interferon may clear HBsAg from the serum, follow-up studies are required to see if this affects long-term prognosis.

There are three aspects to *prevention* of HBV infection (BMA 1987):

Active immunization. Effective vaccines are now offered to all persons in the increased risk groups listed above, including dentists and other clinical dental health care workers, as well as dental laboratory staff who are regularly exposed to blood and saliva-contaminated material. Two types of vaccine are currently available.

The first type is prepared from the plasma of asymptomatic human carriers, and contains only the 22 nm diameter spherical HBsAg particles which stimulate production of protective HBsAb, and does not contain the intact, infective 42 nm diameter virus particles which contain the DNA core. Trials have confirmed the efficacy and safety of these vaccines: they carry no risk of HIV infection.

Immunization involves three injections at 0, 1 and 6 monthly intervals, with a single booster injection after 5 years. 95% of recipients develop HBsAb, which should be tested for 3 months after the last injection, and in these responders there is virtually 100% protection following exposure to HBV. A proportion of the 5% of non-responders may respond to a fourth injection within 1 year. Local reactions occur in less than 20% of subjects, and febrile reactions in only a small number.

The second available type of vaccine is made from cultured yeasts by recombinant DNA techniques (genetic engineering). Trials have shown that this vaccine is also effective and safe, apart from minor local reactions. Other types of vaccine under development include polypeptide vaccines, and recombinant vaccinia or adenovirus vaccines.

Passive immunization. For immediate protection against HBV, anti-HBS immunoglobulin should be given to the following persons at risk:

1. Those who have been acutely exposed to HBsAg-positive blood or other body fluids, especially if highly infective (HBeAg positive). Examples include inoculation, ingestion, or splashing on mucous membranes, conjunctivae or broken skin, and sexual contacts of acute cases. It will be remembered that following needlestick injury with

an HBeAg-positive blood, the risk of HBV transmission is 40%. Immunoglobulin should be given as soon as possible after exposure, preferably within 48 hours, and not more than 7 days after exposure. A second dose is recommended 30 days later.

2. Infants born to HBsAg-positive mothers.

The dose of immunoglobulin given does not interfere with the response to active immunization, which should be given simultaneously but at a different site. If HBV infection has already occurred at the time of first immunization, virus multiplication may not be completely inhibited, but many individuals will be protected from severe illness and from the development of chronic infection.

Prevention of inoculation with infected blood or body fluids. Persons discovered to be carriers of HBV should be counselled and educated concerning their infectivity to others. They should be advised to protect sexual intercourse with a condom, and to limit the number of sexual partners. Sexual partners and spouses should be counselled concerning the risks of infection of themselves and of children, and vaccination offered. Spills of blood and body fluids should be mopped up with disposable tissues and sodium hypochlorite (household bleach) diluted 1 in 10. Carriers should avoid biting or spitting, sharing razors or toothbrushes, tattooing, ear and nose piercing, acupuncture, or bloodletting. They should not inject drugs and never share needles. They and their sexual partners should not donate blood, semen, breast milk, or organs for transplantation. They should be asked to inform any doctor or dentist whom they may attend of their carrier status. Their doctor should inform all health care workers exposed to the patient's blood or body fluids of infectivity, including the patient's dentist: such information is confidential and should not be disclosed to those not directly involved in patient contact. Dentists should take extra precautions against cross-infection in HBV carriers (see below). However since most carriers of HBV are asymptomatic, undiagnosed, and unaware of their condition, and are already being treated by dentists in large numbers, the only safe policy is to take routine precautions with *all* patients.

HEPATITIS D

The hepatitis D virus (HDV, previously known as the delta antigen) is a recently discovered small RNA virus which requires the presence of HBV for its existence. Co-infection with HBV causes a more severe hepatitis in both acute and chronic stages, with a high mortality. In Britain, HDV is currently found most often in intravenous drug abusers. HDV infection can be prevented by measures which prevent HBV infection (see above), and is another reason for stressing the importance of such measures.

HUMAN IMMUNODEFICIENCY VIRUS INFECTION AND AIDS

Epidemiology

This infection was originally defined epidemiologically after a new disease, the acquired immunodeficiency syndrome (AIDS), appeared as outbreaks of unusual diseases in groups of male homosexuals in the United States in 1981–82. The criteria for AIDS were diseases suggestive of acquired cellular immunodeficiency, such as opportunistic infections (e.g. *Pneumocystis carinii* pneumonia) or tumours (e.g. Kaposi's sarcoma), in the absence of other causes of immunodeficiency.

In 1983–84 a new virus was independently discovered in such patients by French and American workers, which was subsequently established as the cause of AIDS and other related diseases (especially neurological diseases including dementia) and named human immunodeficiency virus (HIV). Specific laboratory tests for HIV (antigen and antibody) were soon developed. As with HBV, epidemiological studies using these tests have shown a large number of asymptomatic carriers, estimated as several million worldwide. There is evidence for two types of virus — HIV-1 which is common in western countries, and HIV-2 which is currently less common in western countries.

Although less infectious than HBV, HIV causes disease sooner and in a larger percentage of infected persons; such disease appears to be uniformly fatal within a few years of its appearance. HIV infection is spreading epidemically worldwide and, like HBV, poses a major threat to health. As with HBV, the prevalence of the carrier state varies markedly worldwide. In contrast to HBV, the serum antibody to HIV (HIVAb) does not neutralize the virus, and positive antibody tests denote the carrier state and infectivity.

Central Africa. The occurrence in Belgium and France of many cases of AIDS in patients originating from central Africa led to studies which have shown that AIDS and HIV infection are epidemic in the general population in the Central African Republic, Kenya, Rwanda, Uganda, Zaire, and Zambia. It is likely that HIV originated in this part of the world. In some areas the prevalence of HIVAb is 9% among women attending antenatal clinics, 18% among blood donors, and 29% among adults attending sexually transmitted disease clinics. The sex ratio is equal, and the highest rates of infection are seen in the sexually active age groups and in prostitutes. It therefore appears that the usual route of transmission is by heterosexual intercourse. In central Africa, such transmission may be facilitated by non-availability of condoms and by the high prevalence of other sexually transmitted diseases. Other routes of transmission in Africa include vertical transmission from mother to baby (which can occur during pregnancy); re-use of needles and syringes, which are in short supply; ritual practices involving inoculation of blood, such as scarification; and, theoretically, transmission by bloodsucking insects.

Western countries. Well publicized instances and epidemics of AIDS and HIV infection have occurred in Europe, North America and Australasia in the following at-risk groups:

1. Immigrants and visitors from, and returned visitors to, high-risk areas (e.g. central Africa).

2. *Homosexual or bisexual men.* This group has probably been at increased risk due to multiple partners, non-use of condoms, high prevalence of other sexually transmitted diseases (including HBV), the lower resistance of the thin anorectal mucosa to disruption by trauma compared to the thicker vaginal mucosa, and traumatic practices such as insertion of a hand or fist into the rectum. Recent studies indicate that the number of new AIDS cases is decreasing in this group, possibly due to changes in behaviour following health education, population saturation, changes in reporting, or a decline in the rate of illness. However this group still has the highest prevalence of AIDS in the United States and in England.

3. *Intravenous drug abusers.* The high prevalence of HIV infection and AIDS in this group reflects sharing of contaminated needles and syringes, often in 'shooting galleries', especially if blood is redrawn into the syringe then reinjected ('booting'). Health education measures include advice to drug abusers not to inject, and if they inject not to share needles, syringes or other equipment ('works'). Some cities provide free needles and syringes to drug abusers to prevent sharing, as well as devices to dispose of their contaminated needles to prevent accidental inoculation. This group has the highest prevalence of HIV infection in Scotland, especially in Edinburgh.

4. *Haemophiliacs and other recipients of blood or organs.* Large numbers of haemophiliacs worldwide (about 1200 in Britain) are HIVAb positive, and increasing numbers of these individuals are developing AIDS or HIV-related disease (see Ch. 12). This has resulted from transfusions of infected clotting factor concentrates, especially those imported from the United States. A small number of other recipients of infected blood transfusions, blood products, insemination, or transplanted organs have developed AIDS or HIV infection. These risks have now been substantially reduced by preventive measures:

a. Asking persons in at-risk groups not to donate blood or organs

b. Routine testing of donors for HIVAb

c. Heat treatment of clotting factor concentrates for haemophiliacs.

5. *Prostitutes and sexual partners of the above risk groups.* In western countries, heterosexual transmission is becoming more common and it seems likely that heterosexual transmission will become the main route of spread, as in central Africa. At present the heterosexual epidemic in the United States is largely being driven by transmission from injecting drug users, many of whom turn to prostitution to obtain money for drugs. Among regular female sexual partners of HIV-infected male haemophiliacs, the prevalence of HIVAb is 7–17%. Factors that may increase the likelihood of heterosexual transmission include presence of HIVAg in serum; sexually transmitted diseases causing genital ulceration; anal intercourse versus vaginal; and not using a condom. Health education advice to all sexually active persons includes routine use of condoms and limiting the number of sexual partners, preferably to one. Such meas-

ures should also reduce the incidence of other sexually transmitted diseases, which may be co-factors in the progression of HIV infection in infected persons.

6. *Children of infected mothers.* Because of passive transfer of maternal immunoglobulins, the production of HIVAb by the child can be confirmed only after 3–4 months. Such children have a high risk of progression to AIDS.

Virology

The HIV is an RNA virus which inserts its own RNA into the host cell nucleus; the viral enzyme, reverse transcriptase, produces a complementary DNA copy of the viral RNA genome. Such viruses are called *retroviruses*, and several other examples occur in mammals. A similar virus in humans causes some cases of T cell leukaemia. The DNA copy of the HIV genome integrates into the host cell chromosomes, and infection is probably life-long. HIV infects the subclass of T lymphocytes known as T4 or T helper lymphocytes, macrophages, and certain brain cells. These cells share a receptor (the T4 receptor) to which the virus attaches. When cells are stimulated (e.g. by other infections) to proliferate, new viruses are produced which bud from the cell surface to infect new cells, and the cell dies. Progression of HIV-related disease may therefore occur at any time when immune stimulation occurs: this may be why other sexually transmitted diseases are co-factors in disease progression. Since the virus is lymphotropic and neurotropic, the main clinical features of HIV-related disease result from:

1. Destruction of T4 lymphocytes, causing opportunistic infections due to defective cellular immunity.
2. Destruction of neurones in the central and peripheral nervous systems.
3. Neoplasms resulting from defective cell-mediated immunity, which may normally play a protective role against neoplasms induced by other viruses.

Like HBV, HIV has been found in all body fluids. However unlike HBV, the estimated blood titres are low (100–10 000/ml, compared with up to 10 trillion/ml for HBV during acute hepatitis B). Despite much public concern about the possible risk of transmission by saliva (e.g. kissing, mouth-to-mouth resuscitation, sharing the communion chalice), the concentration of the virus is so low that several litres of saliva would have to be ingested to achieve an infective dose: the risk of infection therefore appears to be very low. Furthermore, HIV is a delicate virus which is readily inactivated by heat (wet heat 56°C for 30 minutes, dry heat 68°C for 24 hours) and by standard disinfectants, detergents, and lipid solvents such as soap. This fragility results from the high lipid content of the virus envelope, which is essential for infectivity. Because of its low titre in body fluids and its fragility, HIV is much less infective than HBV. It follows that preventive measures against HBV infection should be more than adequate to prevent HIV infection. This is borne out by the very low risk of HIV infection in health care workers looking after AIDS patients who use commonsense precautions.

Transmission

HIV transmission is by the same routes as HBV transmission, i.e. transmission from carrier mothers to their babies, by sexual intercourse (heterosexual or homosexual), or by inoculation of blood through the skin or mucous membranes. Due to its low infectivity compared with HBV, transmission by the latter route requires either a large dose, or repeated blood–blood or blood–mucosal contact. There is a proven lack of infectivity by epidemiological studies of health care workers and nonsexual family contacts of persons with HIV infection or AIDS. Single exposure to the virus is unlikely to cause infection. Transfusion of infected blood or blood products or organs, or re-use of syringes by drug addicts, carries the highest risk. Extensive studies of thousands of health care workers with needlestick injuries or mucous membrane exposure to HIV or AIDS have shown only a few cases of HIV infection, usually due to deep injection of a significant amount of blood. There is no evidence of transmission by aerosol spread, food, cutlery, toilets, bedding or clothing. There are no recorded cases of HIV transmission in the dental surgery.

Serology

About four weeks after infection, HIVAg appears in

the blood, before HIVAb. The antibody appears 4–12 weeks after infection, while the antigen disappears. Occasionally HIVAb may take up to one year to appear, or may never appear. In the late stages of HIV-related disease, the antigen may reappear while the antibody may disappear. Patients are most infective in the early and late antigenaemic phases. Blood donors carrying the virus will not be detected in the 'window' period before the antibody appears, and the window will not be closed completely by adding routine donor screening for HIV antigen. It is therefore important to continue to ask persons at risk not to donate blood.

Clinical spectrum of HIV infection

In 1986 the following classification of HIV infection was introduced by the Centers for Disease Control in the United States (CDC 1986b).

Group I: acute infection

A minority of infected persons (10–15%) have transient symptoms and signs at the time of appearance of antigen and antibody, usually 6–8 weeks after exposure. Clinical syndromes include an infectious mononucleosis-like illness (see Ch. 1), viral meningitis, or viral encephalitis (see Ch. 18). Following resolution of clinical features all patients are reclassified into Groups II–IV.

Group II: asymptomatic infection

Most patients remain asymptomatic after infection until they develop HIV-related disease, which may occur after six months or several years (i.e. to the current limits of observation of this new disease). They are diagnosed only when screened by laboratory tests for HIV, usually HIVAb (e.g. when donating blood). Some of these patients have haematological and/or immunological abnormalities, such as lymphopenia, decreased numbers of T4 (helper) lymphocytes, increased numbers of T8 (suppressor) lymphocytes, increased serum immunoglobulins, neutropenia or thrombocytopenia. The increase in immunoglobulins is due to stimulation of B lymphocytes, and the thrombocytopenia is due to immune destruction of platelets by auto-

antibodies (see Ch. 12). The risk of progression to the more symptomatic and life-threatening manifestations of HIV infection (Group IV) is about 10–15% over 3 years: only future follow-up studies will reveal the ultimate outcome.

Group III: persistent generalized lymphadenopathy (PGL)

This is defined as palpable lymphadenopathy (lymph node enlargement of 1 cm or more) at two or more extra-inguinal sites (e.g. neck, axillae), which persists for more than three months, in the absence of an illness or condition other than HIV to explain these findings (e.g. infectious mononucleoses, tuberculosis, syphilis, lymphomas, lymphatic leukaemia; see Chapters 1, 12 and 14). Histology of biopsied lymph nodes shows follicular hyperplasia, presumably as a reaction to HIV infection. As in Group II, some patients may have haematological and/or immunological abnormalities. The risk of progression to Group IV varies from 10–30% with up to five years of follow-up at the present time.

Group IV: other disease

A. *Constitutional disease.* One or more of the following symptoms in the absence of an illness or condition other than HIV to explain the findings:

1. Fever persisting for more than one month
2. Involuntary weight loss of greater than 10% of baseline
3. Diarrhoea persisting for more than one month.

B. *Neurological disease* (see Chapters 18 and 19). One or more of dementia, myelopathy, or peripheral neuropathy in the absence of an illness or condition other than HIV to explain the finding. These are direct effects of HIV on the nervous system. Progressive dementia is common: cerebral atrophy is seen on computerized tomography (CT) scanning of the brain. Myelopathy and peripheral neuropathy cause weakness, unsteadiness, pains, and numbness in the legs.

C. *Secondary infectious diseases.* These result from acquired cellular immune deficiency due to HIV-mediated destruction of T4 lymphocytes.

Some infections are those that occur in the non-immunocompromised, e.g. tuberculosis, salmonellae, although they tend to be more generalized and severe in HIV infection. Other infections are due to unusual organisms which cause disease only in the immunocompromised, e.g. *Pneumocystis carinii*, cryptosporidiosis, isosporiasis. Twelve of the specified infections comprised the original definition of AIDS; six other specified infections are now included in the definition of Group IVC. Most infections involve the lungs, alimentary tract, central nervous system, or skin:

1. Lungs. Pneumocystis carinii pneumonia is a protozoal infection which is the commonest cause of death in HIV infection, and accounts for 85% of pulmonary infections. The usual symptoms are dyspnoea and dry cough. The chest X-ray may be initially normal, but commonly shows general interstitial infiltration which may resemble miliary tuberculosis (see Fig. 1.4). Lung function tests are often abnormal, as are isotope lung scans using Gallium-67. Sputum can be obtained after inhalation of nebulized saline mists, and shows the organism in 50% of cases. In the other cases bronchoscopy with bronchoalveolar lavage and transbronchial lung biopsy is required to show the organism. Open lung biopsy is rarely required. Treatment is with either co-trimoxazole or pentamidine, given by intravenous injection, and high-dose oxygen. These drugs may cause marrow depression and skin rashes. Patients not responding within a week or two have a very poor prognosis: artificial ventilation may be given but at this stage mortality is 90%. Other lung infections include tuberculosis and other 'atypical' mycobacteria, and cytomegalovirus (see Ch. 1).

2. Alimentary tract. Persistent *oral candidiasis* (see Ch. 9) is very common and is seen in about 75% of Group IV patients; it is often the first opportunistic infection and is predictive of more serious infections. Treatment is with nystatin lozenges or paint; lozenges of other antibiotics (amphotericin, miconazole, clotrimazole) are alternatives. Candida infection may spread to the oropharynx, oesophagus (where it may cause dysphagia and is shown by oesophagoscopy or barium swallow, see Ch. 9), or lungs. Systemic treatment with ketoconazole or amphotericin is required for such disseminated infections.

Oral hairy leukoplakia is a recently described condition which presents as totally adherent white lesions on the lateral border of the tongue with irregular hairy surfaces. It is a variant of oral leukoplakia (see Ch. 9) and is probably due to the Epstein–Barr virus (EBV) which also causes infectious mononucleosis (see Ch. 1). Virus particles are seen in biopsies of the lesions. There is no treatment. Other oral infections include herpes simplex, herpes zoster, cytomegalovirus and histoplasmosis (see Ch. 1).

The common intestinal infection is chronic *cryptosporidiosis*, due to another protozoon. It causes persistent watery diarrhoea with fever, abdominal cramps, weight loss, dehydration, and malabsorption. Diagnosis is by finding cysts in fresh stool. The condition is untreatable and miserable, and requires fluid replacement and nutrition. Other gut infections include cytomegalovirus, tuberculosis, and salmonellae (which cause recurrent septicaemia).

3. Central nervous system. Apart from direct HIV infection of the brain, *cryptococcal meningitis*, progressive multifocal leucoencephalopathy (PMLE, due to the JC virus), and encephalitis due to cytomegalovirus, herpes simplex or herpes zoster may occur. *Toxoplasma gondii* (see Ch. 1) is the commonest treatable infection, occurring in about 10% of Group IV patients, and may cause focal neurological signs (see Ch. 18). CT brain scans show multiple lesions surrounded by a ring of oedema. These infections require diagnosis by examination of cerebrospinal fluid or brain biopsy, and some are treatable with antibiotics.

4. Skin. Herpes simplex commonly causes painful perianal lesions and generalized infections. Herpes zoster may cause lesions in several dermatomes. Candida infection of skinfolds (intertrigo) and ringworm (tinea cruris and pedis) are common. Extensive folliculitis and seborrhoeic dermatitis occur, probably due to pityrosporum yeasts. Treatment of these infections is with antiviral or antifungal agents respectively.

D. Secondary tumours. Kaposi's sarcoma was previously very rare in western countries, but is now common in sexually acquired HIV infection. It is much rarer in HIV infection due to contaminated blood (haemophiliacs, drug abusers), hence it may require another co-factor, e.g. another virus spread only sexually. Red-purple lesions which are palpable and painless occur on the head and neck (especially the face), within the oral cavity (especially the hard palate), and on the trunk and limbs. Visceral lesions also occur. Treatment is by chemotherapy, interferon, or radiotherapy. *Lymphomas* are also frequent in HIV infection (see Ch. 12).

Management of HIV infection

The treatment of opportunistic infections and neoplasms (Group IV) has already been outlined. Patients should be educated to avoid co-factors that may hasten progression: sexually transmitted disease (limit partners and wear condoms); other infections (e.g. avoid poultry with its risk of salmonella infection); malnutrition; pregnancy; and immunosuppressive drugs. A positive attitude, healthy lifestyle, and adequate diet should be encouraged. Much research is directed towards antiviral drugs active against HIV. One drug, zidovudine (azidothymidine, AZT, Retrovir®), reduces the incidence and severity of serious infections in Group IV patients. It can cause bone marrow depression and skin rashes. At present, however, AIDS (serious Group IV infections and tumours) appears to be uniformly fatal within a year or two of onset. Terminal care and support are most important, and in view of the increasing numbers of patients this will largely be in the community, e.g. in hospices or at home.

Prevention of HIV infection

Despite intensive efforts, no vaccine is currently available for HIV. Hence prevention is confined to prevention of transmission. General health education of the public concerning sexual intercourse, drug abuse, and care with all blood is the keystone, and has been discussed above. As with carriers of HBV, carriers of HIV should be counselled and educated concerning their infectivity to others. They should be advised to protect sexual intercourse with a condom and to limit the number of sexual partners, who should also be counselled. Other precautions with blood and body fluids are advised, as for carriers of hepatitis B.

Carriers should be advised to inform any doctor or dentist whom they may attend of their carrier status. Their doctor should inform all health care workers exposed to the patient's blood or body fluids of infectivity, including the patient's dentist. Such information is confidential and should not be disclosed to those not directly involved in patient contact. Dentists should take extra precautions in treatment, as with carriers of HBV (see below). However since most carriers of HIV are asymptomatic, undiagnosed, and unaware of their condition, and are already being treated by dentists, the only safe policy is to take routine precautions with *all* patients.

Screening for HIV infection

A positive HIV test can have shattering implications and consequences. People who are usually young and active face lifelong infection with a progressive and often fatal disease, and lifelong infectivity for sexual partners and children. The performance of HIV testing (even if negative) may lead to rejection for life assurance or endowment mortgages. Positive test results are commonly followed by anxiety, depression or even suicide, by stressed or broken relationships, by fears of people finding out and their reaction, by unemployment, and suboptimal medical and dental care. Because of these problems, testing should never be 'routine' and should be preceded by pre-counselling and the person's informed consent, and followed by post-counselling and support.

Because of false-negative tests, HIV testing has a limited role. It is not appropriate to screen patients for 'protection' of health care workers, since precautions against cross-infection in at-risk persons are the same whatever the test results. The main indications for screening are:

1. Screening of donors of blood, semen, organs or breast milk, to protect the recipients.

2. Chronic renal dialysis patients (see Ch. 11) prior to renal transplantation, which should be avoided in HIV infection since immunosuppressive drugs are required to prevent transplant rejection.

3. High-risk women considering pregnancy, which may promote progression of HIV-related disease in infected mothers, and carries a high risk of infection and AIDS in the baby.

4. Persons accidentally exposed to infected blood

(e.g. needlestick injuries), who wish to know whether they have been infected, after pre-counselling and with their informed consent.

GUIDELINES FOR DENTAL PRACTICE

Hepatitis B vaccination

All clinical dental health care workers, including hygienists and surgery assistants, should be offered vaccination against HBV. Testing for seroconversion (HBsAb) should be performed three months after the last dose, and a fourth dose considered in non-converters. Booster doses are given after five years.

Medical history and examination

Always ask about recent or current illness, medications, and hepatitis. Look for:

1. Jaundice.
2. Possible systemic features of HIV infection or tuberculosis (weight loss, fever, cervical lymphadenopathy).
3. Possible oral features of HIV infection (candidiasis, hairy leukoplakia, Kaposi's sarcoma), or tuberculosis or syphilis (mouth ulcers).

Patients with such suspected illnesses should be referred to hospital for dental treatment. They may require prior correction of bleeding tendencies prior to dental procedures (fresh frozen plasma to replace clotting factors in hepatitis; platelets in HIV infection with thrombocytopenia), as well as diagnosis and treatment of their infection. It is inappropriate for dentists to suggest to patients that they may have HIV infection, tuberculosis or syphilis, or to suggest or perform serological testing. Patients should be referred for medical assessment.

Patients who are healthy but volunteer the information that they are carriers of HBV or HIV should be thanked for this courtesy to their dentist. If they are otherwise well (confirm with the patient's doctor) they can and should be safely treated for routine dental procedures in the dental surgery. Dentists unfortunate enough to contract such viral infection themselves would wish prompt treatment of pain and other symptoms by their own doctors and dentists. Likewise, dentists have a responsibility to relieve their own patients' symptoms promptly. They are already treating the majority of carriers of bloodborne viruses, who are asymptomatic, undiagnosed, and unaware of their status. The British Dental Association currently recommends extra precautions for such known carriers (see below).

Routine precautions against cross-infection

Dentists have a duty to ensure the safety of their staff, who should be thoroughly trained in precautions, which should be regularly reviewed. Dental health care workers with exudative skin lesions should refrain from direct patient care and from handling equipment in contact with patients until the condition resolves. Dental health care workers should inspect their exposed skin every morning and cover any cuts or abrasions with waterproof plasters. They should wear disposable gloves routinely when touching mucous membranes (e.g. examining the mouth) or blood, saliva, other body fluids, or items or surfaces contaminated with blood or body fluids. Between patients, hands should be washed with soap and water or surgical handscrub, and gloves changed. Protective glasses and masks (or chin-length plastic face-shields) should be worn when aerosol spray or splashing of blood or other body fluids is likely (e.g. turbines, scalers). Gowns should be worn if clothing is likely to be soiled with blood or body fluids.

High-speed aspirators should exhaust externally, and good ventilation should be provided. Surfaces which may be contaminated by blood or saliva should be covered with impervious, disposable trays or covers, and changed between patients. Surfaces should be cleaned with disposable absorbent cloths (to remove blood and other organic material) and sodium hypochlorite (household bleach, 1 in 10 dilution) or glutaraldehyde if metal since hypochlorite corrodes metals.

Needles and other sharp instruments must be handled with great care to avoid accidental injuries. Avoid recapping, bending or breaking needles; dispose into rigid, puncture-resistant containers as close to the area of use as possible, as soon as possible. Disposable equipment should be used wherever possible, and never re-used (especially needles or local anaesthetic cartridges). Other solid waste contaminated with blood or body fluids should be placed in stout plastic bags, sealed, and incinerated.

Non-disposable equipment should be thoroughly cleaned by scrubbing or ultrasonic cleaners, then sterilized by autoclaving (134°C for at least 3 minutes) or dry heat (hot air ovens, 160°C for 60 minutes without interruption). Boiling and cold sterilization are inadequate for HBV: sterilization should be considered only for instruments which cannot be exposed to heat (soak for 3 hours in 2% glutaraldehyde). Handpieces and ultrasonic scalers which cannot be sterilized should be cleaned and disinfected between patients.

Impressions and appliances should be thoroughly cleaned (or sprayed with glutaraldehyde, then sealed in a bag) before sending to the dental laboratory, with which liaison is required regarding cleaning and handling. Biopsy specimens and swabs should be put in secure, leak-proof containers before sending to the pathology laboratory.

Additional precautions for known carriers of HBV or HIV

These have been outlined in detail by the British Dental Association (1986). Pregnant women should not be involved in treatment. If possible, the appointment should be arranged at the end of the day, with careful cleaning after the procedure. Extraordinary care should be taken to prevent needlestick injury, or splashing of blood or body fluids in the eye or mouth. Gloves, glasses, mask and gown should be worn. If such contamination occurs, the site of contamination should be washed gently but thoroughly, and advice sought immediately from the local hospital (accident and emergency department or infectious diseases department) or dental or medical officer. For hepatitis B exposure, passive and active immunization may be recommended (see above). For HIV exposure, a course of zidovudine may be recommended.

References

British Dental Association (BDA) 1986 Guide to blood borne viruses and the control of cross infection in dentistry. British Dental Association, London

British Medical Association (BMA) 1987 Immunisation against hepatitis B. Report of the Board of Science and Education. British Medical Association, London

Centers for Disease Control (CDC) 1986a Recommended infection-control practices for dentistry. Morbidity and Mortality Weekly Report 35: 237–242

Centers for Disease Control (CDC) 1986b Classification system for human T-lymphotropic virus type III/lymphadenopathy associated virus infections. Morbidity and Mortality Weekly Report 35: 334–339

Greenspan D, Pindborg J J, Greenspan J S, Schiødt M 1986 AIDS and the Dental Team. Munksgaard, Copenhagen (This book illustrates many oral manifestations of HIV infection.)

Pinching A J (ed) 1986 AIDS and HIV infection. Clinics in Immunology and Allergy 6, No. 3

3

Diseases due to infection — surgical aspects

INFLAMMATION

The response of tissue to infection, usually of bacterial origin, is known as inflammation. Bacteria cause inflammation as a result of cellular damage with disruption of the cells and lysozyme release. A complex chain of events is initiated involving both cellular and humoral factors in an effort to destroy the invading microorganisms. Some bacteria secrete toxins (exotoxins); others release toxins as they disintegrate (endotoxins).

The course of the illness produced is the result of the balance between the number, multiplication and virulence of the bacteria and the defence mechanisms of the host. In addition to the immune mechanisms mentioned in Chapter 1, host defences include the intact epithelial linings of the skin, alimentary, respiratory and urinary tracts, and the local acute inflammation which follows breach of the body's defences. Acute inflammation results in vascular dilatation, the passage of exudate into the tissues and the emigration of white cells. The inflamed part becomes red, hot, swollen, tense and painful, and there is some loss of function. Surrounding muscles may go into spasm to protect the part. Thus, in inflammation of the appendix, the abdominal wall muscles are held tense.

The exudate containing natural antibacterial substances and specific antibodies (and administered chemotherapeutic agents) together with the inflammatory cells prevent multiplication or destroy the organisms. These reactions are not as effective in the elderly patient, in the malnourished, if there is severe anaemia, or in some concomitant diseases such as diabetes and renal failure. Poor blood supply to a part is also an adverse factor.

The extent of the original bacterial invasion and the virulence of the bacteria are two important components in determining the outcome, and some bacteria (e.g. *Clostridium tetani*) produce extremely serious effects as a result of exotoxin secretion and yet remain localized at the site of infection.

It is also extremely important to recognize that healthy tissues with a good blood supply do not harbour bacteria readily. On the other hand, in the presence of haematoma, dead tissue or collections of fluid, organisms thrive much more readily. It is an important surgical principle in the prevention of infection to keep such areas to a minimum and to provide drainage following operations that result in collections of serous fluid or haematoma.

Should the body's defences predominate, resolution will be complete. Incomplete resolution is complicated by the formation of scar tissue and fibrosis. On the other hand, the infection may progress, invading venous walls and causing infected clot formation (thrombophlebitis). Bacteria then seed into the bloodstream and the result is the dangerous condition of bacteraemia. This is diagnosed by obtaining culture of bacteria from blood samples.

Cellulitis

Local progression of the infection results in inflammation of the connective tissue, termed cellulitis. This may be subcutaneous (see Ch. 1) but may also occur in other connective tissues such as those in the pelvis, the orbit and the retroperitoneum. Cellulitis is almost always accompanied by a degree of lymphangitis. This can be seen in the skin as red streaks along the lymphatic channels, and the regional glands become enlarged and tender (lymphadenitis).

Abscess

Pyogenic organisms tend to form pus. This is composed of dead and dying leucocytes, tissue debris, and the organisms themselves. The surrounding acute inflammatory reaction walls off the abscess. Septic thrombosis may occur in adjacent small blood vessels and detachment of infected thrombi can result in septic embolization with abscesses forming at distant sites in the body. The abscess is initially hard, red and painful but later, as the result of formation of much pus, it softens and becomes fluctuant. The patient is feverish and there is anorexia, malaise and a polymorphonuclear leucocytosis. If not drained at this stage, the abscess would discharge spontaneously either through the skin, forming a sinus, or internally into a viscus or serous cavity.

The treatment of abscesses is by drainage. Antibiotics without drainage are not only valueless but may be dangerous since the chemotherapeutic agents cannot sterilize the abscess completely, so it remains as a source of toxaemia and becomes surrounded by an increasingly dense mass of reactive fibrous tissue.

A *boil (or furuncle)* is a small abscess arising in a hair follicle and due to *Staphylococcus aureus*. Boils may lead to the formation of distant abscesses and when they occur on the face may spread via the facial veins to the cavernous sinus within the brain, resulting in septic cavernous sinus thrombosis (see Ch. 7).

A *carbuncle* is an area of subcutaneous pyogenic infection resulting in necrosis and discharging to the skin through multiple sinuses. It may commence with the formation of a boil with subsequent spread to surrounding hair follicles. Carbuncles generally occur on the shoulders, the back of the neck, or on the dorsum of the hands, and the condition is more common in diabetic patients.

Acute osteitis

This infection of bone is most often due to *Staphylococcus aureus*. The infection is usually bloodborne but occasionally comes from a compound fracture. The bones most often affected are the tibia and lower end of the femur and the disease occurs mainly in children.

The infection begins at the metaphysis of the long bone and initiates a typical inflammatory reaction. Because of the rigidity of bone the increased tension leads to compression of nutrient vessels and subsequent ischaemia. If the disease process is not promptly arrested, necrotic bone may separate as a sequestrum. The vascular periosteum attempts to reform the shaft of the bone and the sequestrated segment becomes encased in a thick bony involucrum.

The disease is characterized by the sudden onset of severe pain in a limb accompanied by high fever and toxaemia. There is tenderness and swelling over the affected bone, a polymorphonuclear leucocytosis, and blood culture may reveal the causative organism. X-ray is initially normal and osteolytic areas with accompanying periosteal elevation and sclerosis are noted only at a much later stage.

Treatment is by high dosage antistaphylococcal antibiotics and by splintage of the affected limb. If there is not a prompt response then surgical drainage of pus is necessary by incision of the subperiosteal abscess and drilling of the bone through to the marrow cavity.

Failure of complete resolution of acute osteitis is uncommon. It may result in diffuse bone sclerosis and thickening with infected cavities containing sequestrae. There may be multiple sinuses and old puckered scars in the overlying skin. This condition is known as chronic osteitis and although it may be apparently quiescent, it may suddenly become active, even years later. Surgery is the only effective treatment. The bony cavities must be laid open and curetted.

Inflammation in the pulp of a tooth

Inflammation in the pulp of a tooth (pulpitis) results in the same series of changes as those described above and, as in inflammation in the cavity of bone, the resultant swelling of tissue and pressure together with infection results in ischaemic necrosis of the pulp of the tooth. As the inflamed pulp attempts to swell and expand in the confines of the pulp cavity, there is intense pain which persists until the pulp dies. Following death of the pulp, the periapical tissues become involved and a periapical abscess forms. If not drained either by removal of

the pulp or the tooth, it will discharge spontaneously to the surface (dental sinus) or into one of the soft
tissue spaces around the jaws, resulting in a
dangerous spreading cellulitis. This may occur in
the soft tissues on the floor of the mouth (Ludwig's
angina) and spread so as to compromise the airway.

Anaerobic infections

Tetanus

This is caused by the anaerobic spore-forming
Clostridium tetani. Tetanus organism is present in
soil and faecal matter and is a contaminant of dirty
wounds. The organism grows only under anaerobic
conditions and therefore thrives in deeply penetrating wounds where there is much dead tissue. It may
enter the body through quite small penetrating
wounds.

The organism remains confined but secretes a
very powerful exotoxin acting specifically on the
cerebrospinal motor cells resulting in local severe
muscle spasm, particularly in the neck and trunk.
There is a painful trismus and spasm of the facial
muscles (risus sardonicus). The disease progresses
to intense convulsions and death often occurs from
exhaustion, respiratory tract infection, or asphyxiation. Active immunization against tetanus is the
best method of prevention and can be obtained by
the injection of tetanus toxoid. This is carried out
by a course of three injections, the second 8 weeks
after the first, and the third 6−12 months later.
Toxoid is given to children but a booster dose
should be given at five-year intervals and after injuries involving contaminated wounds.

An important part of prophylaxis is the adequate
excision of penetrating wounds, together with
prophylactic antibiotics (penicillin). This, together
with the injection of tetanus toxoid, is considered
adequate prophylaxis and safer than passive immunization with antitetanus serum prepared from
horses, which carries a high risk of anaphylactic
reaction. Human antitetanus globulin is now frequently employed in many centres and given at the
same time as the toxoid.

The treatment of established tetanus involves
care of the wound and nursing in a quiet, darkened
room under sedation. Anticonvulsants are employed and penicillin in high dosage to destroy the
organisms and thus prevent further production of
toxin. Antitetanus serum in high dosage is given.
Tracheostomy and artificial respiration are often
necessary.

Gas gangrene

The *Clostridia welchii*, *septicans* and *oedematiens* are
found in faeces and soil. Like *Clostridium tetani* they
are anaerobic and thrive in dirty wounds. The organisms produce an exotoxin which facilitates their
spread in tissue and which may be haemolytic on
entering the bloodstream. Other Clostridia then
flourish on the dead muscle and break it down into
putrid products.

Clostridial infections tend to complicate large
destructive wounds, but may also occur from contamination arising from the patient's own
gastrointestinal tract after some forms of abdominal
surgery. There is profound toxaemia often associated with septic shock and frequently
haemolysis. The tissues around the wound are
crepitant due to the infiltration of gas (secondary to
fermentation of the muscle carbohydrate) and as
the disease spreads the tissues become discoloured
and gangrenous and a foul smelling discharge
occurs.

Prophylactic treatment is by adequate and extensive excision of dead tissue and the administration
of prophylactic penicillin. For the established disease, large doses of penicillin are given and the
wound is explored and extensively cleaned. Involved muscle is completely excised and amputation of the limb may be necessary. Anti-gas
gangrene serum is administered and blood transfusion is usually necessary.

It cannot be emphasized too strongly that tetanus
and gas gangrene are serious infections with a grave
prognosis and the best method of treatment is the
correct management of contaminated wounds.

Fungal infection

Actinomycosis

Actinomycosis is produced by a mycotic organism,
the *Actinomyces israelii* which is found as a commen-
sal in the mouth. Other strains of Actinomyces
(*Actinomyces bovis*) grow on grasses and are not

pathogenic to humans. The organisms invade usually through a breach in the oral mucosa but infection may occur in the ileocaecal region of the gastrointestinal tract or, following inhalation, in the lungs.

The disease is characterized by the formation of dense fibrous tissue surrounding multiple pockets of pus so that a honeycomb abscess is formed. The pus contains the characteristic 'sulphur granules' (clumps of mycelia) visible in saline suspension or after spreading the pus on a slide. The infection spreads along fascial planes and is difficult to eradicate. Cervico-facial actinomycosis is the most common and is usually seen around the angle of the jaw. The underlying abscesses perforate, forming multiple sinuses exuding thin pus. A similar change occurs in abdominal actinomycosis, which is usually localized in the region of the appendix. In pulmonary actinomycosis the disease spreads to affect the pleura and chest wall. Treatment is by high-dose, long-term administration of penicillin and by local surgery to eradicate slough and abscess cavities.

Hospital and wound infection

A clean surgical wound may become infected. This is more likely if the operation exposes large surfaces and particularly if operation is prolonged. The infection either takes place from an infected focus on the patient himself, from an infected focus or from the nose of a carrier (e.g. one of the attendants) or from the environment (such as infected air disturbed by blankets, or dirty instruments). Some wounds are particularly liable to infection and this occurs when the operation entails opening infected viscera.

Antibiotics have made a vast change in the prognosis of infection but have not prevented hospital infections. Modern surgery has led to more prolonged operations and many seriously ill patients are kept alive by drugs which reduce body reaction to infection (steroids, anticancer drugs). Furthermore, prolonged use of antibiotics in hospital has led to the emergence of bacteria which are often resistant to antibiotics and indeed may be of great virulence.

An outbreak of infection in a hospital must be rigorously investigated and this entails an examination of environmental factors, personnel and procedures such as the carrying out of dressings and the conduct of operations. Such investigations are facilitated by good record-keeping within a hospital so that wound infections are documented, the pus from wounds cultured, and the organisms typed. In this way outbreaks of infection are traced early and can be dealt with.

Wound infection

Wound infection is characterized by malaise, fever and local signs related to the wound. The wound may be swollen, fluctuant and the surrounding skin red. Pus may exude between sutures, or on removal of sutures pus can be located with a sinus forcep and allowed to drain away. If this is done and the pus sent for culture then the organisms can be identified and specific antibiotic sensitivities obtained. Antibiotics are not usually necessary if free drainage is provided.

4

Wounds and surgical operations

A wound may be described as any forcible disruption of the continuity of tissues. A clean cut made by a very sharp instrument is known as an *incised wound*, whereas the ragged wound made by an instrument which tears at the tissue is known as a *laceration*. Surgical wounds are all of an incised nature, the tissue being deliberately opened in a clean-cut fashion. Lacerations may also occur by the forcible stretching of tissue over an underlying structure (such as a tear over the shin following a severe kick). Scrapes against rough surfaces resulting in complete or partial skin loss are called *abrasions*. *Penetrating wounds* occur when a sharp instrument penetrates deeply into the body, or are caused by bullets or other trajectories.

A *haematoma* is an extravasion of blood in the tissues from blood vessels disrupted by a blow. It may be superficial, appearing as an obvious bruise, and is very common after minor injury. However, severe damage may be caused to deeper tissues and viscera, without disruption of the overlying skin, by heavy blows from a blunt object. Examples are rupture of the spleen or deep lacerations of liver following a severe blow in the upper abdomen as in an automobile accident.

Pathophysiology of wound healing

Following disruption of a tissue there is *haemorrhage* into the wound. This may be continuous and severe (see Ch. 5), may be followed by shock, and may lead to death if the bleeding is not stopped. However, once the bleeding has been arrested by a process of contraction of cut vessels and by blood clotting, the wound fills with *haematoma*. An acute inflammatory reaction develops quickly in the surrounding tissue and new blood vessels and fibroblasts begin to grow into the haematoma, which is absorbed. This new tissue is called *granulation tissue* and its presence signifies a healthy healing wound. The haematoma is eventually completely replaced by granulation tissue which then begins to mature, collagen fibres being laid down. As this process continues, epithelium grows in from the sides of the wound to cover the defect. The growing epithelium can be seen as a fine, blue, filmy layer growing in at the edges. Once epithelial continuity is restored, collagen formation proceeds and the new fibrous tissue contracts, drawing the edges of the wound together. This contracted tissue is relatively avascular and covered by firm epithelium and is know as a *scar*. The smaller the area of the wound the less scar tissue formed and consequently the less deformity. Thus an incised wound leaves a much smaller residual deformity than a large lacerated wound which caused much loss of tissue.

Factors affecting healing

Many factors affect healing and these may be local or general. The state of nutrition of the patient, and in particular protein depletion and lack of vitamin C are important. Patients with deep jaundice, liver disease and certain cancers do not heal as well as normal individuals. It has been suggested that environmental temperature may be important and that wounds heal more quickly and easily in warm climates. Local factors are extremely important and good coaptation of the wound margins without intervening dead tissue or foreign bodies are in favour of rapid healing. However, the most important local factors are the presence of a good blood supply and the absence of infection. Fortunately the blood supply is particularly rich in the head and neck and not often affected by disease but it is important in plastic reconstructive procedures about the jaws to ensure that flaps are adequately nourished.

The presence of infection in a wound leads to a continued inflammatory process with the formation of pus. The granulation tissue at the base continues to grow progressively but is impeded by areas of dead tissue (slough). Epithelial growth is inhibited and the wound will not heal until the infection has been treated or subsides. This process of healing can be slow and leads to the production of much deforming scar tissue.

A further local factor affecting wound healing is immobility of the part concerned, and rest is important. Sometimes elevation helps by allowing accumulated transudate and oedema to drain away. This knowledge is made use of in the treatment of wounds of the hand which is often elevated during the healing period.

The treatment of wounds

The treatment of wounds can be considered under the following headings.

Arrest of haemorrhage

Any large bleeding vessels are individually clipped and ligated. Should these vessels be essential to the blood supply of the part and if they are large, then reconstruction must be carried out. The same applies to the severance of large nerves which can be sutured and may regenerate in time.

Wound excision

This refers to the removal of debris and dead tissues from the wound. This is a most important step and the wound must be cut back to reveal clean, viable tissue. The presence of debris within the wound leads to slow healing, the formation of slough, and the danger of tetanus or gas gangrene.

Prevention of tetanus and gas gangrene

This is important in dirty, contaminated wounds, particularly if deep and accompanied by tissue destruction. Wound excision is of the first importance, and then further cleansing of the wound with saline. If the patient has been immunized against tetanus, a booster dose of tetanus toxoid plus an injection of soluble penicillin is adequate. Antitetanus serum carries the risk of allergic reaction but can be used once in conjunction with an initial dose of tetanus toxoid and an injection of antibiotics. Human tetanus immunoglobulin is now available in Britain, and wherever possible should be used instead of antitetanus serum. If the wound is deep then it is best not closed. A secondary suture can, if necessary, be performed at a later date.

Closure of the wound

If the edges can be brought together without undue tension then the wound is closed in layers using catgut in the deep tissues and interrupted everting sutures for the skin. Wounds on the face heal quickly and the skin sutures can be removed by the third or fourth day. For wounds in the mucous membrane catgut is frequently used for suture of all layers as it is absorbable.

Provision of skin cover by skin grafts and skin flaps

Skin grafts and skin flaps are used to provide cover for large open wounds whose margins cannot be coapted or for granulating areas in order to assist and hasten healing and to avoid contracture of tissues as a result of excess scar tissue formation during prolonged healing. In addition, grafts and flaps may be necessary to repair defects originating as a result of trauma or surgical operations. For example, after excision of a portion of the tongue and oral cavity for the treatment of oral cancer, a flap of skin may be rotated from the forehead or from the chest wall in order to provide a lining for the floor of the mouth and to repair the defect left by operation. Similarly, after excision of a portion of the mucosa of the mouth it is possible to place skin within the oral cavity to repair the defect.

Skin grafts refer to skin removed from donor sites and then placed in a new site elsewhere in the body. They are of two varieties. *Split skin grafts* consist of the epidermis and a partial thickness of the dermis and are widely used, especially in the treatment of burns. The resulting defect need not be covered with fresh skin since the skin will regenerate from the remaining dermis of the donor site. Suitable dressings are applied until this occurs.

Full thickness grafts on the other hand consist of the epidermis and the dermis, and the resultant defect can be closed either by direct suture if the donor area is small, by rotational skin flaps created from adjacent areas of skin, or by application of a split skin graft to the area from which the full thickness graft has been removed.

Skin flaps, on the other hand, consist of the epidermis, the dermis and the subcutaneous tissues together with an appropriate blood supply. The latter is important and dictates the length and shape of grafts that can be elevated. Such flaps can be moved on a rotational basis to new sites or can be tubed into the form of a pedicle (Fig. 4.1). The area from which the graft is taken must be repaired and this is usually done with a split skin graft taken from a donor site elsewhere. Skin flaps are extremely useful to repair defects created by surgical manoeuvres, particularly in the head and neck and in the management of large defects elsewhere on the body, and in particular on the limbs.

Similar principles to those used in the creation of skin flaps are used in the creation of plastic repairs

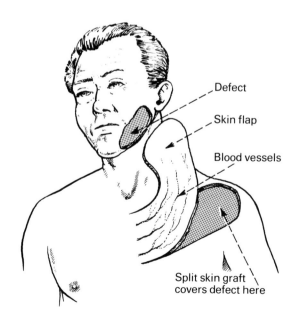

Fig. 4.1 A skin flap raised from the pectoral area to cover a large defect on the face.

to internal organs such as the bladder, the pelvis of the kidney and some other internal organs. The dentist may occasionally be called upon to form a small rotational flap of oral mucosa to close a persistent oral-antral fistula.

Dressing the wound

A minimum of dressings is desirable and usually of the dry variety. Antibiotics are used only in the prophylaxis of tetanus as described above and sometimes in the prevention of gas gangrene after amputation of the thigh in elderly patients with poor peripheral circulation.

Burns

Burns are a special kind of wound and may be caused by chemicals, by heat, and by electricity. A burn is classified as superficial if all layers of the skin are not damaged so that regrowth of skin is possible. Deep burns destroy all the layers of the skin, which cannot regrow from skin elements remaining but must heal from the edges or the defect must be closed by a skin graft. Following a severe burn there is a complex initial phase of shock. This is caused partly by the pain of the burn but largely as a result of loss of tissue fluid from the surface of the burn and by destruction of tissue such as muscle. If infection supervenes this can be a major additional factor.

Treatment of burns is directed towards relief of the pain and the replacement of the vast quantities of fluid that can be lost. Attempts are made to prevent infection and the burned area is either treated with a moist dressing or allowed to form a dry eschar. Skin grafting can be done either early or later after the dry crusted eschar separates.

SURGICAL OPERATIONS

Surgical operations are carried out to correct deformity, to remove diseased tissue or to repair defects in tissues caused by trauma or disease.

Incisions are made, if possible, along lines in the skin that will leave a minimum of scarring and will not lead to limitation in the movement of joints or muscles. Incisions in the abdominal or chest wall are made in such a way as to cause minimum muscle damage and allow healing with maximum strength.

A number of terms are used to describe various types of operations. Thus the suffix -otomy is used to describe operations in which an incision is made into a cavity for exploration without necessarily removing anything. Examples are laparotomy (exploration of the abdomen), thoracotomy (exploration of the chest), craniotomy (opening and exploration of the skull). The suffix -ectomy is used to describe operations in which some part of the body is removed. Examples are appendicectomy, cholecystectomy (removal of the gallbladder), partial thyroidectomy (partial removal of the thyroid gland), glossectomy (removal of the tongue). The suffix -ostomy is used to describe operations in which an orifice is made either between an internal organ and the surface or between two internal organs. Examples are, cholecystduodenostomy (creation of an opening between the gallbladder and the duodenum), colostomy (creation of an opening between the colon and the skin — used to relieve intestinal obstruction).

Examples of reconstructive and reparative surgery have already been given (the use of skin grafts) but there are many other examples. Thus, a damaged head of femur can be replaced by a metal prosthesis and of course there are many examples in dentistry from the filling of a cavity in a tooth and the provision of a denture through to the complex reconstructive procedures used to repair defects of the mandible as a result of loss by trauma or surgical removal. Repair of congenital defects such as cleft lip and cleft palate are other well-known examples involving the use of plastic surgical techniques. Indeed, this form of reconstructive or reparative surgery is common in the head and neck, and elaborate dental prosthesis is often necessary. The plastic surgeon and dentist work as a team.

Excisional and incisional surgery has a very wide range and can be used to treat a variety of disorders of most parts of the body. The operations used include drainage of pus from abscess cavities, selective division of nerves in order to produce specific effects, removal of cancerous growths, and total or partial removal of diseased organs. Some structures can be removed with almost total impunity. Thus the spleen can be sacrificed without undue

ill effect and one kidney can be removed provided the other is normal. Indeed the remaining kidney hypertrophies and the patient suffers no significant defect in renal function. On the other hand, the liver cannot be totally removed, although large portions can since it has extraordinary regenerative capacity and the remaining liver tissue will grow to reconstitute the original mass and support life. Large portions of the small bowel may be removed and partial or total gastrectomy can be performed. Removal of some organs leads to a necessity for replacement therapy. Examples of this are the necessity to supply vitamin B_{12} to patients who have had gastrectomy since they lack intrinsic factor and the necessity to supply corticosteroids to patients who have had the adrenal glands removed.

Abdominal operations are frequently used for diseases of the stomach or gut. For example, division of the vagus nerves (vagotomy) is used in the treatment of peptic ulceration because this cuts down gastric acid secretion and allows a duodenal ulcer to heal. Similarly, partial or total gastrectomy can be carried out for gastric ulcer or gastric cancer respectively and the same applies to the colon. Defects in the continuity of the intestinal tract are repaired by direct reconstruction (anastomosis) between the divided ends.

Pre- and postoperative care

It may seem too simple to state that no operation should be carried out unless it is necessary and has a good chance of success. It is, however, important to emphasize that good operative judgement depends on accurate diagnosis. Given precise diagnosis, good judgement and expert technique, the success of an operation depends on the care with which a patient is prepared, the skill of anaesthesia and the attention to detail in the postoperative period.

Preoperative preparation

A history must always be taken. No matter how minor the procedure the surgeon should always enquire as to the patient's general health and previous illness. The presence or absence of a productive cough, chest pain or dyspnoea reflecting cardiorespiratory disease must be sought and any medical history of hypertension or myocardial infarction ascertained. A personal and family tendency to bleed easily is of importance and especially bruising or continued haemorrhage from minor wounds. It is also important to take a drug history and to enquire as to allergy regarding particular drugs (for example, a patient on anticoagulant drugs may bleed heavily if subjected to surgery and a patient sensitive to penicillin may well die of an anaphylactic-type reaction if given further penicillin).

Postoperative deep vein thrombosis can complicate any operation involving bed rest (see below). A history of a previous episode of pulmonary embolism is sought and since the contraceptive pill predisposes to deep vein thrombosis enquiries should be made as to whether the patient is taking such a preparation. If this is the case, and the patient is to be submitted to general anaesthesia and so lie recumbent on an operating table for any length of time, she should cease taking the drug for at least one month before surgery and take alternative contraceptive measures.

A full physical examination is carried out with particular reference to cardiac and respiratory status. A chest X-ray and an electrocardiogram may be required, if indicated by the history. At least a haemoglobin estimation but usually a full blood count is carried out and anaemia corrected before operation. Estimation of the blood urea and electrolytes is performed, especially for operations that are likely to be followed by disturbances in fluid balance or by blood loss.

In the case of diabetics receiving insulin or hypoglycaemic drugs, appropriate precautions are taken, usually consisting of the administration of insulin and glucose infusion (see Ch. 15). Should the patient have a bleeding tendency or a disease which predisposes to this then a full coagulation screen is performed and appropriate precautions taken on the basis of the result. Thus, for instance, in obstructive jaundice, vitamin K_1 is administered before operation (see Ch. 12).

The anaesthetist is consulted in advance so that an appropriate assessment can be made of the best form of anaesthesia. It is important for the surgeon to select a form of anaesthesia which will allow him to proceed in an adequate manner and not be limited by inadequate anaesthesia as for instance

may occur where a local anaesthetic is inappropriately used.

Postoperative management

In the immediate postoperative period the patient must be closely observed until fully recovered from anaesthesia so that obstruction to the airway or inhalation of vomit or foreign bodies or of pharyngeal secretion does not occur. Respiratory function is of the greatest importance and in some patients who have respiratory embarrassment assisted ventilation by means of an indwelling endotracheal tube or even tracheostomy may be necessary for several days.

The patient's respiratory rate, pulse and blood pressure are monitored. The earliest sign of postoperative bleeding is a sustained rise in the pulse rate and this occurs before obvious signs of circulatory collapse occur. Urine output is carefully observed and is the best index of adequate renal perfusion and of adequate fluid intake.

In some patients operations on the gastrointestinal tract necessitate postoperative nasogastric suction in order to keep the gastrointestinal tract, and particularly the stomach, empty, and fluids must be supplied by means of intravenous therapy. Blood transfusion is administered as required and based on repeated estimations of the haemoglobin or haematocrit. The temperature of the patient is measured at least four hourly and a rise in temperature is investigated (see below).

The patient is carefully observed for postoperative complications and these may be specific to the operation performed or more general and likely to complicate any procedure.

Postoperative complications

Respiratory deficiency

Patients with pre-existing respiratory disease (e.g. chronic bronchitis) are more prone to postoperative respiratory problems, and operations upon the chest itself or involving upper abdominal incisions also predispose to postoperative chest problems. Inhalation of vomit, pharyngeal secretions or foreign bodies (e.g. an inhaled tooth) are certain to be followed by postoperative chest complications (Fig. 4.2 and Ch. 8).

Fig. 4.2 Tooth (upper arrow) in left lower lobe bronchus with collapse of left lower lobe (lower arrow) and mediastinal displacement.

In severe cases the patient is clearly dyspnoeic after operation and cyanosis is evident. The respiratory rate is rapid. Measurement of blood gases is helpful both in assessing severity and progress and in diagnosis of the respiratory defect.

The commonest chest complications are atelectasis (collapse of a portion of the lung due to plugging of a bronchus) and bronchopneumonia which is particularly liable to occur in the basal areas of the lung in old people confined to bed. Occasionally lobar pneumonia complicates the postoperative period. A chest X-ray is helpful in differentiating these conditions but they may coexist and are usually accompanied by a rise in temperature. Pulmonary embolism is a further severe postoperative complication which is discussed below.

Management is in the first instance by means of vigorous physiotherapy and encouraging the patient to cough. This must be done together with the provision of adequate analgesia. A specimen of sputum is sent for culture and the patient may then be commenced on antibiotics although many prefer to await the result. It is often found that in the intervening period the condition resolves spontaneously as a result of the simple measures outlined above.

Occasionally, bronchial secretions must be removed by means of aspiration through a bronchoscope, and very occasionally assisted respiration is necessary. This is also needed in severe chest injuries with disruption of a portion of the chest wall (flail chest) so that paradoxical respiration occurs. In this situation an endotracheal tube is passed and connected to a ventilator. The patient is paralysed with appropriate drugs and ventilated by the machine until such time as he is fit to breathe again himself. Whilst the endotracheal tube is in place the bronchial secretions are aspirated at regular intervals with sterile catheters and humidified gases are provided so that the bronchi do not become dried with the formation of crusting which also threatens respiration. An endotracheal tube can be left in place for several days provided that a low pressure cuff is used to avoid pressure necrosis of the tracheal wall. Should assisted ventilation be necessary for a prolonged period, tracheostomy must be performed.

Tracheostomy. This is an important operation and one which the dentist must understand. It consists of an opening in the trachea below the cricoid cartilage and through the second, third and fourth rings of the trachea to allow the insertion of an artificial airway which bypasses the upper respiratory tract. The advantages of tracheostomy are: (i) any obstruction to the respiratory tract in the pharynx or larynx is bypassed; (ii) the dead space is greatly reduced so that respiration is much easier for the patient; and (iii) there is access to the trachea and bronchial tree for toilet and suction as described above.

It is sometimes necessary to perform the operation as an emergency, but rarely before adequate facilities are at hand. The procedure is not easy and should not be attempted without due preparation unless absolutely essential.

An incision is made in the skin in a transverse manner about two fingers below the lower margin of the thyroid cartilage. Dissection is then proceeded with in the midline, and the strap muscles of the neck are retracted or divided. The best guide to the correct position for a tracheostomy is the isthmus of the thyroid gland, which usually requires division. The trachea is then exposed and either a disc removed from it or a flap hinged forwards and stitched to the lower skin incision. An appropriate tracheostomy tube is inserted and the cuff is then inflated and either connected to a respirator or left open to humidified air.

Wound infection

Any wound may become infected. This may arise from pre-existing infection within the patient such as the infection of an appendicectomy wound or may follow secondarily as a result of contamination. Wound infection is characterized by a red, painful and sometimes swollen wound, and fluctuation may be present. The patient has an elevated temperature and often an elevated pulse rate. Probing the wound and the removal of stitches results in the drainage of free pus and this should be sent for culture. Antibiotic therapy is not always necessary.

Wound disruption

Failure of the wound to heal may occur for reasons outlined previously. This is treated either by allowing the wound to granulate or by secondary suture.

Other postoperative infections

Apart from infection of the chest and of the wound, which are the most common varieties, infection can also occur elsewhere. Thus, urinary tract infection is common particularly if catheterization has been necessary. Infection of body cavities also occurs and this is particularly common after intra-abdominal operations on infected organs. The usual sites are beneath the diaphragm (subphrenic abscess) or deep within the pelvis (pelvic abscess). These conditions present with fever and local signs of inflammation and are treated by prompt drainage of the accumulated pus to the exterior.

Bacteraemia and septic shock

Very occasionally bacteria enter the bloodstream and multiply, producing toxins and leading to profound shock. Septic shock is discussed in the next chapter.

Deep vein thrombosis and pulmonary embolism

It has been shown that almost 30% of all patients submitted to elective major surgery develop deep vein thrombosis: the elderly, patients with cancer, and women on the pill are at increased risk. A proportion of patients who develop such thrombi within the legs shed these as emboli which pass in the venous circulation through the right side of the heart and lodge in the lung. A large pulmonary embolus results in sudden death but multiple small emboli present as chest pain, dyspnoea or syncope, often accompanied by a pleural rub, haemoptysis and fever.

Deep vein thrombosis may occur with minimal or even without obvious physical signs although leg swelling due to oedema and pain in the calf sometimes occur. An unexplained fever may be the only suggestion of the condition.

Preventive measures are extremely important. All patients at significant risk of venous thromboembolism should receive either measures to maintain calf blood flow (fitted elastic stockings or pneumatic compression leggings) or low-dose anticoagulants (subcutaneous heparin or oral warfarin). Suspected cases should be confirmed by venography or lung scanning, then anticoagulated (see Ch. 7).

Risks of operation to the surgeon

It is of importance, particularly in dental practice, to recognize that operations carry some risk to the operating surgeon. Of these the most important is the risk of contracting hepatitis B, HIV infection or syphilis (see Ch. 2) as a result of contamination by the patient's blood. In addition to these factors penetration of the eyes of the surgeon by infected material or sharp debris is not uncommon and may occur in dental practice.

5

Acute haemorrhage, shock, and severe injury

Haemorrhage may occur as a result of injury or from pathological processes resulting in damage to vessel walls. In addition, severe bleeding may result from apparently trivial injuries in patients who suffer from a haemorrhagic disorder or who are taking anticoagulant drugs.

The haemorrhage may be external and visible on the surface or from one of the orifices of the body, or internal as when bleeding occurs into a body cavity, into the lumen of hollow viscera, or into tissue spaces.

The haemorrhage may be primary and occur at the time of injury, or reactionary and occur 4–6 hours later usually as a result of displacement of a clot, dislodgement of a ligature or movement of a dressing. It may be secondary, occurring 7–14 days later associated with infection or separation of a slough.

PATHOPHYSIOLOGY OF HAEMORRHAGE AND HYPOVOLAEMIC SHOCK

Following damage to a blood vessel, blood escapes and comes into contact with damaged tissue, platelets become adherent and aggregate, and clot formation is initiated (see Ch. 12). Complete division of a vessel, particularly an artery, results in retraction of the vessel with a tendency to seal off but this does not occur if the vessel is partially divided. As a result of the loss of blood, the blood volume is reduced and consequently the venous return and central venous pressure fall. There is a tendency for the blood pressure to fall but baroreflexes operate resulting in tachycardia and peripheral vasoconstriction as a result of sympathetic activity. These factors tend to maintain the blood pressure. Should haemorrhage continue unchecked, a stage of hypovolaemic shock results. In this condition, despite an increase in the heart rate and maximal peripheral vasoconstriction, the blood pressure falls. In other words, decompensation has occurred. The patient is pale and sweating with a cold clammy skin, there is a rapid pulse rate, hypotension, and rapid shallow breathing. Unless haemorrhage is checked and the blood volume replaced, death results. It should be noted that in a case of progressive haemorrhage, the initial abnormal signs may be only tachycardia and pallor. Once a low blood pressure is present, decompensation has already taken place.

Management of haemorrhage and hypovolaemic shock

Arrest of haemorrhage

Arterial haemorrhage is to be recognized by the red colour of the blood and the fact that the bleeding occurs in spurts. In venous haemorrhage, on the other hand, the blood is much darker in colour and the bleeding is continuous in nature. Capillary haemorrhage is characterized by an ooze of bright red blood from a broad surface.

The arrest of haemorrhage depends on its nature. Temporary control of arterial bleeding may be obtained by the application of a tourniquet but the only certain way of obtaining control is to ligate both ends of the divided vessel or the main supplying vessel at a proximal point. Thus for severe bleeding from the mouth or face it may be necessary to ligate the external carotid artery. Arterial haemorrhage occurring during operation can be controlled by ligation or clamping of vessels, by firm pressure (packing), or by electrocoagulation.

Venous haemorrhage can be very difficult to control. It may be possible to ligate both ends of a large vein that is bleeding but more often venous haemorrhage is controlled by pressure, combined if possible with elevation of the wounded part. In the case of venous and arterial haemorrhage, large vessels may sometimes be controlled by patching or suture repair. Capillary haemorrhage usually offers no problem in control unless there is an associated coagulation defect. Bleeding from a ruptured viscus can sometimes be controlled by excision (e.g. splenectomy for splenic rupture).

After extraction of a tooth or operation within the mouth, haemorrhage may occur from vessels in the mucous membrane, periosteum, or from within the cancellous bone of the jaws. Control is usually obtained by the insertion of sutures, but occasionally packing may be necessary. Where haemorrhage is anticipated the construction of special splints for the application of gentle pressure may be necessary.

Replacement of blood volume

In addition to arrest of haemorrhage, the management of the patient demands prevention and treatment of shock. The blood pressure and pulse are observed at regular intervals and in the severely ill patient a catheter is inserted to record central venous pressure. This central venous pressure line is of value in monitoring rapid transfusion of fluids used to replace blood volume.

The ideal method of restoring the blood volume is by the transfusion of whole blood compatible with that of the recipient. Donor blood is grouped and cross-matched against that of the recipient and must be carefully checked before administration.

While blood is being grouped and cross-matched, the patient may be transfused with an electrolyte solution such as isotonic saline or may be given plasma protein solution (PPS) or a plasma substitute such as dextran. If dextran is used, blood must be taken for grouping and cross-matching before its administration. The urine output is monitored and should be maintained at a minimum of 50 ml per hour.

Often surprisingly large quantities of fluid and blood must be transfused in the treatment of haemorrhagic shock and the quantities administered are best guided by reference to the central venous pressure, the heart rate and the urine output.

Blood transfusion

Transfusion of whole blood is wasteful, and only the specific components required are given. Packed red cells are given to correct anaemia or blood loss, the remaining volume in blood loss being replaced by plasma protein solution (PPS) which is largely albumin. Plasma is reserved for treatment of coagulation defects (see Ch. 12), either as fresh frozen plasma, or as clotting factor concentrates (factor VIII or factor IX) for haemophilia. Surplus plasma is then made into PPS or albumin solution. Platelet concentrates are given in thrombocytopenia.

The recipient blood must be compatible with that of the donor or agglutination and haemolysis occur with dire results. The ABO blood group system contains four primary blood groups based on two antigens denoted A and B (to which antibodies occur naturally). The antigens are found singly, together, or may be entirely absent (Table 5.1). The four blood groups which result are given the symbols group AB, A, B and O, and the blood groups are inherited as autosomal dominant conditions.

Table 5.1 The ABO group system

Group	Cells	Serum
O	neither A nor B	anti A, anti B
A	A	anti B
B	B	anti A
AB	AB	neither anti A nor Anti B

Many other blood grouping systems have been discovered. In addition to belonging to one of the four primary blood groups, every individual has or has not in their blood a factor known as Rhesus (Rh). Rh incompatibility can lead to transfusion reactions and whenever possible Rh grouping is undertaken before transfusion is given. Since sensitization to Rh factor can occur, Rh negative patients should whenever possible receive only Rh negative blood.

Complications of blood transfusion

Blood transfusion may be complicated by the dangers associated with the transfusion of any fluid such as infection, fever, allergic reactions, thrombophlebitis, overtransfusion with resultant heart failure and air embolism.

Dangers especially associated with the transfusion of blood include the following:

1. Hypothermia — a rapid transfusion of large quantities of cold blood may lead to reduction in body temperature.

2. Clotting defect — storage of blood results in reduction in platelets and loss of clotting factors. Large transfusions may result in dilution of the recipient's own platelets and coagulation factors and a clotting defect.

3. Infection — bacterial contamination or contamination with viruses may result in infection. Thus hepatitis B and non-A, non-B, HIV, syphilis and malaria may be transmitted by transfused blood.

4. Biochemical upset — hyperkalaemia or hypocalcaemia may occur in massive blood transfusion.

5. Serological incompatibility — the reactions seen are the result of agglutination and haemolysis. Often the first complaint is of pain in the loins. There may be tachycardia associated with pallor and vasoconstriction of the skin vessels but this may be replaced by flushing. There may be rigors, severe dyspnoea, and the patient may collapse. Acute renal failure and also jaundice may develop as a consequence of intravascular haemolysis.

If any of the signs and symptoms referred to above occur, or indeed if there is a brisk reaction to the transfusion in the form of pyrexia, the transfusion should be stopped and samples of the transfused blood and of the patient's blood saved for later investigation.

Other forms of shock

In addition to hypovolaemic shock, which has been dealt with in some detail, the student should be aware of other forms of shock. Some of these are referred to in other chapters.

1. *Cardiogenic shock*. This occurs in myocardial infarction due to failure of the heart as an efficient pump (see Ch. 7).

2. *Septic shock*. This is an important form of shock and has shown an increased incidence in recent years, probably due to the increased use of an-

tibiotics (with the development of resistant strains of organism), the fact that operations are conducted on a more extensive scale, occupy longer periods of time, and are frequently carried out in the elderly. In addition, surgery is often performed in immunosuppressed patients. The increasing incidence of severe trauma is also a factor.

The condition is due to toxins, usually endotoxins, released from the walls of small bacteria and, in particular, Gram-negative organisms such as Esch. coli. It is characterized by fever, sometimes by the development of a classical form of shock but more frequently by development of warm, dry extremities associated with a decrease in the peripheral resistance, a fall in blood pressure, and early hyperventilation. These features are accompanied by an increased cardiac output in the face of a falling blood volume and it is characteristic that the patient may have an elevated central venous pressure. Arteriovenous shunting occurs in the lungs and there is a decreased peripheral utilization of oxygen due to the direct effect of the toxins. Blood begins to pool in the periphery and, indeed, clotting may occur in the vessels themselves. Renal function is impaired as a result of hypoperfusion, also possibly as a result of intravascular coagulation.

The condition of septic shock is especially likely to follow procedures on organs that are already infected, e.g. the urinary tract, the biliary tree, or after surgery on the large bowel.

Treatment of the condition is by early institution of antibiotic therapy, a good combination being gentamicin and metronidazole, the two antibiotics together coping with most Gram-negative organisms including the Bacteroides. Attempts are made to maintain or even increase the cardiac output and the use of appropriate drugs to stimulate the myocardium, of which dopamine is the most frequently used, is instituted. Fluid is replaced and red cells are administered if necessary.

It should be emphasized that septic shock is a highly dangerous condition and the mortality is high, this being inevitable if sepsis is not controlled. Survival depends upon early recognition and appropriate treatment. As mentioned above, the initial therapy is directed at maintaining blood volume and treating the underlying bacteraemia, support of respiration, monitoring of renal function and treatment of the failing myocardium. One of the most important features is the early identification and surgical drainage of abscess collections and of infective fluid. This is mandatory and must be carried out as soon as the initial measures of resuscitation have been instituted.

The important points to emphasize are the following:

a. The possibility of preventive measures by the use of prophylactic antibiotics (as, for example, in operations on the infected biliary tree).
b. The early recognition of the physical signs.
c. The prompt institution of broad-spectrum antibiotic cover (without waiting for sensitivities obtained from culture) and supportive measures.
d. Adequate drainage of collections of pus (e.g. within the peritoneal cavity) if there is to be any real hope of recovery.

3. *Anaphylactic shock.* This results from antigen-antibody reactions in previously sensitized individuals and is the result of the release of a variety of vasoactive substances, mainly histamine. These substances cause intense dilatation of small vessels causing shock, together with increased permeability and constriction of bronchioles resulting in bronchospasm. Anaphylactic shock usually follows injection of drugs (e.g. penicillins, local anaesthetics) or blood products, or insect stings. Treatment is discussed in Chapter 16.

4. *Neurogenic shock (vasovagal attack).* This is the simple faint and is often precipitated by sudden fright, fear, or by pain. It is described fully in Chapter 7. It is important to recognize that fainting may occur during anaesthesia and for this reason the administration of anaesthetics in the upright position in the dental chair is associated with danger of cerebral anoxia.

5. *Adrenal failure.* Lack of glucocorticoids and mineralocorticoids due to absence or disease of the adrenals can lead to a clinical state indistinguishable from shock. A similar problem may occur in patients who have been receiving long-term steroid therapy with prednisolone or similar preparation; in such individuals atrophy of the adrenal cortex is likely to occur so that the patient is unable to respond in the normal way to the stress of infection, injury, anaesthesia and surgical procedures. In these circumstances patients on steroid therapy may become collapsed, hypotensive and gravely ill. Prevention and treatment are discussed in Chapter 13.

Assessment and management of severe injury

Severe injury in civilian life is usually due to the effects of road traffic accidents. Multiple injury is frequent with damage to the head, chest, abdomen and limbs. The situation is often complicated by drunkenness in the victims of accidents or in the drivers, and perhaps by prior consumption of drugs. Immediate threats to life are usually from obstruction to the airway, haemorrhage and rapidly advancing intracerebral haemorrhage.

The assessment of such injuries and their appropriate management is a complex matter. In general, injuries can be divided into:

1. Those injuries which are immediately life-threatening. The haemorrhage may be so gross and so rapid that life will be lost if operation is not carried out within a few minutes and there may be obvious obstruction to the airway and impending asphyxia. In such instances immediate control of the airway with, if necessary, the insertion of an endotracheal tube or even an immediate tracheostomy are essential. Haemorrhage must be arrested immediately and blood replaced if life is to be saved. Operation, therefore, may have to be carried out as a dire emergency and possibly even within the casualty department or at the site of the accident.

2. In other injuries, there is no immediate threat to life and there is some time to assess the situation. Most such patients, usually with injury to the chest or abdomen, require surgery within one or two hours, but there is an opportunity to assess the degree of damage, to group and cross-match blood, and to take essential X-rays. Antibiotics are administered if necessary and the patient is then taken to the operating theatre for appropriate surgery to control haemorrhage and for the removal of damaged tissues or repair of ruptured organs.

3. Occult injuries may develop slowly and quietly and there may even be few signs of damage. A high index of suspicion is necessary in the detection of such injuries, which usually involve the abdomen after blunt injury, but also occur in some forms of head injury (see Ch. 18). In such instances there is time for more extensive tests and for assessment of a

planned course of action. An example is the delayed presentation which occurs in some ruptures of the spleen and liver. In such instances, the use of angiographic methods or isotope studies may reveal the diagnosis.

In summary, the assessment and management of severe trauma is as follows:

1. Make sure that the airway is clear. Remove broken teeth, mucus and foreign bodies from the mouth.
2. Arrest obvious haemorrhage.
3. Set up intravenous line for replacement of lost blood.
4. Assess associated injury, particularly:
   a. to the head;
   b. occult injury to the chest and the possible presence of pneumothorax;
   c. injuries to the limbs (compound fractures should be immediately covered with a sterile dressing and temporarily splinted);
   d. assess the presence or absence of haematuria.
5. Pass a catheter to monitor urinary output.
6. Make an assessment of the presence of intoxication, drug consumption or associated disease.

It is important in injury to obtain a good history from the patient, if possible, but also from the ambulance driver or police who accompany the patient to the hospital and from any relatives who are either with the patient at the time of admission or who are available at a later stage.

6

Tumours and their management

New growths arising from and resembling the tissues of the body are referred to as tumours or neoplasms. They are distinguished from the phenomena of hypertrophy and hyperplasia in that they continue growing independent of the growth or well-being of the host and even after the stimulus which initiated them has been removed. Indeed our understanding of tumours is handicapped in that we know so little of the initiating stimuli. In some instances specific aetiological factors such as hereditary predisposition, chronic mechanical or chemical irritation, infections such as syphilis or HIV, or response to hormonal stimulation are known to be partially responsible. In most cases, however, the causative factors are obscure.

Neoplasms are classified according to their structure and their behaviour into two groups, benign and malignant. Most tumours can be easily allocated to one or other of these groups but occasionally the distinction is difficult to make and some benign tumours are prone to undergo malignant change.

Differences between benign and malignant tumours

Benign tumours resemble in consistency and in histological characteristics the tissues of the body. In general, they are encapsulated by a compressed layer of connective tissue and displace the surrounding tissues without evidence of invasion. As a result of this, they are well defined and do not readily become attached to surrounding structures. They are generally not dangerous to life but they may grow to a considerable size and thus interfere with vital structures. In addition, benign tumours may rupture and cause life-threatening haemorrhage or they may secrete abnormal quantities of hormones and thereby cause significant disease.

It is important to recognize that benign tumours do not spread either by direct invasion or by the development of daughter growths to distant parts of the body and are therefore capable of cure by local excision. This is what separates them more than anything else from the malignant tumours which do invade and destroy local tissues and also spread to distant parts of the body by a process known as metastasis.

Malignant tumours, although broadly resembling normal tissue histologically, usually differ considerably from the normal body tissues both in the structure of individual cells and in the architecture of the tissue so that it may be extremely difficult to determine the tissue of origin. Such dedifferentiation is termed anaplasia and the greater it is, the higher the degree of malignancy. The tumours are not encapsulated and have an indefinite growing edge which may involve local blood vessels, nerves, or other vital structures. Malignant growths may also compress adjacent tissues or produce abnormal hormone secretion.

In addition, malignant neoplasms are often associated with a progressive deterioration in general health and wasting, referred to as cachexia. The mechanism of malignant cachexia is obscure but may be due to the fact that malignant tumours metabolize excessive quantities of nutrient material at the expense of the host. In addition, they may bleed giving rise to anaemia, they may have an effect on the appetite of the host and, by their situation (e.g. cancer of the stomach), they may lead not only to decreased food intake but also to increased protein loss through the gut. Furthermore, secondary infection is undoubtedly an important factor and contributes significantly to a general decline in health.

Spread of malignant tumours

As stated above, malignant tumours invade local tissues and this is referred to as *spread in continuity*. Closely adjacent structures may also be affected and this is referred to as *spread in contiguity*. Thus, a carcinoma of the bronchus may affect the surrounding lung tissue and might invade the heart or the nearby oesophagus.

Spread of the tumour to form secondary growths in other parts of the body takes place by a number of methods. Firstly, tumour cells may enter the lymphatics and grow along the lymphatic pathways by a process known as *permeation*. Alternatively, tumour cells that have entered the lymphatics pass in the lymph flow to the nearest lymph node where they become arrested. This is known as *lymphatic embolism*. This process is repeated successively until tumour cells pass not only to other local lymph nodes but also to subsequent groups of nodes and finally enter the bloodstream.

Secondly, tumour cells may directly invade local blood vessels and such invasion is followed by the growth of tumour cells in cords along local blood vessels, but more commonly they become detached and embolize along the venous pathways until arrested in the nearest capillary bed. It is for this reason that tumour cells spreading by the bloodstream from cancers of the gut pass in the portal vein and are arrested in the liver, this being the commonest site for daughter growths from the alimentary cancer. On the other hand, tumours associated with or draining into the peripheral venous system shed tumour cells which are arrested in the lungs, which are also a common site of secondary deposits. Not all tumour cells escaping into the lymphatic system or bloodstream survive and some tumours seem to have a special predilection for metastasis to certain organs. For instance, secondary tumours in bone tend to be associated with primary growths in the bronchus, thyroid, breast, kidney, and prostate gland. Some small emboli may succeed in traversing the capillary bed and are then carried from the liver or lungs via the arterial stream to other parts of the body. The process of formation of metastases is of great importance because prevention of such daughter growths would be a major advance in the treatment of malignant disease.

Thirdly, tumour cells may spread across body cavities by a process known as *transcoelomic spread*. Thus, a cancer of the stomach may penetrate the wall of the stomach and seed cells into the peritoneal cavity which come to rest on the ovaries within the pelvis. Similar spread takes place in the pleural cavity. Tumours of the central nervous system are a rather special case in that they do not spread outside the meninges but may form daughter growths elsewhere within the central nervous system by spreading within the cerebrospinal fluid.

Fourthly, tumours may grow along pre-existing tubular structures within the body, as for example the growth of a cancer of the renal pelvis down a ureter. Finally, tumour cells contaminating surgical instruments may occasionally be embedded in wounds and grow at their site of implantation.

It is important to differentiate secondary daughter growths from completely new primary tumours within the same organ.

TYPES OF NEOPLASM

Neoplasms are described depending on the nature of the tissue from which they arise.

Epithelial growths

Such growths may be benign or malignant and originate either in surface epithelium or in glandular structures. The neoplastic tissue is epithelial but there is usually a supporting stroma of connective tissue containing blood vessels and frequently nerve fibres. Benign growths that arise from surface epithelium are known as papillomata and are extremely common. Such small papillomata may occur on the face or in the mouth.

Malignant tumours arising from the epithelium are of importance to the dental surgeon. They may arise from squamous or glandular epithelium.

Squamous epithelium

Basal cell carcinoma (rodent ulcer, Fig. 6.1) occurs commonly on the lateral side of the nose or at the

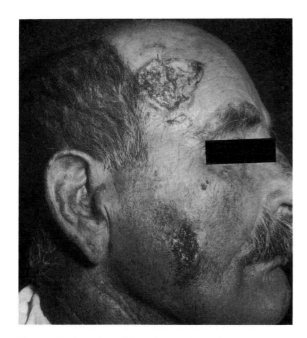

Fig. 6.1 Rodent ulcer of right cheek and right forehead.

lateral canthus of the eye. The lesion presents as a small nodule which ultimately forms an ulcer with a rolled, pearly edge.

Squamous cell carcinoma (epithelioma) occurs widely on the skin of the body and also occurs at the anal canal, on the glans penis, in the squamous lining of the oesophagus, and commonly on the lips or in the oral cavity. In this latter situation, it is recognized by the fact that it is commonly ulcerated and has a raised, rolled, everted hard edge with an indurated base.

Glandular epithelium

Carcinomata arising from glandular epithelium are known as adenocarcinomata. Such cancers may arise in solid glandular structures such as the thyroid and adrenal glands but more commonly arise from the glandular lining of the gastrointestinal tract (adenocarcinoma of the stomach or colon) or within the breast.

Connective tissue growths

Connective tissue growths may be benign and arise from fatty tissue (lipoma), fibrous tissue (fibroma),

bone (osteoma) or cartilage (chondroma). They may contain neural or vascular elements (neurofibroma, haemangioma). Tumours such as simple lipomata are ubiquitous and may be found in relation to the head and neck. Haemangiomata may bleed excessively with trauma and are of importance to dental surgeons since they occur within the oral cavity or even within bone. There is also a group of giant cell tumours known as osteoclastomata which are common in the long bones in the young and are composed of osteoclasts. A variety of benign tumours may arise from tissues of dental origin.

The *malignant* neoplasms of mesodermal origin are referred to as sarcomata and, unlike the carcinomata, are relatively common in children and in the young adult. Like their benign counterparts, they may arise in cartilage, bone, fat or muscle (e.g. liposarcoma).

Such sarcomata are highly malignant and prone to bloodborne metastases, especially to the lungs. They tend to be anaplastic lesions consisting of round or spindle cells. They are common in relation to bone (osteosarcoma) and are highly vascular. Tumours arising from the lymphoid organs (lymphomas) are highly anaplastic growths.

Melanoma

Melanomata arise from the melanin-containing cells of the body and may occur as simple pigmented moles which are extremely common. These moles may be found scattered on the body surface and are quite benign. On the other hand, the malignant melanoma is highly dangerous and metastasizes readily. Should a benign pigmented naevus show an increase in size, change in colour, the development of a surrounding halo of pigment, or bleed, it should be suspected of having undergone malignant change. Malignant melanoma not only occurs in the skin but is also found in the bed of the nails, in the oral cavity, in the oesophagus, and may occur within the eye. Spread is via the lymphatics and also by means of the blood, multiple liver metastases being very common.

Teratomata

These are neoplasms which contain mixed elements of both epithelial and mesodermal origin. Benign teratomata are extremely rare but occur on occasion; the dermoid cyst of the ovary is an example. It may contain such diverse elements as thyroid gland, cartilage, and even teeth and hair. Malignant teratomata, which lead to the formation of metastatic deposits, also occur.

Dermoid cysts, which are simple growths found at the lines of embryological fusion such as at the lateral canthus of the eye, must be distinguished from the teratomata referred to above.

PRESENTING FEATURES OF TUMOURS

Local mass

All tumours, whether benign or malignant, may present as a local swelling. The mass may be small so that in the case of malignant tumours the presenting symptom may be from a secondary deposit rather than the primary growth. On the other hand, the local mass may be of considerable size. Careful examination of the characteristics of the mass is important since benign tumours remain mobile and are not attached to the skin or underlying deep tissues. They tend to grow slowly. Malignant neoplasms, on the other hand, form local masses which grow steadily in size, are invasive, and consequently are attached to the surrounding structures and so become progressively fixed. These characteristics can be demonstrated on physical examination. Thus, an invasive carcinoma of the breast produces distortion of the breast and retraction of the nipple or skin tethering due to local invasion and cannot be readily moved on the underlying pectoral muscles when these are contracted.

As the tumour grows, it may produce signs and symptoms from pressure on neighbouring structures. Thus, a tumour of the thyroid gland may compress the trachea or oesophagus causing dyspnoea or dysphagia. Such compression may become suddenly more severe if necrosis and haemorrhage occur in the centre of the tumour with consequent rapid increase in size.

The local mass may ulcerate with consequent secondary infection or local abscess formation (Fig. 6.2). In addition, such secondary infection leads to a reactive change in the draining lymph nodes which should not be mistaken for spread of tumour. The presence of ulceration or central necrosis may be accompanied by local pain.

Fig. 6.2 Ulcerating secondary carcinoma involving lymph nodes of the neck. The patient died later from exsanguinating haemorrhage following involvement of the carotid artery.

As the tumour extends locally, the invasive process may involve blood vessels with consequent exsanguinating haemorrhage; this is not uncommon as a terminal event in advanced tumours of the head and neck. Similarly, local nerves may be involved with the production of pain which may be referred to distant sites. The growing tumour may also cause perforation of hollow viscera or fistulate into neighbouring viscera or to the skin. In the case of bone tumours, the local mass may so erode the bone as to result in pathological fracture.

Metastatic tumour

The outstanding characteristic of malignant tumours is the production of metastases (Fig. 6.3) which may be the presenting feature. For example, a patient with primary adenocarcinoma of the colon may present with a painful enlarged liver due to secondary deposits, or a patient with osteosarcoma of bone may be found to have large secondaries in the lung fields on chest X-ray.

Hormonal effects

Benign and malignant tumours may produce abnormal secretion of hormones and present with the

Fig. 6.3 Involvement of the shoulder with lytic deposits from a primary carcinoma of the prostate gland.

clinical effects of excessive hormone production. Thus, for example, patients with insulin-producing tumours of the pancreas may first present with the features of hypoglycaemia. In a similar way, patients with tumours of the adrenal cortex may present with the clinical features of Cushing's syndrome.

General effects

In addition to the deterioration in general health which has been referred to above, further, more specific systemic effects may be produced in association with tumour growth. Thus, for example, some tumours of the kidney may be associated with fever of unknown origin or with polycythaemia, and ill-understood neurological deficits may occur in association with some carcinomata of the bronchus in the absence of demonstrable secondary deposits in the brain.

PRINCIPLES OF TREATMENT

In the case of benign tumours, the indications for treatment are the production of pressure effects, abnormal hormone production, or unsightly appearance of the tumour. In addition, many benign tumours are excised for the purposes of histological examination since their nature is in doubt.

In the case of malignant neoplasms, death will result unless the lesion is completely eradicted.

Surgical removal

Removal of a benign tumour results in cure unless small portions of the tumour are left behind, in which case it may recur. Removal is in general not difficult since a tissue plane between the normal and the abnormal tissue can generally be defined. Occasionally, surgical removal is effected by diathermy destruction, the use of cryosurgical methods, or laser therapy.

The surgical removal of malignant tumours is not simple since the plane between normal and abnormal tissue cannot be seen with the naked eye. For this reason, wide excision is practised removing a generous portion of surrounding normal tissue. Because of the possibility of spread to local lymph nodes, these are usually excised in continuity although in some instances secondary excision of the lymph nodes is practised if they later show signs of involvement. Local surgery, even with wide excision of the tumour and the related lymph nodes, is bound to be unsuccessful if distant bloodborne metastases or involvement of distant lymph nodes has already occurred. This is the limiting factor in the practice of excisional surgery and much effort is directed towards the definition of the extent of the disease in cancer and in particular to assessment of the primary growth and related nodes and to the possibility of the involvement of distant organs.

The wide areas of normal tissue excised along with cancerous growths result in defects which are made good by reparative surgery.

Radiotherapy

Radiotherapy may be applied by irradiation from an external source such as supervoltage machine or linear accelerator, or less frequently by irradiation from radioactive material inserted into the tumour substance or administered orally or by injection.

A sufficiently high dosage of X-rays is lethal to all tissues, including all tumours. The use of radiotherapy depends on the fact that firstly some tumours are especially radiosensitive, their cells being destroyed by radiation dosage which is tolerated by normal tissues, and secondly that the X-rays are directed at the tumour as a target. Conventional radiotherapy machines operate at voltages up to 250 kilovolts but supervoltage machines generate radiation of very short wavelength and these have great penetrating powers and thus can be used to deliver larger dosages of the radiation to deeply seated lesions with less risk of damaging overlying tissues. A radioactive isotope of cobalt can provide an alternative source of irradiation, the gamma rays produced being therapeutically effective.

The dosage of radiation is measured in units known as grays (Gy), the gray being related to the quantity of absorbed energy in the tissues irradiated. Interstitial irradiation is used in the treatment of some tumours by the insertion of radioactive material in the form of radium needles, radon seeds, or by other methods. These procedures are not used as frequently nowadays, having been superseded by better methods of external irradiation, but they still have a place in the treatment of tumours of the tongue, pharynx, bladder and cervix. Radioactive iodine (^{131}I) can be administered orally or by injection for the treatment of carcinoma of the thyroid gland, but only for tumours that can be shown to take up iodine.

Indications for radiotherapy

In the treatment of primary tumours, radiotherapy may be used in an attempt to effect a cure and is the treatment of choice for most epitheliomata of the skin, uterine cervix, lip and oral cavity, and for basal cell carcinoma of the skin. In addition, radiotherapy and surgical excision can be practised in combination. Thus, in some clinics cancer of the oesophagus is irradiated before surgical excision and the same approach is under investigation in the treatment of carcinoma of the rectum. In the same way, radiotherapy can be used in an attempt to eradicate cells possibly left behind after surgical excision. Thus, for example, in carcinoma of the breast, radiotherapy can be applied to the healed skin flaps and, where there are secondary deposits in the axilla, to the entire remaining lymphatic drainage of the breast in the axilla, supraclavicular and mediastinal nodes.

In the palliative treatment of advanced cancer, radiotherapy is extremely valuable not only for the relief of symptoms from inoperable tumours but for the treatment of metastases. Thus, for example, it is extremely common for patients to develop very painful secondary deposits in bone and the pain can be completely relieved by the skilled application of radiotherapy.

Chemotherapy

Many cytotoxic agents have anticancer effects due to their ability to damage actively dividing cells. They are not specific for malignant tissue and their use therefore produces toxic side-effects. These drugs are currently used mainly for the palliation of advanced malignant disease but they are being employed as adjuvants in cancer surgery or radiotherapy in the hope of yielding a greater cure rate.

The most important toxic effects result from haemopoietic depression (see Ch. 12) but gastrointestinal ulceration and alopecia also occur. Therefore monitoring of treatment is necessary and frequent estimations of the haemoglobin, white cell count and platelet count are necessary. Severe stomatitis, vomiting or diarrhoea may necessitate discontinuing therapy. It is important to bear in mind that the effects of therapy must not be allowed to become more severe than the symptoms of the disease.

Four main groups of cytotoxic agents are in common use:

1. Alkylating agents
2. Antimetabolites
3. Alkaloid drugs
4. Products of microorganisms.

Alkylating agents cause cell death by alteration in essential cellular constituents. Examples of such drugs are the nitrogen mustards or nitrogen mustard analogues such as chlorambucil and cyclophosphamide. The antimetabolites depend on the blocking of enzymatic reactions and fall into two groups, the antipurine drugs and the folic acid antagonists. The best known examples of these are 6-mercaptopurine which is used in the management of leukaemia, and 5-fluorouracil which is finding increasing use in the treatment of metastatic large bowel cancer. The alkaloid drugs such as vinblastine and vincristine have considerable cytotoxic effects and are used in the treatment of certain leukaemias and lymphomas.

Chemotherapy using cytotoxic agents may be applied by oral or intravenous injection but high concentrations of anticancer drugs may be delivered to the tumour by intra-arterial perfusion. Such intra-arterial methods have been used in the management of advanced lesions of the head and neck.

Endocrine therapy

Some tumours are sensitive to changes in their hormonal environment. Such tumours are said to be hormone-dependent and modifications in their growth can be achieved either by additive therapy whereby hormones are administered parenterally or orally in an attempt to control the growth of the tumour (e.g. oestrogens in the form of stilboestrol can be given to men with cancer of the prostate) or by ablative therapy whereby major endocrine glands are surgically removed or destroyed by means of irradiation (e.g. hypophysectomy or adrenalectomy in advanced breast cancer). Not all tumours of a particular type are sensitive to their hormonal environment in the same way and research is being directed towards the assessment of sensitivity prior to treatment.

Immunotherapy

The theory that an immune response to cancer occurs is being investigated in many centres and attempts are being made to exploit any possible host reaction to the tumours. The fact that spontaneous regression has been noted in some tumours, particularly in malignant melanomata, has encouraged the investigation of immunotherapy, but such methods are not yet established.

Nonspecific therapy

It should be remembered that patients suffering from tumours, particularly malignant lesions, require expert nursing, psychological support and, in the advanced stages of the disease, relief from pain. Such measures are of equal importance to attempts at cure. In addition, during the terminal stages of illness, skilled counselling of the patient and family are of considerable importance. This terminal care is increasingly performed in cancer hospices, or in the patient's home with visiting support from the hospice.

SOME IMPORTANT TUMOURS

It is important that the dentist has a clear appreciation of carcinoma of the tongue, of the lip and, to a lesser extent, of carcinoma of the oesophagus, and these are described below. Carcinoma of the breast is an important tumour which illustrates well many of the points outlined above and is therefore described in some detail.

Tumours of the breast

Both benign and malignant tumours of the breast must be differentiated from cysts of the breast, which are common.

Benign tumours

Papillomata of the ducts of the breast tissue may occur and present with a blood-stained or watery discharge from the nipple.

Fibro-adenoma is a benign tumour with epithelial elements derived from the ductules and acini and set in a fibrous stroma. This tumour occurs frequently in young women and is a lump of firm consistency and smooth surface which is well demarcated and very mobile (breast 'mouse').

Breast cancer

This is the commonest malignancy in women in Britain. The disease causes over 10 000 deaths annually. Nearly all cancers of the breast arise from the epithelial lining of the duct system. The tumour grows into the breast tissue locally, involving the overlying skin and causing retraction of the nipple and distortion of the breast. Finally the skin ulcerates and satellite nodules may occur involving the whole chest wall. The tumour grows deeply and involves the pectoral muscle with deep attachment. Lymphatic spread extends to the regional nodes of which the axillary nodes are extremely important but, in addition, the mediastinal and supraclavicular nodes become involved. Blood spread tends to occur early in the disease and the cancer may spread to any tissue. However, the bones are commonly involved, as are the lungs and liver. Metastases to bone are commonly osteolytic and may be seen on skeletal X-ray but early bony deposits may not be visible although they can be demonstrated by means of radioisotopic scanning techniques.

Diagnosis is based on the clinical finding of a lump in the breast, which may be small and difficult to distinguish from a benign tumour but may be large, with tethering and dimpling of the skin as described above. A lump in the breast must never be regarded as benign on clinical examination alone and excision biopsy is necessary.

Treatment. There is debate as to the treatment of choice for early cancer of the breast. In Britain, simple mastectomy and biopsy of the axillary nodes is at present the most common form of treatment, and radiotherapy is given should the axillary nodes be involved with tumour. However, these methods of treatment should not be employed if distant metastatic spread is already evident. In this connection, it should be remembered that cancer of the breast may present with a metastasis, the primary tumour being very small. Thus, the patient may complain of a lump in the axilla or may even present with a pathological fracture of a long bone, or indeed of the mandible.

Palliative treatment. In advanced breast cancer, the disease can cause extreme pain and discomfort and effective palliation is extremely important. Radiotherapy can be of great value in treating local recurrence for relief of pain. However, widespread metastatic disease demands more general treatment and alterations in the hormonal environment may affect the course of the disease beneficially. Surgical removal of the ovaries, adrenal, or even the pituitary gland, or the administration of sex hormones or tamoxifen (which blocks oestrogen receptors), may be effective.

Cytotoxic chemotherapy is generally reserved for treatment of the disease when it has not responded to the above measures, and can give striking palliation in some patients.

Carcinoma of the tongue

Cancer of the tongue is more likely to be found in patients with poor oral hygiene and has been said to occur more frequently in patients who smoke ex-cessively, who have suffered from syphilis, or who have some form of chronic oral irritation. Leukoplakia consists of patches of thickened white mucosal epithelium which are easily recognized and which, on biopsy, have a characteristic appearance. Such leukoplakic patches have a definite precancerous tendency. It is most important that the dentist recognizes such areas and their potential malignancy.

A common site for carcinoma of the tongue is in the anterior two-thirds and frequently at its edge (Fig. 6.4). The lesion usually presents as a typical malignant ulcer although it may be nodular and occasionally papillary or fissured before becoming ulcerated. The lesion is usually a squamous cell carcinoma and spreads locally to the floor of the mouth, eventually involving the alveolar margin and, in the posterior part of the tongue, the tonsil and palate. Lymphatic dissemination occurs to the submental, submandibular and deep cervical lymph nodes. For tumours at the edge of the tongue, the node involved is generally ipsilateral but in more centrally placed tumours in the posterior third of the tongue, lymph node involvement may be bilateral. Continuing lymphatic spread involves the mediastinum. Blood spread is unusual.

The presenting symptom is of *a nodule or an ulcer* on the tongue which soon becomes infected and painful. The pain may be referred to the ear or in the distribution of the auriculotemporal nerve. Excessive salivation and halitosis are common and, in the later stages, dysphagia and slurring of speech result from fixation of the tongue. The ulcer is a

Fig. 6.4 Squamous carcinoma of the tongue. Ulcerated lesion with rolled, everted edges. Note the stitch at the site of biopsy.

typical malignant lesion with everted edges and an indurated base. Repeated small haemorrhages, toxic absorption from the infected area, and anorexia result in debility and anaemia.

It is essential to examine the neck for palpable lymph nodes which may be enlarged as a result of tumour or infection or both. Indeed, in some growths, glandular involvement in the neck may be the first sign of malignancy.

Death results from general inanition, broncho-pneumonia as a result of aspiration of infected material, and in the late stages sudden haemor-rhage from involvement of large vessels.

The differential diagnosis is from other forms of oral ulceration and in particular syphilis and tuber-culosis. Suspicion of malignancy is confirmed by biopsy.

Initial management is by good oral toilet, and dental extractions may occasionally be required before definitive therapy is commenced. The treat-ment of choice to the primary lesion is radiotherapy which may be administered in the form of radium needles implanted into the tumour. In the posterior one-third of the tongue, cobalt or supervoltage therapy is preferable.

Surgery is reserved for radioresistant growths and for tumours that recur after irradiation. In addition, in some cases with extensive bone involvement, radiotherapy is impractical and radical surgery is employed. The operation involves removal of the affected tongue following prelimi-nary ligation of the external carotid artery. The excision may need to include a portion of the floor of the mouth and related mandible and suitable prosthetic replacement. Prophylactic surgical or radiotherapeutic treatment of cervical lymph nodes is not necessary if they are impalpable. If, however, on follow-up, lymph nodes become palpable, the treatment of choice is ipsilateral block dissection of the cervical lymph nodes including the sternomas-toid muscle, internal jugular vein and posterior belly of the digastric. Should lymph glands in the neck be clearly inoperable, surgery is contraindicated but radiotherapy may afford some palliation.

Cancer of the remainder of the oral cavity presents, in general, the same pathological features, and is managed in a similar fashion although, when surgery is required in carcinoma of the floor of the mouth, block dissection with removal of the primary lesion, related mandible and cervical lymph nodes is more frequently necessary.

Carcinoma of the lip

Cancer of the lip is especially common in in-dividuals who smoke very heavily. It is also very much more common in Caucasian individuals ex-posed to especially strong sunlight. Management is similar to that of carcinoma of the tongue, consisting of good oral hygiene and treatment of the lesion by means of radiotherapy or by surgery. Operation in-volves removal of affected lymph nodes, but it is im-portant to be sure that enlarged nodes are not simply the result of lymphadenitis consequent on infection of the primary lesion. As for carcinoma of the tongue, prophylactic removal of lymph nodes is not necessary but should be carried out if such nodes become palpable during follow-up.

The prognosis is worse for lesions on the upper lip and at the angle of the mouth, but in general is better than that for lingual cancer.

Carcinoma of the oesophagus

This disease is common in elderly men. Some countries have a high incidence, notably among the Bantu populations of South Africa and in South-East Asia and Japan. Smoking and alcohol are causal factors.

The growth is usually squamous cell carcinoma, but near the lower end of the oesophagus adenocar-cinoma may be encountered. The growth infiltrates the submucosa and forms an ulcer in the mucous membrane. The malignant stricture progressively tightens and the cardinal symptom is therefore dys-phagia, persistent and progressive, until eventually even fluids cannot be swallowed and are regur-gitated. Rapid weight loss results with cachexia, and death follows from inhalation pneumonia or per-foration of the growth into the pleural cavity.

Barium examination shows the lesion, which has a rigid, irregular outline, and oesophagoscopy with biopsy confirms the diagnosis (Fig. 6.5).

Treatment is by surgery in the distal half of the oesophagus but more proximally radiotherapy is commonly advised. A plastic tube may be inserted to permit continued swallowing.

Fig. 6.5 Barium swallow examination showing a carcinoma of the lower end of the oesophagus. There is hold-up of barium in the dilated oesophagus above the tumour.

BONE TUMOURS

Bone tumours (Table 6.1) may arise from the cells forming the supporting structure of bone (osteo-cytes, chondrocytes, fibrocytes of the periosteum), from the bone marrow elements, or they may be secondary to malignant tumours elsewhere.

Benign bone tumours

Osteomata

These tumours are composed of hard and compact bone and are termed 'ivory osteoma'. They are commonly found in the skull, and very rarely cause symptoms. Osteomata also occur in the mandible

and may occasionally compromise dental extraction or the fitting of dentures.

Chondromata

These may be single or multiple. If a chondroma occurs within the bones, it is known as an enchondroma and these are commonly found in the phalanges. Chondromata growing from the surface of bone (ecchondromata) may become very large and are not uncommon on the rib cage. They seldom cause symptoms but by virtue of their size may need treatment. Multiple chondromata are part of an hereditary abnormality known as diaphyseal aclasis. Small caps of cartilage cells become separated from the edges of the growing metaphysis. These continue to grow, forming large exostoses bearing cartilaginous caps. Such exostoses may cause symptoms from pressure and occasionally need removal. Because of the bony element contained within such growths, they are known as osteochondromata.

Solitary bone cysts

Such cysts usually occur in long bones (humerus or femur). They contain a browny fluid and slowly expand the bony structure, and often present as a pathological fracture (see Ch. 17). The cause of such bone cysts is not known but they may originate following trauma. They are treated by curettage but, if the bone structure is weak, bone grafting with bone chips may be necessary.

Osteoclastomata

These tumours are mostly benign but occasionally malignant forms occur. The tumour is metaphyseal in origin, usually occurs in young adults, and more

Table 6.1 Bone tumours

Tumour	Age group	Situation in bone
Osteoma	—	Skull, mandible
Chondroma	35+	Epiphysis, fingers
Bone cyst	—	Metaphysis, diaphysis
Osteoclastoma	20–35	Metaphysis (near knee joint)
Osteosarcoma	10–20 (the elderly in association with Paget's disease)	Metaphysis (region of knee common)
Chondrosarcoma	35–50+	Flat bones (pelvis, scapula)
Ewing's tumour	Childhood	Diaphysis

than 70% of cases occur in the region of the knee joint (femur or tibia). Histologically the tumour is characterized by large multinucleated giant cells of similar appearance to osteoclasts lying in a spindle cell stroma. Haemorrhagic areas are common. There is pain and swelling of the bone, sometimes with pathological fracture. The lesion must be distinguished from osteitis fibrosa cystica (see Ch. 13) in which the serum calcium is raised and the lesions are multiple, and from metastatic tumour. As the tumour grows, the cortex becomes thin and, on palpation, so-called 'eggshell crackling' can be elicited and there is a characteristic radiological appearance. The tumour is usually localized and metastases are uncommon.

A similar enlarging bony mass with eggshell crackling occurs in the jaws, in association with *adamantinoma*. This tumour arises from the enamel organ, is not malignant, but grows in a similar manner to the osteoclastoma. It may present with a swollen jaw, loosening of teeth, or pathological fracture of the mandible.

Treatment of osteoclastoma and adamantinoma consists of excision of the tumour, together with an area of normal bone, and a graft of bone placed across the gap. Surgical curettage accompanied by X-ray therapy is less mutilating and is effective in many instances.

Malignant bone tumours

It is important to realize that most malignant bone tumours occurring in adults are secondary to malignancy elsewhere. However, there are some important primary malignant tumours of bone, particularly in children and young adults.

Primary malignant bone tumours

Osteosarcoma

This tumour occurs usually in the second decade of life and usually near the actively growing metaphysis of the bone. Occasionally it may occur in late life as a complication of Paget's disease of bone (see Ch. 17). The tumour arises from osteoblasts with extension along the shaft and through the cortex inwards into the medullary cavity and outwards, raising the periosteum which provides a temporary barrier to the tumour spread.

The epiphysis also acts as a barrier to tumour growth. The tumour is composed of numerous tiny spindle-shaped and round cells lying in a stroma consisting of osteoid and fibrous or cartilaginous tissue. The tumour is very vascular and spread is initially by the bloodstream to the lungs.

The clinical presentation is of a painful, often warm, swelling related to bone and near a joint. The knee joint is most commonly affected. On examination, the swelling is bony in texture and tender. Dilated veins may be seen in the overlying skin. The clinical picture may be confused with osteomyelitis.

There are characteristic radiological changes with osteolytic and osteosclerotic areas along the shaft and extending into the soft tissues. Where the periosteum is raised at the edges, there is a characteristic deposition of bone (Codman's triangle) and as the tumour extends outwards, spicules of bone become laid down as the periosteum is pushed away ('sunray' appearance). X-ray of the chest frequently demonstrates secondary deposits. Biopsy is necessary for precise diagnosis. The prognosis is poor and pulmonary metastases may be visible at the time of initial diagnosis. Treatment is by amputation including the whole length of the affected bone. Since amputation followed by subsequent early development of metastases is an avoidable tragedy, it is often advised that radiotherapy be given initially. If three months later metastatic spread is not apparent, then amputation is proceeded with. More recently preliminary results of combined chemotherapy followed by amputation have suggested an increased survival in some patients. Adriamycin and methotrexate in combination appear to be the most effective drugs.

Chondrosarcoma

This growth arises usually in the pelvis and ribs but may occur in long bones. The growth is often lobulated and, although consisting largely of cartilage, cystic degeneration and haemorrhage within the tumour are not uncommon. Cartilage cells are apparent but the tumour may be very anaplastic in appearance. The tumour is slow-growing with local destruction, and blood spread is much less common than in osteosarcoma. It is important to note that a combination of osteosarcoma and chondrosarcoma (osteochondrosarcoma) may occur.

The tumour occurs in an older age group than the osteosarcoma, usually in adults. Treatment is by wide local excision, and amputation may be required. Radiotherapy is not utilized since the tumour is radioresistant.

Ewing's tumour ('onion tumour')

This is a tumour of childhood composed of many small round cells so similar in appearance to the neuroblastoma that for many years the two tumours were confused. Indeed, it is important to make sure that, in cases of apparent Ewing's tumour, there is no neuroblastoma within an adrenal gland. Clinical presentation is with pain and swelling but the tumour is rapidly growing and fever may occur. Like the osteosarcoma, the lesion can be confused with osteomyelitis although it should be noted that the latter condition is more common near the metaphysis of the bone. The characteristic X-ray appearance shows deposition of layers of bone beneath the raised periosteum. These layers give an onion appearance and biopsy confirms the diagnosis.

The prognosis is poor but the tumour is very radiosensitive, so radiotherapy is the treatment of choice.

Secondary tumours of bone

The common tumours that metastasize to bone are breast, lung, kidney, prostate and thyroid but bony deposits may occur in any carcinoma. The metastases are more common in the vertebral bodies, pelvis, upper ends of the femora or humeri, the ribs, or in the skull. Occasionally the mandible is involved.

The initial presentation of the primary tumour may be with a secondary lesion in bone. Presentation is with pain at the site of involvement and X-ray often reveals a destructive lesion, although occasionally osteosclerotic lesions (for instance, secondary deposits from carcinoma of the prostate) may be seen. Sometimes lesions are not visible on X-ray and scanning of the skeleton after injection of a suitable isotope may reveal the bony deposit.

Treatment is by palliation only. For localized lesions, radiotherapy is useful but chemotherapy or hormonal therapy may be needed for widespread deposits. Pathological fractures may be treated by suitable support or by fixation in combination with radiotherapy or chemotherapy.

Final comments

Only some of the tumours that may affect humans have been described in this chapter but the general classification and understanding of the mode of spread, the method by which malignant tumours kill, and the broad principles of management described are applicable to nearly all tumours. Perhaps the most important factor to appreciate is that accurate assessment of the extent of spread of disease in cancer allows planning of rational treatment.

7

Disorders of the heart and blood vessels

ANATOMICAL AND PHYSIOLOGICAL CONSIDERATIONS

The heart lies to the left side of the thorax, being well protected from external damage by the sternum, the ribs, the vertebrae and the chest muscles.

Chambers

The walls of the ventricles, especially the left, are thick and muscular, while the atrial walls are relatively thin. The prime function of the atria is to collect blood while that of the ventricles is to pump the blood into the pulmonary and systemic circulations. The ventricles are divided one from the other by the intraventricular septum, the atria by the intra-atrial septum.

Valves

The flow of blood into and from the various chambers is regulated by the four heart valves, which are formed by folds of endocardium strengthened by fibro-elastic tissue (Fig. 7.1). All the valves have three cusps except the mitral which has only two. The tricuspid valve regulates the blood flow from right atrium to right ventricle, the pulmonic valve that from the right ventricle into the pulmonary trunk, the mitral valve that from the left atrium to the left ventricle, and the aortic valve that from the left ventricle to the aorta. The pulmonic and aortic valves are attached directly to the walls of the pulmonary trunk and the aorta respectively. The tricuspid and mitral valves have delicate cord-like structures, the chordae tendineae, which pass from the free borders of the valves to the inner walls of the respective ventricles.

Walls of the heart

The walls of the heart are composed of three layers. The inner layer, or endocardium, is a smooth membrane of endothelium which lines the heart chambers and is folded over on itself to form the heart valves. The middle layer, or myocardium, is a very specialized involuntary muscle which, unlike the skeletal muscles, never rests but contracts rhythmically more than once a second from birth to death. The outer layer, or pericardium, is formed by the visceral layer, which is closely attached to the myocardium, and the outer parietal layer.

Conducting system

The heart muscle is intrinsically capable of conducting nervous impulses but there is in addition a very specialized conducting system which forms a pathway through the heart for the rapid trans-

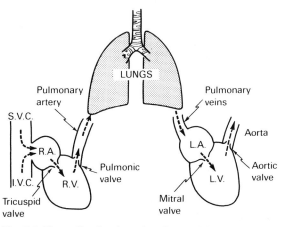

Fig. 7.1 The cardiac chambers, the valves, and the lungs showing the circulation of blood from the right side of the heart to the left.

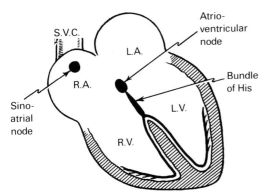

Fig. 7.2 The principal components of the conducting system of the heart.

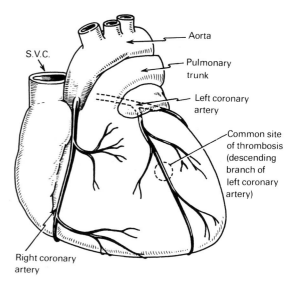

Fig. 7.3 The coronary arteries.

mission of impulses (Fig. 7.2). The starting point of this pathway, the sino-atrial node or pacemaker, is situated in the right atrium near the orifices of the great veins. It initiates each heart beat and regulates the rate and the rhythm of the heart's action. From the sino-atrial node impulses pass down over the atrial walls and are gathered at the atrio-ventricular node which lies between the atria and the ventricles. It acts as an intermediate collecting and transmitting station from which impulses pass to the bundle of His. In its first part this is a single pathway but it soon divides into the two main branches which go down the left and right side of the intraventricular septum and then ramify over the ventricular walls.

Nerve supply of heart

A cardiac centre lies in the floor of the fourth ventricle and from it impulses are transmitted to the heart by parasympathetic (vagal) and sympathetic nerve pathways. Vagal stimulation leads to slowing and sympathetic stimulation to acceleration of the heart.

Nutrition of the heart

The heart receives its blood supply from the two coronary arteries which arise directly from the aorta near the aortic valve (Fig. 7.3). They fill during cardiac diastole. The left is the more important as it is responsible for the blood supply to the greater part of the left ventricle and, in addition, it is more frequently affected by coronary artery disease.

The cardiac cycle

The cardiac cycle occupies three phases:

1. During *atrial systole* the atria contract simultaneously and discharge their contained blood into the ventricles through the open tricuspid and mitral valves.

2. At the beginning of *ventricular systole* the tricuspid and mitral valves close, the ventricles contract, and, when the ventricular pressure has risen sufficiently, the aortic and pulmonic valves are forced open and the blood is ejected into the aorta and pulmonary arteries respectively. The aortic and pulmonic valves then close to prevent a reflux of blood into the ventricles.

3. During the third phase of the cardiac cycle, termed *diastole*, the cardiac muscle rests, the coronary arteries fill with blood, the right atrium receives deoxygenated blood from the great veins, and the left atrium simultaneously fills with oxygenated blood from the lungs.

INVESTIGATION OF CARDIOVASCULAR DISORDERS

The remarkable technological advances of recent years are of considerable value in the investigation of patients with cardiovascular disorders, but the student should remember that a careful history and physical examination are still of paramount importance.

History

The history that the individual with cardiovascular disease gives in response to an intelligent and patient enquiry is more important than any other single method of investigation. In no other system is the adage more true: 'Listen to the patient; he is telling you the diagnosis'. The most important symptoms are breathlessness, chest pain, ankle swelling, joint pains, haemoptysis, and palpitation. Regarding past history, enquiry should be made about rheumatic fever, chorea, heart murmurs and hypertension.

General examination

Much information may be gained from a general examination of the patient before a study is made of the cardiovascular system. The presence of cyanosis, oedema, neck vein overfilling (Fig. 7.4), dyspnoea, and finger clubbing can be quite readily detected in the ambulant patient without any special skill.

Fig. 7.4 Neck vein congestion.

Pulse

The pulse is normally examined by palpation of the radial artery at the wrist. The student should first become proficient at counting the rate of the pulse and then at determining whether it is regular or ir-

regular. Appreciation of alterations in the quality of the pulse require more experience but the dentist should be able to recognize the poor quality, thready pulse associated with shock.

Blood pressure

Estimation of the blood pressure is an essential step in the examination of the cardiovascular system. The patient must be relaxed both physically and mentally or falsely high readings may be obtained. The sphygmomanometer consists in essence of an inflatable cuff connected to a mercury manometer. The empty cuff is placed comfortably but firmly round the upper arm and the pressure increased until the radial pulse disappears. This gives an approximate estimate of the systolic blood pressure. The cuff is allowed to empty and, after a few moments, reinflated to a point just above the estimated systolic pressure. The examiner auscultates over the brachial artery in the antecubital fossa and, as he gradually allows the pressure to fall, a distinct beat is heard when the systolic pressure is reached; the pressure is allowed to fall further and on reaching the diastolic blood pressure the sounds quickly fade and become inaudible.

Examination of the heart

Clinical examination of the heart by means of inspection, palpation, percussion and auscultation requires a degree of clinical skill which the dental student is not expected to acquire. He should appreciate, however, that by means of these techniques the doctor can obtain valuable information regarding the heart size, the quality of the heart sounds, and the presence of heart murmurs.

Mention may be made of the apex beat which is normally produced by the apex of the left ventricle impinging against the chest wall during systole. It lies in the fifth left interspace within a line drawn vertically from the midpoint of the clavicle and its position is, in the absence of mediastinal displacement, a good guide to the heart size.

Radiology

The size of the heart is shown more accurately by a chest X-ray, which may also show pulmonary congestion and oedema in left-sided heart failure. Radio-opaque material may be injected into the aorta, heart or coronary arteries enabling their precise delineation, prior to cardiac surgery.

Electrocardiography

The changes in electrical potential which occur when the heart muscle contracts and relaxes may be recorded by means of electrocardiography. This method of investigation is widely used in the study of coronary artery disease and it also yields valuable information in the arrhythmias.

Echocardiography

Cardiac scans with ultrasound visualize the heart chambers and valves, often giving useful information rapidly and non-invasively.

Cardiac catheterization

The pressure in the great vessels and heart chambers, and the oxygen saturation of the blood, can be measured via a cardiac catheter inserted via a peripheral vein or artery.

CAUSES OF HEART DISEASE

A simple outline of the main causes of heart disease is set out in Table 7.1. The great majority of cases seen in ordinary clinical practice are accounted for by the first four causes listed — coronary artery disease, hypertension, rheumatic heart disease and, in industrial areas, pulmonary heart disease.

COMMON SYMPTOMS AND SIGNS

Dyspnoea

Dyspnoea literally means difficult or disordered breathing. It is an extremely important symptom of cardiac disease as it is often the earliest indication that cardiac function is impaired. Dyspnoea also occurs in various lung disorders, in anaemia, in obesity, and where there is abdominal enlargement.

Cardiac causes

Cardiac dyspnoea is caused by pulmonary venous congestion due to left-sided heart failure, and may take one of two forms:

1. The breathlessness may be felt only on *exertion* and be relieved by rest. Thus it is common to obtain a history in cardiac patients that they are breathless on hurrying and on climbing hills or stairs and that the breathlessness disappears in a relatively short time once they rest. As cardiac decompensation becomes more severe the degree of effort required to provoke dyspnoea becomes less until eventually the patient is breathless even at rest. At this stage he is invariably more comfortable in a propped-up or sitting position (orthopnoea) as the heart has less work to do in this posture.

2. The second variety of cardiac dyspnoea, which is termed *paroxysmal nocturnal dyspnoea*, occurs in cases of acute left ventricular failure (e.g. in hypertension or in coronary artery disease) and in cases of mitral stenosis with severe pulmonary hypertension; it is due to *acute pulmonary oedema*. The patient is wakened from sleep with a sense of suffocation or choking, the respirations are extremely laboured, he becomes cyanosed, is intensely dis-

Table 7.1 The causes of heart disease

Type	Frequency	Maximum age incidence
Coronary artery disease	COMMON	Middle age onwards
Hypertension		Middle age onwards
Pulmonary heart disease*		Middle age onwards
Rheumatic heart disease		Children to middle age
Thyroid heart disease	UNCOMMON	Middle age
Congenital heart disease		Infancy to early adult life
Syphilitic heart disease		Middle age

* Especially in industrial areas.

tressed, and he coughs up frothy sputum which may be tinged with blood.

Lung disorders

Pulmonary causes of dyspnoea are discussed in the chapter on respiratory diseases.

Anaemia

A substantial fall in the haemoglobin level causes impaired oxygenation of the tissues and resultant dyspnoea even when there is no intrinsic cardiac or pulmonary disorder. Dyspnoea is more likely to occur if the anaemia has developed quickly as compensatory mechanisms develop in anaemias of gradual onset.

Abdominal enlargement

Considerable abdominal swelling, e.g. from ascites, late stages of pregnancy, large cysts or tumours, causes elevation of the diaphragm with resultant pulmonary embarrassment and dyspnoea.

Cardiac pain

The most important variety of cardiac pain is that resulting from myocardial ischaemia which is usually a consequence of coronary artery disease. The pain may take one of two forms:

1. *Angina pectoris* is the term given to the sensation of tightness or pain experienced behind the sternum when there is *transient myocardial ischaemia*. It tends to radiate across the chest and into the shoulders and arms. It is typically brought on by exertion, relieved by rest, and usually lasts not more than a few minutes.

2. The pain associated with *myocardial infarction* has the same pattern of distribution but it is usually much more intense and of considerably greater duration. Its onset is not determined by exertion and it is not relieved by rest.

Central chest pain may also be due to pericarditis, dissecting aortic aneurysm, and reflux oesophagitis or oesophageal spasm (see Ch. 9). The latter may be difficult to distinguish from angina pectoris.

Mention must be made of the musculoskeletal chest pain complained of by the nervous, introspective individual who fears that he has cardiac disease. The pain is commonly described as sharp or stabbing in nature; it is located principally below the left breast, and it bears a poor relation to effort. In all these respects it is different from the pain of myocardial ischaemia.

Palpitation

Palpitation means an awareness of the heart's action. Some individuals describe the symptom as a 'thumping', others as a 'fluttering' in the chest. In the majority of instances there is no serious condition present.

Palpitation is experienced by normal individuals when the heart is acting forcibly as a result of exertion or emotional upset. Some nervous individuals experience the symptom after trivial exertion or emotional upset and it may be interpreted by them as an indication of heart disease. In some of these cases the cardiac rhythm is regular while in others there may be occasional extrasystoles. Once it is ascertained that no cardiac disease is present these individuals can be safely reassured.

Palpitation may occasionally be the presenting symptom of a significant cardiac disorder, e.g. the palpitation associated with an uncontrolled atrial fibrillation or paroxysmal tachycardia.

Oedema

Oedema is the term given to the accumulation of an excessive amount of fluid in the tissues of the body. It occurs in congestive cardiac failure, in some forms of renal and hepatic disease, in beriberi, in starvation, and as a local phenomenon in certain circumstances.

Cardiac oedema

In right-sided cardiac failure the site of the oedema is largely determined by gravity, being most evident in the legs, particularly around the ankles, in cardiac patients who are ambulant, and in the lumbosacral region in patients who have been in bed for a period of time. In gross cardiac failure fluid may also accumulate in the serous cavities of the body giving rise to ascites and pleural effusion; this is termed *anasarca*.

The oedema fluid, which is slightly yellowish in colour and relatively low in protein, is formed as a passive transudate from the blood vessels. It is due to decreased excretion of sodium and hence chloride and water; the retained fluid is then localized to parts of the body where venous hydrostatic pressure is increased, behind the failing heart (Fig. 7.5).

The earliest indication of oedema is an increase in weight which, in an average adult, must rise by about 4.5 kg (10 lb) before visible changes occur. When swelling of the legs or of the lumbosacral region does develop it may be demonstrated to be due to fluid by the simple clinical test of producing pitting by pressure with the ball of the thumb or finger.

Renal oedema

In acute glomerulonephritis a slight or moderate degree of oedema is commonly present; the earliest indication is often a puffiness of the face especially in the mornings. Gross oedema is a characteristic feature of the nephrotic syndrome (see Ch. 11) where the sequence of events is protein loss in the urine — fall of plasma proteins — fall in plasma oncotic pressure (see Fig. 7.5).

Fig. 7.5 Simplified representation of the relationship between the hydrostatic pressure (B.P.) and the oncotic pressure (O.P.) in a capillary.
Arterial end — fluid passes from vessel.
Venous end — fluid passes to vessel.

Hepatic oedema

Hepatic cirrhosis (see Ch. 10) is due to reduced hepatic synthesis of plasma albumin, which again reduces plasma oncotic pressure.

Starvation oedema

This is rarely seen in western countries except under such grossly abnormal conditions as prevailed in concentration camps. It is common in many Third World countries. Dietary deficiency leads to low plasma protein levels and thus to a fall in the plasma oncotic pressure.

Local oedema

Oedema is seen as a local phenomenon in inflammatory states, and the dentists frequently encounter examples of this in the buccal cavity. Obstruction to venous or lymphatic drainage also produces oedema. Examples of this are the oedema seen in deep venous thrombosis, most commonly of the calf, and in lymphatic obstruction by malignant growths.

Cyanosis

Cyanosis is the term given to bluish discoloration of the skin and mucous membranes due in most cases to the presence of an excessive amount of haemoglobin in the reduced or deoxygenated form (at least 5 g per 100 ml of reduced haemoglobin must be present before cyanosis is clinically apparent) and, less commonly, to the presence of certain abnormal haemoglobin derivatives.

Consideration of the causes given below shows that in many cases of cyanosis due to cardiac disease two factors are responsible — the central one of impaired pulmonary oxygenation and the peripheral one of increased conversion of oxyhaemoglobin to reduced haemoglobin.

Inadequate pulmonary oxygenation

This may result from pulmonary congestion due to cardiac failure, mitral stenosis of long standing, or extensive lung disease.

Increased peripheral deoxygenation

The conversion of oxyhaemoglobin to reduced haemoglobin may be increased peripherally because of general or local slowing of circulation. Examples are cardiac failure, shock, Raynaud's phenomenon, and local venous obstruction.

Cardiovascular shunts

In certain forms of congenital heart disease some deoxygenated blood may pass directly from the right to the left side of the heart without traversing the pulmonary circulation.

Abnormal blood pigments

Cyanosis may be caused by the presence of sulphaemoglobin, or methaemoglobin, this usually being a toxic effect of certain drugs.

DISTURBANCES OF CARDIAC RATE

The average cardiac rate in the healthy resting adult is about 70 beats per minute but it should be appreciated that there are considerable individual variations. The cardiac rate of the child is faster, in infancy being about 120 beats per minute, and at the age of 10 years about 90 per minute.

Tachycardia

When the cardiac rate in the adult is above the arbitrary level of 100 per minute tachycardia is said to be present. Tachycardia occurs physiologically after exertion and emotional upset. It is also seen as a normal reaction to fever, shock, haemorrhage, administration of adrenaline, and it is a characteristic feature of thyrotoxicosis. Tachycardia occurring in a person with organic heart disease is usually an indication that cardiac function is decreasing.

Paroxysmal tachycardia

This is a common condition characterized by the sudden development of tachycardia (e.g. 160 beats per minute) which may last from a few minutes to several hours and then as suddenly cease. The individual usually seeks advice because of the associated palpitation. In some cases the attack may be terminated by vagal stimulation, e.g. pressure on the carotid sinus. In other patients, antidysrhythmic

drugs are required to terminate the attack, or else the passing of an electric shock across the heart of the anaesthetized patient (cardioversion).

Bradycardia

When the cardiac rate falls to 60 per minute or less bradycardia is said to be present. It is seen physiologically in certain athletes, particularly highly trained distance runners. It is a typical feature of treatment with beta-adrenergic receptor blocking drugs, or myxoedema; it occurs in association with jaundice and increased intracranial pressure; and it is one of the manifestations of excessive dosage with digoxin. Its occurrence otherwise should suggest the presence of heart block (see below).

DISTURBANCES OF CARDIAC RHYTHM

The cardiac rhythm is normally regular due to the activity of the sino-atrial node or pacemaker.

Sinus arrhythmia

This, the simplest form of cardiac arrhythmia, is seen physiologically in children and in many young adults. It consists of a quickening of the cardiac rate during inspiration and a slowing during expiration, and it is thought to be caused by alterations in vagal tone. Many students may personally demonstrate the condition by feeling their pulse during deep breathing. The condition does not produce any symptoms.

Extrasystoles

An extrasystole is a beat of the heart which is initiated in a focus of abnormal excitation outwith the sino-atrial node. Depending on the site of origin they may be classified as atrial, ventricular, or nodal (atrioventricular node); the distinction is made on electrocardiographic evidence.

The individual who has extrasystoles may experience no symptoms or may have palpitation. On feeling the pulse the basically regular rhythm is interrupted from time to time by the occurrence of a premature beat which is weaker than normal and is followed by a longer pause (Fig. 7.6). Extrasystoles may be infrequent or so numerous as to mimic atrial fibrillation. Occasionally a premature beat occurs regularly after each normal beat producing coupling of the pulse (pulsus bigeminus); this is most often due to digoxin overdosage.

In most instances the presence of extrasystoles does not signify organic heart disease. Thus anxiety, or overindulgence in tobacco, coffee or tea, may be responsible and all that is required is correction of the faulty habit and reassurance. Extrasystoles may also result from organic heart disease or from digoxin overdosage.

Atrial fibrillation

In atrial fibrillation the sino-atrial node no longer controls the heart rhythm. The atria beat very rapidly (about 400 per minute) and irregularly by a process of excitation arising in the atria, the precise details of which are not fully understood. The atrioventricular node can transmit to the ventricle only about 140–160 of these irregular impulses per minute.

The most important causes of atrial fibrillation are chest infection, ischaemic heart disease, rheumatic heart disease (particularly mitral stenosis), thyrotoxicosis, and alcoholic heart disease.

The pulse is completely irregular and, in the absence of treatment, usually rapid. At this stage palpitation is commonly experienced. The heart rate, determined by auscultation, is often considerably greater than the radial pulse rate because many of the ventricular beats are too feeble to produce a radial pulse; this phenomenon is known as a pulse deficit and it may number 20–30 beats per minute. The electrocardiographic pattern is characteristic (see Fig. 7.6).

Atrial fibrillation throws an added strain on an already damaged heart and, in addition, embolization may occur. Clots tend to form in the atria because they are not emptying completely and a portion of clot may become dislodged and cause blockage, e.g. of a cerebral vessel producing a stroke, or of a limb vessel leading to gangrene.

Treatment consists in the use of digoxin to reduce the ventricular rate to the normal range (it does not produce a return to normal rhythm) and management of the basic cause whether it be a chest infection, cardiac lesion or thyrotoxicosis. In some patients the dysrhythmia can be terminated by electrical cardioversion. In others, long-term oral anticoagulants are given to reduce the risk of thromboembolism.

Atrial flutter

Atrial flutter is closely related to atrial fibrillation but the atrial rhythm, although very rapid, is regular. The atrioventricular node transmits every second, third or possibly fourth atrial impulse so that the ventricular rate is one-half, one-third, or one-quarter

Fig. 7.6 Electrocardiograms showing the normal pattern, extrasystole (E.S.), atrial fibrillation, and early myocardial infarction. P represents the wave of excitation through the atria, Q R S and T the changes in the ventricles.

that of the atrial rate (2 to 1, 3 to 1, or 4 to 1, atrial flutter). The pulse is therefore regular, although rapid. Causes and treatment are as for atrial fibrillation.

Heart block

Interference with transmission of the impulse from the atria to the ventricles may be caused in younger individuals by rheumatic fever, in older individuals by ischaemic or degenerative changes in the conducting mechanism, or it may result from digoxin overdosage at any age.

Heart block may be potential, partial, or complete. The potential variety is detectable only by electrocardiography. In partial heart block some atrial impulses do not produce a ventricular response and the pulse is irregular due to 'dropped beats'. In complete heart block no impulses from the atria reach the ventricles and death occurs if idioventricular rhythm is not initiated within a few seconds. During these critical few seconds the individual usually loses consciousness, his colour becomes deathly pale and then cyanosed, and he is pulseless; this is termed an Adams-Stokes attack. Treatment is with a battery-operated cardiac pacemaker. Temporarily this is performed by passing a wire up a peripheral vein into the right ventricle; permanently the pacemaker is implanted under the skin of the chest wall.

CONGENITAL HEART DISEASE

In early fetal life the heart is represented by a simple tube-like structure which, by an extremely complicated process, evolves into the delicately regulated four-chambered structure that we know as the human heart. It is not surprising that sometimes this process is not completely flawless and a form of congenital heart disease results. An aetiological factor in certain cases is infection of the mother, in the early weeks of pregnancy, with the virus responsible for rubella (see Ch. 1). Some babies have Down's syndrome (see Ch. 19).

Congenital heart disease may be classified according to whether cyanosis is present or not. In the cyanotic group (the 'blue babies') there is flow of some venous blood from the right side directly to the left side of the heart without traversing the pulmonary circuit. In general, the cyanotic forms have a graver prognosis.

Congenital heart disease is of importance to the dentist in two ways. Firstly, these patients may be high risks for dental anaesthesia or dental surgical procedures because of impaired cardiac function; secondly, they may develop subacute bacterial endocarditis after dental extractions unless appropriate prophylactic measures are taken.

Until relatively recently no basic treatment was possible for any of the forms of congenital heart disease, but advances in cardiac surgery and anaesthesia now permit a striking benefit to be achieved in carefully selected cases.

Acyanotic congenital heart disease

Some of the less rare anomalies merit a brief description.

A defect may exist in the atrial or ventricular septum and, if it is the sole abnormality and is small, may cause relatively little upset in cardiac function. In other instances the *septal defect* is associated with other anomalies, as in Fallot's tetralogy.

The ductus arteriosus, which in fetal life allows blood to pass from the pulmonary trunk to the aorta without traversing the lungs, may remain patent after birth permitting a flow of blood from aorta to pulmonary trunk and producing a characteristic murmur at the base of the heart. Ligation of a *patent ductus arteriosus* is relatively speaking, one of the simpler operations that the cardiac surgeon may be asked to perform.

In *coarctation of aorta* the thoracic aorta is narrowed, causing a decreased blood supply to the lower part of the body associated with a compensatory hypertension in the upper part. The arteries of the intercostal region become enlarged and tortuous in an attempt to provide a collateral circulation to the lower part of the body. From the dental point of view an increase in size of the mandibular arteries and the arteries leading to the individual teeth has been reported and, in consequence, there is a tendency to haemorrhage after dental extraction.

In *dextrocardia* the heart lies on the right side of the thorax. No symptoms are produced if dextrocardia is the sole defect and the condition may remain undetected until the individual undergoes some routine medical examination or has a chest X-ray.

Cyanotic congenital heart disease

The majority of infants with cyanotic congenital heart disease who survive the early months of life suffer from *Fallot's tetralogy* which comprises pulmonary stenosis, right ventricular hypertrophy, ventricular septal defect, and dextroposition of the aorta. The presence of these defects permits the passage of unoxygenated blood from the right to the left side of the heart and the individuals affected show marked cyanosis, finger clubbing, dyspnoea, and retarded development. The buccal mucosa is often intensely cyanosed and has been likened to the colour of a ripe Victorian plum. There is delayed eruption of both deciduous and permanent teeth. An increase in the number of red cells occurs (polycythaemia) as a compensatory mechanism to offset the poor oxygenation of the blood. Cardiac surgery is used to correct the defect in a considerable portion of these unfortunate children and even very severe defects are now amenable to operation.

RHEUMATIC FEVER

Incidence

Rheumatic fever has its highest incidence in the autumn and winter months in countries with damp, temperate climates. The disease is now less common than it was but in Britain it is still an important cause of heart disease in children and young adults. The maximum age incidence is 5–15 years.

Aetiology

Rheumatic fever is an abnormal immunological response to infection with the haemolytic streptococcus. The infection is usually in the throat and a history of an upper respiratory infection, or of scarlet fever, some 10–21 days before the onset of rheumatic fever is often present.

Pathology

The inflammatory reaction affects the connective tissues of the heart, the joints, and the subcutaneous tissues. The pathological changes are of greatest importance in the heart where the valves (endocarditis), the myocardium (myocarditis), and the pericardium (pericarditis) may be affected in greater or lesser degree. The valves are swollen and small; firmly adherent vegetations develop along the lines of contact of the cusps. After the acute stage has settled fibrous tissue reaction may produce permanent deformity and impaired function of the heart valves, and impaired efficiency of the myocardium. The mitral valve is most frequently affected, the aortic valve comes next in frequency, while the valves on the right side of the heart are rarely involved due to the low mechanical pressures acting upon them.

Clinical picture

The patient is usually a child or a young adult in whom it is often possible to obtain a history of an upper respiratory tract infection some two or three weeks before. The onset of the rheumatic fever is usually manifested by the development of arthritis which causes flitting pains particularly in the larger joints. The affected joints are tender to touch, painful, hot, swollen and red. The temperature is elevated, the pulse rapid, and the skin hot and sweating. The throat may still be inflamed from the previous streptococcal infection.

When the heart is seriously involved, cardiac enlargement occurs, the heart sounds are softer than normal, and murmurs develop. Active pericarditis causes audible pericardial friction followed by pericardial effusion.

The erythrocyte sedimentation rate is accelerated and the level does not usually return to normal until the rheumatic process is quiescent (normal level is up to 20 mm in one hour by the Westergren method). Electrocardiography may yield evidence of potential heart block. Antistreptococcal antibodies are usually present.

Diagnosis

In a typical case, such as described above, there is no diagnostic problem, but in some instances pain is much more prominent in one limb suggesting, for a time, a diagnosis of local inflammatory lesion, or joint pains may be slight or absent, the picture being that of a child who is vaguely unwell, has a poor appetite and abdominal discomfort. Sometimes the symptoms are so mild that the child never comes under medical care.

Prognosis

Death in the acute stages of rheumatic fever due to cardiac failure is fortunately now rare. Many patients make a complete recovery and are left with no clinical evidence of any cardiac lesion. A substantial number, including some of the atypical or 'missed' cases, suffer permanent cardiac damage and this group is discussed further in the section on mitral and aortic valve disease.

Treatment

The individual with rheumatic fever is confined to bed until the process is deemed inactive by the absence of symptoms and a return of pulse, temperature and erythrocyte sedimentation rate to normal levels. The duration of bed rest is, on an average, about six weeks. Salicylates are given in full dosage either as sodium salicylate or as aspirin. Salicylate therapy leads to a fall in the temperature (antipyretic effect), relief of joint pains (analgesic effect), and is generally believed to reduce the incidence and severity of permanent cardiac damage.

Steroid therapy, although it has a marked anti-inflammatory effect, does not lessen the incidence of permanent cardiac damage.

The after-care of the patient who has had rheumatic fever is important. The individual should take commonsense precautions to avoid as far as possible the development of upper respiratory infections. As a prophylactic against further throat infections many favour long-term sulphonamide or penicillin therapy. In this respect mention must also be made of tonsillectomy; if the tonsils are diseased and the individual has frequent sore throats he may benefit considerably from tonsillectomy, but healthy tonsils should never be removed in the hope of preventing further sore throats.

Chorea (Sydenham's chorea)

This is a less common manifestation of acute rheumatism. The maximum incidence is in children. It is characterized by oedema and focal changes in the brain especially the basal ganglia.

The main clinical features are involuntary jerky, purposeless movements of the limbs, facial grimacing, and 'jack-in-the-box' movements of the tongue. The risks of cardiac damage are as in rheumatic fever.

VALVULAR DISEASE OF THE HEART

For practical purposes we need consider only the mitral and aortic valve since the tricuspid and pulmonic valves are rarely affected. In the case of the mitral valve, rheumatism is the only aetiological factor, but with aortic valve lesions consideration must also be given to the possible role of syphilis (see Ch. 1) and degenerative changes.

If the valve is deformed in such a way that its aperture is narrowed, the term *stenosis* is used, while if the deformity results in incomplete closure of the valve we use the term *incompetence*.

Pathological effects of valvular lesions

In mitral stenosis the valve cannot open properly, causing obstruction to the flow of blood from the left atrium to the left ventricle. The pressure in the left atrium rises, the left atrium enlarges and hypertrophies, pressure increases in the pulmonary circuit producing pulmonary congestion, and the right ventricle hypertrophies.

In mitral incompetence the valve cannot close properly and when the left ventricle contracts some blood passes back through the mitral valve to the left atrium instead of all passing into the aorta. The left ventricle attempts to pass into the systemic circulation a normal quantity of blood and consequently hypertrophies.

In aortic stenosis the valve cusps become fused together so that the valve cannot open fully and there is obstruction to the free passage of blood from the left ventricle to the aorta; left ventricular hypertrophy results.

In aortic incompetence the valve does not close properly at the end of ventricular systole and there is a reflux of blood from the aorta to the left ventricle leading to left ventricular hypertrophy.

Clinical features

The majority of cases are seen in young adults. A

past history of rheumatic fever, scarlet fever, or chorea is obtained in about 50%. In the case of aortic lesions consideration must also be given to a past history of syphilis (aortic incompetence) and to the question of degenerative changes.

At first there are no symptoms, but later, when cardiac decompensation occurs, the individual experiences breathlessness on effort which becomes progressively worse. Palpitation may also be noted. Haemoptysis secondary to pulmonary engorgement is a feature in mitral stenosis and the patient may also have attacks of paroxysmal nocturnal dyspnoea.

The presence of mitral stenosis may be suspected by a malar flush due to cyanosis of the cheeks. In aortic incompetence the diastolic blood pressure is lowered as a result of reflux of blood to the left ventricle while the systolic pressure is often elevated because of more forcible left ventricular action, e.g. a blood pressure of 140/40 mmHg is common. The high pulse pressure produces the characteristic collapsing pulse of aortic incompetence. The pulse meets the examining fingers abruptly and forcefully but the impact is of very short duration as the pressure falls away quickly (Fig. 7.7).

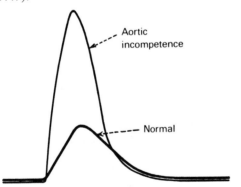

Aortic incompetence

Normal

Fig. 7.7 Comparison between the normal pulse wave and that in aortic incompetence; the latter is sharply rising, sharply peaked, and sharply falling.

Clinical examination of the heart may reveal enlargement and the presence of various heart murmurs which, from their time, site and quality, indicate which form of valvuar lesion is present. Echocardiography usually confirms the diagnosis, but cardiac catheterization is sometimes also required, especially when considering surgery.

Combination of valve lesions

In many cases more than one valve lesion is present,

e.g. both mitral stenosis and incompetence, or both aortic stenosis and incompetence, or a combination of mitral and aortic lesions. Double or multiple valve lesions obviously throw a greater strain on the heart.

Complications of valvular disease

The individual with rheumatic valvular disease of the heart may suffer three main complications and, as a result, the majority do not survive beyond middle age unless surgical correction of the valvular lesion is possible.

1. *Atrial fibrillation* is particularly common if mitral stenosis is present. Fibrillation brings with it the danger of embolism.
2. *Congestive cardiac failure* is likely to occur if the valve deformity is producing considerable interference with cardiac function.
3. *Subacute bacterial endocarditis* may develop at any time.

Treatment

Until recently treatment was in effect for complications, using digoxin for the control of atrial fibrillation, diuretic drugs to relieve congestive cardiac failure, and antibiotics for the prophylaxis and treatment of subacute bacterial endocarditis. However, surgical treatment has now advanced considerably. Mitral stenosis can be treated by mitral valvotomy but other valvular disease is managed by open heart surgical methods using a temporary heart/lung bypass machine, and valves may be replaced either by prostheses or by grafting of tissue valves. Such patients remain at risk of thromboembolism and may require long-term oral anticoagulants. They also remain at risk of infective endocarditis and require prophylaxis.

INFECTIVE ENDOCARDITIS

Infective endocarditis is infection of the heart valves or endocardium with bloodborne organisms, usually bacteria but sometimes *Candida albicans*, rickettsiae, mycoplasmas or chlamydiae. The valves may be normal, especially if the organism is virulent (e.g. *Staphylococcus aureus* or *Streptococcus pyogenes*). The infection is often acute, and is a common complication of intravenous drug abuse. However abnormal heart valves (congenital or rheumatic heart disease, artificial valves) or indwelling pacemakers are more prone to infection, often with less virulent bacteria causing *subacute bacterial endocarditis*.

Aetiology and bacteriology of subacute bacterial endocarditis

In this bacterial infection, heart valves that are damaged or abnormal as a consequence of replacement by a prosthesis, rheumatic disease or congenital anomaly are affected.

The infecting organism is, in the great majority of dental cases, the *Streptococcus viridans* which is a normal inhabitant of the buccal cavity. After many dental procedures, but especially extractions, there is a transient bacteraemia which in the healthy person is of no consequence but in a patient with damaged endocardium the organisms may gain a foothold on the damaged area resulting in bacterial endocarditis. All cases of subacute bacterial endocarditis are not the consequence of dental procedures. In some instances dental sepsis, other operative procedures in the mouth or throat (e.g. tonsillectomy) or upper respiratory infections may be responsible. Subacute bacterial endocarditis may also follow surgery or instrumentation of the alimentary or genitourinary tracts (*Streptococcus faecalis*) or cardiac surgery (*Staphylococcus albus* or *Candida albicans*).

Pathology

Vegetations, which are composed of blood platelets, round cells, bacteria, and fibrin, are formed on the heart valves. These outgrowths are, in contrast to the vegetations of rheumatic fever, friable, and small fragments may become detached and pass in the circulation to produce embolic phenomena in many parts of the body.

Clinical features

The condition may occur at any age. There may or may not be a history of underlying heart valve disease. The presence of the underlying rheumatic or congenital heart disease may or may not have been known previously. A history of dental treatment, which may not necessarily include extractions, may be obtained. When subacute bacterial endocarditis does follow some dental procedure there is usually a

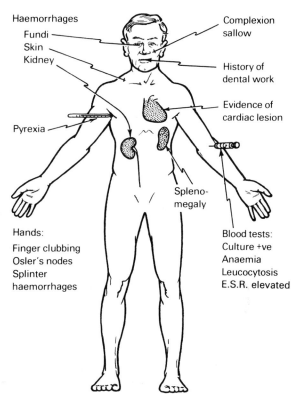

Fig. 7.8 The principal features in subacute bacterial endocarditis.

latent period before symptoms and signs develop. The principal features are depicted in Figure 7.8.

The patient complains of loss of energy, loss of appetite, possibly of undue sweating, and he may have noted that he has become paler than normal. The skin and mucous membranes are pale and in advanced cases the skin has a light brownish tint sometimes described as an earthy pallor or a *café-au-lait* colour. The temperature becomes elevated but the degree of fever is usually slight and the fever is not constant; thus a single normal temperature recording by no means rules out the diagnosis. Finger clubbing develops but it is seldom gross and thus requires to be looked for carefully. Small petechial haemorrhages may be seen in the skin, the buccal mucosa, the conjunctivae, and the nail bed (splinter haemorrhages). These haemorrhages, as well as painful little swellings in the pulps of the fingers and toes (Osler's nodes), microhaematuria, and mental changes, are due to inflammation of small blood vessels (*vasculitis*). Enlargement of the spleen, again of slight or moderate degree, is a common finding, since the spleen is part of the body's defence mechanism against infection. Examination of the blood confirms the presence of anaemia and reveals a leucocytosis and elevation of the erythrocyte sedimentation rate. Several blood cultures may be required to isolate the organism.

Examination of the cardiovascular system reveals tachycardia, and the doctor may note heart murmurs which may change with time due to increasing deformity of already damaged valves.

The effects of embolism can be very diverse but the organ most frequently affected is the kidney, causing frank haematuria and pain in the loin. Obstruction of limb arteries may cause gangrene, while cerebral arterial occlusion may cause stroke.

Diagnosis

Subacute bacterial endocarditis should be suspected when any patient known to have rheumatic or congenital heart disease, cardiac surgery, artificial heart valves or pacemakers, or to be an intravenous drug abuser, suffers deterioration in health. Careful enquiry regarding the symptoms outlined above should be made, followed by a detailed clinical examination, and examination of the blood and urine.

Repeated blood cultures should be made before starting antibiotics to identify the organism and its drug sensitivity. No organism is identified in about one-third of patients. Echocardiography may show abnormal heart valves or vegetations.

Treatment and prognosis

Until the introduction of penicillin the prognosis was hopeless. The outlook is now favourable provided the case is diagnosed reasonably early, the heart is not badly damaged, and appropriate and adequate antibiotic treatment is given. Antibiotics are given according to the drug sensitivity of the known or suspected organism. They should be bactericidal, and are often given in combination to prevent drug resistance. Examples are penicillin and gentamicin for *Strep. viridans*; ampicillin and gentamicin for *Strep. faecalis*; and flucloxacillin and gentamicin for *Staph. albus*. They are initially given intravenously for four weeks to achieve adequate blood levels (measured by the bacteriologist) and to kill all organisms. Oral antibiotics are then given for a further 6−8 weeks. Patients should be carefully monitored during treatment. After eradication of

infection, cardiac surgery may be required to replace damaged valves, and dental extractions (with antibiotic cover) for dental sepsis.

Prophylaxis in dental practice

Close co-operation between dentist, doctor and patient is essential to avoid bacterial endocarditis. The doctor should warn patients and their dentists that antibiotic prophylaxis is required, and give them an appropriate warning card to show the dentist. All dental procedures that cause gingival bleeding (and hence bacteraemia) should be covered in all patients with congenital or rheumatic heart valve disease or artificial valves. Antibiotics should be bactericidal, given 30−60 minutes before the procedure, and their administration supervised and recorded in the case-sheet. The following recommendations are from the British National Formulary (1987); however the guidelines are revised every few years and the dentist should follow the current guidelines and liaise with the patient's doctor before treatment.

Local anaesthesia, no previous endocarditis. 3 g oral amoxycillin should be given 1 hour before the procedure or, if the patient is allergic to penicillin, 1.5 g oral erythromycin stearate 1 hour before the procedure, then 500 mg 6 hours later.

General anaesthesia, no previous endocarditis or prosthetic valve. Either 1 g intramuscular amoxycillin before induction should be administered, then 500 mg oral amoxycillin 6 hours later, *or* 3 g oral amoxycillin 4 hours before induction then 3 g oral amoxycillin as soon as possible after the procedure, *or* 3 g oral amoxycillin and 1 g oral probenecid (which reduces renal excretion of penicillins) 4 hours before procedure.

General anaesthesia and prosthetic heart valve; patients with previous endocarditis (local or general anaesthesia). 1 g intramuscular amoxycillin and 1.5 mg intramuscular gentamicin per kg bodyweight should be administered immediately before induction, then 500 mg oral amoxycillin 6 hours later.

Patients in the last two groups who are allergic to penicillin or already taking a penicillin. 1 g intravenous vancomycin should be infused over 60 minutes, then 1.5 mg intravenous gentamicin per kg bodyweight before induction.

It should be noted that dentists cannot prescribe

gentamicin or vancomycin, so patients requiring such prophylaxis must be hospitalized and treated in collaboration with a doctor.

HYPERTENSION

Hypertension is said to be present when the arterial blood pressure is consistently higher than normal and requires treatment. In healthy young and middle-aged adults the systolic blood pressure should not, at rest, be higher than 140 mmHg and the diastolic pressure greater than 90 mmHg. The upper limits of normal are rather higher in older people, e.g. 160/100 mmHg in persons aged over 60 years. Since considerable increases of blood pressure may result from emotional upset or exercise, these factors should be excluded before a person is considered to be hypertensive. In most cases of hypertension both the systolic and diastolic pressures are high.

Causes of hypertension

1. In the great majority of cases the hypertension appears to exist as a primary disorder and this variety is termed *essential hypertension*.

2. Hypertension results from bilateral renal disease such as glomerulonephritis or pyelonephritis and it also may follow unilateral affections of the kidney. It is important that unilateral renal lesions are not overlooked as surgical treatment of the renal abnormality leads in some cases to cure of the hypertension.

3. Less common causes of hypertension include endocrine abnormalities such as phaeochromocytoma, Conn's syndrome and Cushing's syndrome, and these also may be cured by surgical means. Coarctation of the aorta is a further rare cause of hypertension which is amenable to surgical therapy.

4. Hypertension may appear during pregnancy.

Essential hypertension

Incidence

Essential hypertension is a common condition in people of middle age and over. It is often associated with obesity and with a family history of hypertension.

Aetiology

Despite much experimental work the basic causation of essential hypertension is still unknown. There appears to be increased tone in the small blood vessels which causes an increased peripheral resistance, but the basic abnormality producing this deviation from normal has not yet been elucidated.

Pathology

Once hypertension has been present for some time it produces characteristic changes in the blood vessels, the heart, and the kidneys. The walls of the arteries become thicker and harder due to hypertrophy of the middle coat, while the lumen becomes narrower due to changes in the intima. These arterial changes are of greatest pathological import in the heart, the brain, and the kidney. The left ventricle enlarges and hypertrophies because it has to pump blood against a higher pressure but the arterial changes noted above lead to diminished blood supply to the myocardium and in time result in cardiac decompensation. The changes in the small blood vessels of the kidney produce ischaemia which in turn aggravates the already existing hypertension; a vicious circle of hypertension–arterial change–renal ischaemia–further hypertension is thus set up. Hypertension causes small aneurysms in the arteries at the base of the brain, which may rupture causing cerebral haemorrhage.

Clinical picture

In the early stages there may be no symptoms, the elevation of the blood pressure being discovered incidentally during some routine examination, e.g. for insurance purposes. When symptoms do occur they include headache, which may be throbbing in character, breathlessness on exertion, chest tightness or pain on exertion, deterioration in visual acuity, and epistaxis. Troublesome bleeding after dental extractions is not a common complication. Attacks of paroxysmal nocturnal dyspnoea due to acute left ventricular failure occur in severe cases. Congestive cardiac failure develops late in the course of the illness.

Blood pressure readings around 200/120 mmHg are common while much higher levels are seen not infrequently. The arterial changes may be noted in the arteries of the retina by use of the ophthalmoscope. Haemorrhages, exudates, and swelling of the optic nerve head (papilloedema) may also be noted in the retina in advanced cases. The simplest clinical indication of left ventricular enlargement is displacement of the apex impulse downwards and to the left from the normal position; it may thus come to be left in the sixth left interspace as far out as the anterior axillary line. Left ventricular hypertrophy is confirmed by electrocardiography.

Prognosis

With increasing arterial blood pressure there are increasing risks of stroke, ischaemic heart disease, heart failure, renal failure, and visual damage.

Treatment

Patients should be advised to lose weight if obese, and to restrict their intake of salt, alcohol and tobacco. If the blood pressure remains elevated antihypertensive drugs are employed. In many patients effective control of the hypertension can be achieved by the use of a thiazide diuretic (e.g. bendrofluazide) or a beta-adrenergic receptor blocking drug (e.g. propranolol or atenolol) either alone or in combination. In more severe cases additional drugs may be required, e.g. vasodilators such as nifedipine, or angiotensin-converting enzyme inhibitors such as captopril. Long-term follow-up by the general practitioner or hospital clinic is required since compliance is often poor. Treatment reduces the risks of stroke, heart failure or renal failure, but not ischaemic heart disease. The value of treatment is greatest in patients aged over 60 years. Some antihypertensive drugs cause hypotension, especially on standing or after anaesthesia.

Malignant hypertension

This term is used when the hypertension is very marked (e.g. diastolic blood pressure 130–140 mmHg) and is associated with severe fundal changes and rapid deterioration in renal function. It necessitates vigorous antihypertensive therapy.

CORONARY ARTERY DISEASE

Incidence

Coronary artery disease is a very common disorder which has become increasingly common this century in developed countries, although the incidence is now falling. It is more common in males. Those of middle age and over are mainly affected although cases in younger individuals, especially men, are not infrequent. Smoking, hyperlipidaemia, hypertension, diabetes mellitus and myxoedema are predisposing factors. Epidemiological surveys suggest that the incidence is higher in those engaged in sedentary work and in lower social classes.

Aetiology and pathology

The reasons for the high incidence of coronary artery disease are obscure. Considerable attention has been paid to the possible role of the animal fat content of the diet, to the sugar content of the diet, and to the hardness of the water supply, but there is no general agreement on these factors. Cigarette smoking is now firmly accepted as an important and preventable factor in the aetiology of coronary artery disease and obesity is also a significant factor. Reduction of high blood pressure does not prevent ischaemic heart disease. Reduction in cholesterol by diet or drugs has been shown to prevent nonfatal heart attacks, but not mortality. In patients with premature coronary artery disease (under 50 years) the serum cholesterol should be measured to exclude *familial hypercholesterolaemia*. Such patients may have fatty deposits in the cornea (arcus), eyelids (xanthelasmas) or skin (xanthomas). Treatment is by low cholesterol diet and drugs (cholestyramine, gemfibrozil).

Whatever the precise cause, the discernible pathological lesion is atheroma of the coronary arteries, which causes narrowing and irregularity of the lumen of the vessel and leads to fibrous tissue replacement of the medial coat. The blood supply to the myocardium is reduced by the arterial narrowing, and thrombus formation may develop suddenly on atheromatous patches which ulcerate. These changes are seldom confined to the coronary vessels and involvement of the arteries of the limbs, the brain, and the kidney may materially affect the ultimate course of the disorder.

Coronary artery disease may become manifest by angina pectoris, myocardial infarction, ventricular or atrial fibrillation, and cardiac failure secondary to fibrotic changes in the conducting mechanism and myocardium.

Angina pectoris

Angina pectoris, which literally means a strangling pain in the chest, is caused by transient myocardial ischaemia. The usual cause is coronary athero-sclerosis, but spasm of the coronary arteries is also a factor in some patients.

Clinical features

The characteristic story is that the individual feels a retrosternal tightness or pain which tends to spread across the chest and to the shoulders and arms especially on the left side, and often to the neck and lower jaw. Breathlessness is commonly associated. Angina pectoris is experienced when the heart is given extra work to do as on exertion, emotional excitement, after a meal, or after exposure to cold. An attack may be precipitated by the emotional reaction to a dental procedure. Angina due to spasm may have no such precipitating factors. The pain is gripping in nature and may be severe. With rest it decreases in intensity and passes off within a few minutes. The symptom has been graphically described as 'the cry of the heart for oxygen'. The diagnosis may be supported by ischaemic changes on the electrocardiogram, either at rest or during a standard exercise test.

Treatment

The patient should be advised to rest when the pain comes on. Prompt *symptomatic relief* follows the sublingual administration of a spray or a tablet of glyceryl trinitrate, a vasodilator which quickly dilates the coronary blood vessels, and also peripheral vessels, reducing cardiac workload and thus relieving myocardial ischaemia. The tablet should be allowed to dissolve under the tongue as absorption from the buccal mucosa is very rapid.

Prevention of anginal attacks can be achieved by several drugs. Long-acting nitrates can be given orally or as skin patches. Beta-adrenergic blockers (e.g. propranolol, atenolol) prevent the increases in rate and force of heart contraction induced by exercise and emotion. Calcium antagonists (e.g. nifedipine) prevent coronary spasm and pool blood in peripheral veins, reducing cardiac workload. If obesity is present it should be corrected. The patient is advised to stop smoking. Hypertension should be treated.

In recent years surgical treatment has become possible for stenosis of the coronary arteries. The methods include percutaneous transluminal angioplasty, or bypass procedures on the coronary arteries. This is usually done by carrying a bypass graft (using a segment of vein or the internal mammary artery) from the aorta to the coronary artery beyond the block. Coronary artery bypass grafting (CABG) is preceded by coronary arteriography to define the stenosed vessels, and is performed by open-heart surgery using heart–lung bypass. It is now the commonest major operation in Britain. The indications are: (i) failure of medical treatment to control angina; and (ii) severe angiographic coronary artery disease, in which surgery increases life expectancy. Aspirin is frequently prescribed to reduce the risk of graft thrombosis, by reducing platelet aggregation.

Myocardial infarction

Myocardial infarction results when an area of the myocardium has its blood supply markedly and suddenly reduced. It commonly follows thrombus formation on an ulcerated atheromatous patch in a coronary vessel, haemorrhage into such a patch, and it may also result from obliteration of the lumen without actual thrombus formation. The descending branch of the left coronary artery is a common site for thrombosis to develop (see Fig. 7.3). A mural thrombus may form on the endocardium underlying the zone of infarction in the heart wall and pericarditis may develop overlying it (Fig. 7.9).

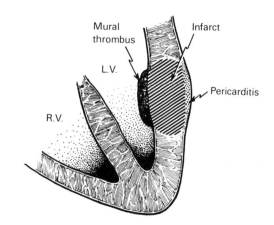

Fig. 7.9 Diagrammatic representation of a section through the wall of the left ventricle in a case of myocardial infarction.

Myocardial infarction may occur in a patient known to have had angina pectoris for some time or it may be the first indication of coronary artery disease.

Clinical features

In its most characteristic form there is a sudden onset of severe, crushing chest pain. The pain is felt behind the sternum and tends to radiate across the chest into the shoulders and into the arms. The onset is not determined by effort. The pain may last for hours unless relieved by morphine and is often associated with evidence of shock. The patient frequently collapses and may lose consciousness for a period. The skin is cold, clammy and pale, the lips and fingers cyanosed, the breathing shallow, the pulse of poor quality, the blood pressure low, and vomiting is common. The heart sounds are faint and, after a day or two, pericardial friction may be audible.

The picture is not always so typical. Pain may be slight or absent or it may be felt largely in the abdomen raising the question of an acute abdominal emergency. In other cases there is more or less instantaneous death without time to indicate whether pain was present or not. This is due to cardiac arrest from ventricular fibrillation. Some patients who sustain a sudden cardiac arrest following myocardial infarction may be successfully resuscitated (see below).

Diagnosis

As a reaction to the tissue necrosis there is commonly slight pyrexia, leucocytosis, elevation of the sedimentation rate, and increase in the level of certain enzymes in the blood (creatine kinase, transaminases, and lactate dehydrogenase). These changes are often of diagnostic help. The diagnosis may be further substantiated by the characteristic changes in the electrocardiogram (see Fig. 7.6), which are of particular value where the clinical features are not straightforward. Many patients with typical history do not show evidence of myocardial infarction by electrocardiography and cardiac enzymes (*unstable angina*); the management is similar to myocardial infarction.

Course and prognosis

About one-third of patients die following myocardial infarction and most of these deaths occur in the first few days from uncontrollable shock, left ventricular failure, or a serious cardiac arrhythmia. One-half of all deaths occur in the first hour from ventricular fibrillation, so that the hospital mortality is about 15%; it increases with age. Other hazards are arterial embolism to the brain or leg from the mural thrombus and pulmonary embolism from peripheral deep vein thrombosis. Right-sided heart failure may also supervene or the heart may rupture.

In patients who recover from the initial attack of myocardial infarction the average expectation of life depends on age, size of infarct, and the extent of underlying coronary disease.

Treatment

The first priority is pain relief by intravenous or intramuscular diamorphine or morphine. Patients should be admitted to a coronary care unit as soon as possible for electrocardiographic monitoring to detect and treat dysrhythmias and heart block (by drugs, pacers or electrical cardioversion). Intravenous injection of streptokinase often lyses the thrombus by activating the fibrinolytic system, reduces infarct size, and hence reduces death from heart failure or heart rupture. It is of most benefit in patients presenting within 6 hours of onset, with large infarcts. Following streptokinase, patients are anticoagulated with heparin, then oral warfarin for 3 months. Patients are mobilized in hospital for 7–10 days, carefully observing for complications. Once home, progressive return to normal activities over several weeks is advised. Smokers should stop smoking, which halves the risk of recurrence. Recurrence is also reduced by long-term aspirin (300 mg daily) and by beta-adrenergic blocking drugs (e.g. propranolol, atenolol). Surgery should be deferred for 6 months if possible, since general anaesthetics may cause dysrhythmias and hypotension.

PULMONARY HEART DISEASE

Interference with the flow of blood through the

lungs most commonly results from chronic bronchitis and emphysema. Right ventricular hypertrophy occurs and cardiac failure may ensue. This form of heart disease is commonly termed *cor pulmonale*. It may also result from the pneumoconioses or dust diseases.

The clinical picture is partly determined by the underlying lung disease and partly by the secondary cardiac failure. The individual will likely give a history of cough and spit associated with exertional dyspnoea. When cardiac failure supervenes, dyspnoea is increased, cyanosis intensified, and oedema develops.

Treatment of the cardiac failure (with diuretics) is often only partially successful because the underlying lung disease is irreversible.

THYROID HEART DISEASE (see Ch. 13)

Thyrotoxicosis in young individuals is seldom associated with any evidence of cardiac failure, but when the disorder occurs in middle-aged or elderly individuals cardiac complications are common. Extrasystoles or atrial fibrillation may occur and, in severe cases, congestive cardiac failure may follow. The diagnosis of thyrotoxicosis is frequently overlooked in such instances because eye signs and thyroid gland enlargement may be slight or absent. The cardiac failure will respond poorly to treatment until the thyrotoxicosis is controlled.

There is an increased incidence of coronary artery disease and of myocardial ischaemia in myxoedema. For this reason, when thyroxine is given the initial dose should be small and the dosage should be increased gradually.

CARDIAC FAILURE

The commonest causes of cardiac failure are coronary artery disease, hypertension, and rheumatic heart disease. The condition is usually considered under the headings of left heart failure and right heart failure, but pure examples of either variety are less common than combinations of the two types.

Left heart failure is seen most often in hypertension and coronary artery disease. It is characterized by accumulation of blood in the *pulmonary* veins, causing dyspnoea. Attacks of paroxysmal dyspnoea, often nocturnal, are due to acute pulmonary oedema. The administration of a diuretic together with a small dose of morphine usually produces quick symptomatic relief. Inhalations of oxygen in high concentration are commonly given; digoxin may be required.

Right heart failure is commonly seen in cases of pulmonary heart disease, alcoholic cardiomyopathy, and rheumatic heart disease particularly once atrial fibrillation is established. Frequently it develops subsequent to left ventricular failure. The dominant feature of the condition is accumulation of blood on the *systemic* venous side of the circulation.

Clinical features

The main symptom is breathlessness. At first this is experienced only on exertion but in severe cases it is present at rest and the individual cannot lie flat without acute distress. Oedema is most prominent around the feet and ankles of the ambulant patient, especially in the evenings. In the patient who has been confined to bed for some time it should be looked for in the lumbosacral region. Cyanosis of the lips, cheeks, ears and fingers is present and becomes more marked if the patient is exercised. The neck veins are engorged (see Fig. 7.4) and they may be made even more prominent by pressure over the liver (hepatojugular reflux), which is enlarged and tender because of its increased content of venous blood. Ascites (excess fluid in the peritoneal cavity) develops in severe cases. The lungs are congested especially at the bases and in severe cases pleural effusion develops. The urinary output is low; the urine is concentrated and commonly contains albumin. The findings in the cardiovascular system depend on the basic cause but frequently the heart is enlarged and the rhythm irregular. There is a high risk of deep vein thrombosis and pulmonary embolism.

Treatment

The patient invariably finds it easier to be nursed in a propped-up position as this lessens dyspnoea. After the acute stage has passed he may with advantage sit in a comfortable chair for part of the day. Inhalations of oxygen may be required in severe cases. Subcutaneous heparin is given to prevent venous thromboembolism.

The oedema may be quickly reduced by repeated administration of a *diuretic* such as one of the thiazide drugs or frusemide. *Digoxin* is useful in atrial fibrillation since it slows the ventricular rate and increases cardiac output. It also increases the force of contraction of the failing ventricles and may be used in patients without atrial fibrillation. However toxicity is common (nausea, vomiting, and dysrhythmias including extrasystoles which are often coupled). In recent years *vasodilators* have replaced digoxin. They reduce cardiac workload by dilating peripheral arteries and veins. These drugs include nitrates and angiotensin-converting enzyme inhibitors (e.g. captopril). The latter group of drugs reduces mortality in chronic heart failure. In a few younger patients, *heart transplants* have given a new lease of life, but few donors are available.

SYNCOPE

Syncope means transient loss of consciousness due to insufficient blood supply to the brain. The cerebral ischaemia may result from a simple fainting attack, from postural hypotension, from severe blood loss, or from a cardiac disorder such as heart block or myocardial infarction.

Simple fainting attack

This is the commonest form of syncope. The medical term for the condition is a *vasovagal attack* since it is due to the combined effects of increased vagal tone, which leads to slowing of the heart, and vasodilatation, which leads to lowering of the blood pressure; these changes produce cerebral ischaemia especially on standing or sitting.

Fainting attacks may be precipitated by prolonged standing or by some emotional shock which, in susceptible individuals, may be relatively slight. Examples are hearing bad news, witnessing an accident, seeing blood, or going through some form of medical or dental treatment particularly if pain is experienced or anticipated. The individual feels lightheaded, giddy, nauseated, and then loses consciousness. If this happens quickly he may fall to the ground and sustain injury. Due to compensatory adrenergic activity, the skin is cold, pale, and clammy because of the profuse vasoconstriction and sweating that occurs. The pulse is slow (e.g. 40–50 per minute), weak, and the blood pressure is low. The pupils are dilated and the breathing is shallow. The duration of the attack is commonly a few minutes but it may last up to half an hour or so.

If consciousness is lost the individual should be laid flat on the floor or on a couch since a low position of the head improves cerebral blood flow; should a fainting attack affect a patient in a dental chair the chair should be tilted so that the head is as low as possible. Any tight clothing around the neck should be loosened and it should be ascertained that the airway is patent. Adequate ventilation around the individual should be ensured. Once consciousness is regained, a cup of tea is usually found to be beneficial. Alcohol should not be administered.

Postural hypotension

Most people have experienced the cerebral effects of postural hypotension in a minor form. A feeling of giddiness or lightheadedness is experienced on suddenly assuming the erect posture after sitting or lying flat for a period of time. In severe cases transient unconsciousness may occur. In the recumbent position blood tends to pool in the abdominal vessels and it is redistributed, by a reflex mechanism, on standing; before the redistribution is complete there may be temporary cerebral ischaemia.

Postural hypotension may be seen in patients who are receiving antihypertensive drugs which produce peripheral vasodilation.

Severe blood loss

This results in reduction in the blood volume leading to oligaemic shock. Consciousness may be lost as a result of cerebral ischaemia but in contrast to vasovagal attacks the pulse is usually rapid in this variety of syncope.

CARDIAC ARREST AND RESUSCITATION

Cardiac arrest describes the situation where there is no spontaneous cardiac output. It can be due to either cardiac standstill (asystole) or ventricular fibrillation. Both have the same presentation, and differentiation between them requires electrocardiography. Cardiac arrest can be due to:

1. Primary cardiac causes such as acute myocardial infarction.
2. Pulmonary embolism.
3. Sensitivity to drugs such as adrenaline or to local and general anaesthetics.
4. Respiratory obstruction due to inhalation of vomit or the tongue falling back to occlude the airway.

Fig 7.10 Mouth-to-mouth breathing to inflate the lungs in cardiac arrest.

Clinical features

The patient is unconscious, pulseless (feel the carotid artery, see Fig. 7.10) and cyanosed. To begin with respiration is stertorous but spontaneous respiration soon ceases and the pupils become dilated.

Management

It is essential to establish effective first-aid measures at once since irreversible brain damage due to hypoxia may occur as little as three minutes after cardiac arrest. The following measures are recommended:

1. *Summon help.* Note the time and summon help immediately. It is possible for one person to undertake mouth-to-mouth breathing and external cardiac massage but it is easier when another person is there to help.

2. *Institute mouth-to-mouth ventilation (Fig. 7.10).* Lay the patient down on a flat surface and clear the airway. Extend the neck to open the nasopharynx and help the tongue forward. Pinch the patient's nostrils shut and blow into the mouth. Make sure that the chest wall moves with the force of expiration. Repeat this 12 times per minute. It is recommended that a simple airway be available in the dental surgery for insertion over the tongue.

3. *Initiate external cardiac massage* (Fig. 7.11). A vigorous blow on the front of the chest may produce spontaneous cardiac activity. If this is not immediately effective, do not delay starting external cardiac massage. The heels of the hands should be placed on the lower sternum and sharp downward presses administered. These should be sufficiently

Fig. 7.11 External cardiac compression in management of cardiac arrest.

forceful to depress the sternum by $1-1\frac{1}{2}$ inches. The heart is compressed between sternum and spine and adequate cardiac massage will produce a palpable carotid or femoral artery pulse. External massage should be done approximately 60 times per minute. The ratio of four massages to one ventilation should produce an adequate circulation of oxygenated blood until hospital facilities are available.

PRACTICAL DENTAL CONSIDERATIONS

The following points summarize the main practical considerations which the dentist should bear in mind when dealing with cardiac patients:

1. Patients with cardiac disease should be con-

sidered as poor risks for any major surgical procedure. If multiple extractions or removal of a dental cyst or tumour is required prior consultation with a doctor is desirable. Multiple extractions should take place in several stages.

2. A local anaesthetic is usually preferable to a general in these patients but if general anaesthesia is required it should be undertaken by a fully trained anaesthetist.

3. Particular care should be taken to minimize emotional stress prior to any dental procedure and pain during it if the patient has coronary artery disease, or angina may be induced. Mild sedation for a day or two before the dental procedure may be helpful in severe cases.

4. In patients with rheumatic or congenital heart disease it is imperative that prophylactic measures be taken to prevent subacute bacterial endocarditis.

5. Rarely a patient with coronary artery disease may present initially with a dental problem because atypical angina is experienced only in the jaws and teeth. The relationship of the discomfort to exertion and emotional upset is important.

6. The dentist should be capable of carrying out first aid measures for cardiac arrest and should have in the surgery a simple airway to facilitate mouth-to-mouth respiration.

DISORDERS OF THE PERIPHERAL ARTERIES

Raynaud's disease

This is a disorder of the peripheral circulation which mainly affects young women. A family history is often present. There is paroxysmal vasoconstriction of the digital arteries associated with vasodilatation of the skin capillaries, in which the blood is stationary and cyanosed. The fingers, which are cold, may be white for a short period at the beginning of an attack but they quickly become blue. Attacks usually follow exposure to cold or emotional upset. As the vasoconstriction wears off the fingers tingle and throb and regain their normal colour. People working with vibrating tools may develop Raynaud's disease as an occupational disorder.

Cases of moderate severity are often controlled by avoidance of cold, the wearing of gloves, and abstinence from tobacco. Vasodilators (e.g. nifedipine) may be effective. In some patients there is an underlying connective tissue disease, e.g. systemic sclerosis or systemic lupus (see Ch. 17).

Peripheral arterial disease

Atherosclerosis of the peripheral vessels, especially those of the legs, is a common feature of elderly people and, if marked, causes a decreased blood supply to the tissues, hence the term *obliterative or occlusive vascular disease*. Hypertension, smoking, and diabetes mellitus are predisposing factors. Similar changes are frequently present in the arteries of the brain, the heart, and the kidneys.

The main complaints are of cold feet plus a cramping discomfort or pain in the calf muscles when walking, with relief on rest. The latter symptom is termed *intermittent claudication* and is a direct result of muscle ischaemia. Examination reveals the feet to be cold and the skin smooth with loss of hair. The peripheral arterial pulses are weak or absent.

In severe cases the impairment of blood supply is sufficient to cause pain in the muscles even when the patient is at rest and especially at night. This condition of night pain at rest is important as it is a sign of impending gangrene which occurs when the blood supply is sufficiently impaired to cause death of tissues. Such gangrene is initially confined to a toe or toes but later the foot or even the leg may become involved. As gangrene sets in pain becomes extremely severe and the affected parts become cold, blue, and finally black. If the limb remains dry when the tissue becomes desiccated, and a line of separation develops at the point where the healthy tissues have enough blood supply to maintain viability, the condition is known as *dry gangrene*. However, if infection supervenes then the gangrene tends to spread. This is a dangerous condition known as *wet gangrene*.

Considerable improvements may occur in the early stages if the patient wears warm footwear and avoids injury and direct contact of the skin with heat. Abstinence from tobacco is important. Vasodilator drugs have been tried but it is extremely doubtful if they have much action on organically narrowed blood vessels. The toenails should be cut by a chiropodist.

Lumbar sympathectomy often improves the blood supply of the superficial tissues and is still an important surgical measure. However, the effect on muscle blood supply is poor and, although skin nutrition is frequently improved, intermittent claudication is seldom alleviated for long periods.

Sympathectomy may be performed either by injection of the lumbar sympathetic chain with phenol or by open surgical methods. Surgical bypass using autogenous vein or artificial materials is widely used with considerable success in selected cases. Even the aorta and iliac vessels may be replaced by such means. Long-term aspirin is given to prevent graft occlusion.

The carotid artery may be affected by obliterative vascular disease resulting in strokes and sometimes in unilateral blindness. Treatment is with aspirin, with or without removal of atheromatous plaque (carotid endarterectomy, see Ch. 18).

Arterial aneurysms

Damage to the wall of the major blood vessels by atherosclerosis can lead to weakening so that the arterial wall expands to form a saccular or fusiform distension known as aneurysm. This becomes partly filled with thrombus but the area is weak and the end-result of such aneurysms is rupture. Large vessels are often involved (e.g. the aorta and the iliac vessels). Patients with abdominal aortic aneurysms complain of pain in the abdomen and back; a pulsatile abdominal swelling is palpable. The aneurysm is confirmed by ultrasound or angiography. Treatment is by surgery, bypassing the aneurysm by a synthetic Dacron graft.

Peripheral arterial thromboembolism

This is a surgical emergency. Thrombosis may occur on a ruptured atherosclerotic plaque or following arterial catheterization. Embolism can occur from the heart in atrial fibrillation, rheumatic heart valve disease, infective endocarditis, or mural thrombus in acute myocardial infarction. The limb suddenly becomes painful, pale, pulseless and paralysed. The occlusive thrombus may be visualized by angiography, then removed surgically by a Fogarty embolectomy catheter. This is passed beyond the occluding thrombus, then a balloon is inflated and withdrawn with the thrombus. In some patients, the thrombus may be lysed by local infusion of streptokinase through an arterial catheter, or the occlusion may be bypassed by a graft. If such measures are unsuccessful gangrene will occur, requiring amputation.

VENOUS THROMBOSIS

Superficial thrombophlebitis

In this disorder the superficial veins, particularly of the legs, become inflamed and thrombosed. The affected vein is red, tender, painful and hot. Varicose veins predispose to thrombophlebitis and the condition sometimes follows an infection such as a sore throat. Superficial thrombophlebitis is unpleasant but seldom dangerous.

Treatment consists of rest and the administration of antibiotics if there is an infective basis. Anticoagulants are usually given if extension to the deep veins is confirmed by venography.

A frequent cause of superficial thrombophlebitis, particularly in the arms, is the use of intravenous therapy. Treatment is simple and consists of removal of the intravenous infusion at that site.

Deep vein thrombosis

Thrombosis in the veins which lie deep in the calf and thigh muscles is liable to occur in surgical patients after operation (see Ch. 4), in medical patients on bed-rest, and in obstetric patients after confinement. Details of the presentation of deep vein thrombosis and its management are discussed with postoperative complications (see Ch. 4).

Recurrent venous thromboembolism

Recurrent superficial or deep venous thromboembolism may be associated with underlying cancer (e.g. bronchus, pancreas), with polycythaemia (see Ch. 12), or with congenital deficiency of one of the natural plasma inhibitors of blood coagulation — antithrombin III, protein C, or protein S. These disorders are collectively known as *thrombophilia*; there is usually a family history of premature venous thromboembolism. Patients with recurrent, spontaneous, or premature venous thromboembolism should be referred to a haematologist for screening for thrombophilia. Family members should be screened: the inheritance is autosomal dominant. Long-term anticoagulation with oral warfarin is required to prevent thrombosis, especially after surgery or during pregnancy.

Cavernous sinus thrombosis

This is a special variety of venous thrombosis of direct dental interest. It usually arises from spread of infection from the face and the buccal cavity, and a dental condition particularly dangerous in this respect is sepsis in the region of the third upper molars. Infection is likely to spread via the pterygoid plexus to the cavernous sinus if some surgical procedure such as extraction is performed when the infection is acute.

In a fully developed case the patient is extremely ill with a swinging temperature, oedema of the eyelids and the conjunctivae, prominence of the eyeballs (exophthalmos), severe headache, vomiting, and leucocytosis. The infection and thrombosis may spread to the other intracranial sinuses and veins. Treatment consists of intensive antibiotic therapy plus the administration of anticoagulants.

8

Disorders of the respiratory system

ANATOMICAL AND PHYSIOLOGICAL CONSIDERATIONS

Anatomy

The principal anatomical components of the respiratory system are depicted in Figure 8.1 which is largely self-explanatory. The nose, air sinuses, pharynx, and larynx are usually termed the upper respiratory tract while the lower respiratory tract comprises the trachea, the bronchial tree, and the lung tissue.

The trachea can normally be readily palpated in the suprasternal notch in the midline; if deviated it indicates mediastinal displacement. At the level of the second costal cartilage the trachea divides into the right and left main bronchi which soon sub-divide into a bronchus for each lung lobe and

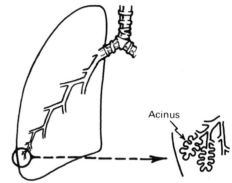

Fig. 8.2 The division of the bronchial tree into the terminal air spaces.

thereafter subdivide again and again until very small bronchioles, each ending in a cluster of thin-walled air spaces or alveoli, are formed (Fig. 8.2). The right lung has three lobes (upper, middle and lower) while the left lung has only two lobes (upper and lower).

The pleura, or covering membrane, of the lungs is in two parts —the visceral pleura which is closely applied to the surface of the lungs, and the parietal pleura which lines the chest wall, diaphragm and mediastinum. Between the two layers is a thin film of fluid.

Chest movements

The lungs are kept expanded in the thoracic cavity by the difference between the positive pressure in the respiratory passages and alveoli (atmospheric pressure) and the negative pressure present between the pleural layers.

During inspiration the chest wall moves outwards and upwards (the ribs are hinged at the

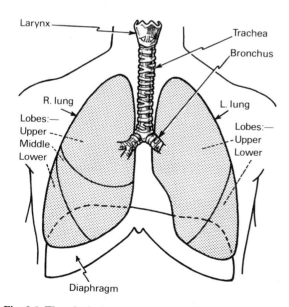

Fig. 8.1 The principal components of the respiratory system.

vertebrae), the diaphragm moves downwards, the negative pleural pressure increases and, in consequence, the lungs expand further. Expiration is largely a passive process dependent on the elastic recoil of the lungs.

The amount of air that can be expired from the lungs by maximum expiration after maximum inspiration (vital capacity) varies from about $3\frac{1}{2}$ to $5\frac{1}{2}$ litres but, under ordinary conditions, only $\frac{1}{2}$ litre is breathed in and out with each respiration; this illustrates the large reserve of respiratory tissue which exists for use in emergency.

Functions of the lungs

The prime function of the lungs is to provide the circulating blood with oxygen and to remove from it carbon dioxide. The alveolar walls, which are only one cell thick, have a very large surface area and they are covered with a rich network of thin-walled capillary blood vessels so that conditions are ideal for the rapid diffusion of oxygen and carbon dioxide. The air which is drawn into the alveoli with each inspiration is rich in oxygen (approximately 20 per cent) and low in carbon dioxide while the expired air contains a lower percentage of oxygen and a higher percentage of carbon dioxide. The respiratory rate rises from the normal level of 16–18 per minute when there is an increased demand for oxygen, as on exertion or when some of the lung tissue is out of action, e.g. in lobar pneumonia.

The excretion of carbon dioxide by the lungs is an extremely important factor in the control of the acid–base balance of the body. When there is an increase of carbon dioxide (as carbonic acid) in the blood the respiratory centre in the medulla is stimulated and the breathing becomes deeper, quicker, and may have a hissing quality (Kussmaul's respiration); this is a characteristic feature of uraemia.

The lungs play a part in the fluid balance of the body. In temperate climates about 500 ml water are lost from the lungs each day by the process of insensible evaporation.

Defences of the air passages

We inhale many thousands of litres of far-from-sterile air each day and yet only relatively rarely does infection of the respiratory passages or lung tissue arise. This is because the lungs have a very efficient protective mechanism which is constantly on guard.

1. In the nose, air sinuses and nasopharynx, dust particles and microbes are trapped on a sticky 'fly-paper' of ciliated epithelium and are then propelled towards the exterior by the movement of the cilia. The efficiency of this barrier is apparent if we examine the material blown from the nose on a foggy day.

2. A further defence is provided by the larynx, which closes reflexly if it is irritated.

3. The cough reflex, initiated by irritation of the respiratory mucosa, helps to keep the bronchial tree clear.

4. Infected material from the nasopharynx is often swallowed and rendered harmless by the powerful bactericidal activity of the gastric juice.

5. Organisms that penetrate the above defences do not necessarily cause lung disease as many of them are dealt with by the local defences of the lung (macrophages and polymorphs)

INVESTIGATION OF RESPIRATORY DISORDERS

History

In addition to a full account of the patient's immediate symptoms specific enquiry must always be made regarding cough, spit, haemoptysis, chest pain, dyspnoea, weight loss, occupation, smoking habit, and family history. The more common symptoms are discussed in the next section.

Examination

On general examination we should look for cyanosis, dyspnoea, and finger clubbing; no special skill is required for their detection.

Examination of the chest by means of inspection, palpation, percussion and auscultation is a matter for the doctor but as an illustrative example the characteristic physical signs of an extensive pleural effusion may be mentioned. On the affected side there is impaired movement, a dull percussion note, and absence of breath sounds; the effusion displaces the mediastinal contents to the opposite side, shown by deviation of the trachea (felt in the suprasternal notch) and of the apex beat.

Sputum

Examination of the sputum is an important step in investigation of respiratory disorders. The presence of pus or blood is usually obvious on naked-eye examination. A very large volume of purulent sputum should always raise the suspicion of bronchiectasis. Microscopic examination of a stained smear is of value in defining the bacteria present; if tuberculosis is suspected the Ziehl-Nielsen staining technique is employed and several specimens must be examined before a firm negative answer is given. Culture of the organisms present and determination of their sensitivity to antibiotics is a valuable guide to treatment. Cytological examination of the sputum for malignant cells is a very important investigation if bronchogenic neoplasm is suspected.

Radiology

Radiological examination of the lungs (chest X-ray) is an essential step as it detects many cases of tuberculosis and carcinoma at a stage when clinical examination is quite negative, and it also gives much more precise information than physical examination in following the progress of lesions. Special techniques may be required, e.g. bronchography in bronchiectasis, pulmonary angiography or isotope lung scanning in pulmonary embolism.

Bronchoscopy

Direct visualization of the mucosa of the upper part of the bronchial tree through a bronchoscope is of great importance in the diagnosis of bronchogenic carcinoma. A biopsy may be taken at the time of the examination.

COMMON SYMPTOMS AND SIGNS

Epistaxis

The vast majority of nose bleeds result from erosion of the vascular plexus in the anterior nasal septal mucosa. This is usually easily controlled by sustained pressure. However, should the bleeding become persistent or recurrent local electrocautery or chemical cautery under topical anaesthesia may be required.

Bleeding from the posterior part of the nose is much less common and may be more severe and difficult to control. Nasal packing may be necessary if the precise bleeding point cannot be identified and dealt with. Recurrent nose bleeds may be due to hypertension (see Ch. 7), hereditary haemorrhagic telangiectasia (see Ch. 12), or to platelet disorders (see Ch. 12).

Cough

A cough is a defensive reflex set up by irritation of the mucosa lining the respiratory tract; it protects against the entrance of foreign material into, and expels secretion from, the respiratory tract. The term dry cough is used when no spit is produced and loose, or productive, cough when there is sputum.

Cough is a very common symptom of respiratory disease. A dry, irritating cough occurs in simple upper respiratory tract infections while if there is a more marked inflammatory reaction purulent sputum is produced. The commonest cause of chronic cough in this country is undoubtedly chronic bronchitis; characteristically the cough is worse in winter months. Cough is an important symptom of pneumonia and is usually associated with pleuritic chest pain. Pulmonary tuberculosis is seldom forgotten as a cause of cough but it should be remembered that many early cases of the disease have no respiratory symptoms. In bronchiectasis the cough, and associated sputum, is most marked in the morning on rising. Carcinoma of the bronchus is a serious cause of cough in those of middle age and over.

Haemoptysis

Haemoptysis, which means the coughing up of blood from the respiratory tract, is a symptom that usually causes the patient great alarm and leads him to seek medical advice. The blood is commonly frothy and bright red in colour (oxygenated) due to admixture with air but, if the blood is small in amount, the sputum may be rusty in colour as in pneumonia, while if bleeding is copious, clots may be produced. The main causes of haemoptysis are:

1. Pulmonary tuberculosis either in the early exudative stages, or in the late stages due to erosion of a blood vessel in a cavity.
2. Lobar pneumonia — characteristic rusty sputum.
3. Bronchial carcinoma.
4. Bronchiectasis.
5. Pulmonary infarction, e.g. from peripheral deep vein thrombosis.
6. Heart disease
   a. mitral stenosis where the haemoptysis is due to pulmonary hypertension;
   b. acute left ventricular failure.
7. Haemorrhagic disorders.

Dyspnoea

Dyspnoea, which is more fully discussed in the chapter on cardiac disorders (see Ch. 7), may arise from any pulmonary disorder that is extensive enough to cause impaired oxygenation of the blood passing through the lungs. Common examples are chronic bronchitis and emphysema, pneumonia, asthma, lung collapse, and pleural effusion.

Chest pain

The pain associated with cardiac disease has already been described (see Ch. 7). Pain arises from respiratory disorders when the pleura is involved, as for example over an area of pneumonia, or if there is pressure on bony structures by tumour growth. Pleuritic pain is characteristically increased by coughing or deep breathing.

Hoarseness

The main causes of hoarseness of the voice are:
1. Laryngitis secondary to the common cold.
2. Chronic laryngitis due to excessive smoking or excessive shouting (e.g. newsvendors).
3. Tuberculous laryngitis — this is always secondary to pulmonary tuberculosis.
4. Syphilitic laryngitis—now rarely seen.
5. Neoplasm of the vocal cords, either papilloma or carcinoma.

6. Paralysis of the recurrent laryngeal nerve which supplies all the intrinsic muscles of the larynx with the exception of the cricothyroid. On the right side the nerve arises from the vagus in the root of the neck but on the left it arises from the vagus in the upper part of the thorax and is closely related to the arch of the aorta and the left main bronchus in its ascent to the larynx. The left recurrent laryngeal may be compressed in the mediastinum by secondary carcinomatous lymph nodes or aortic aneurysm, while either nerve may be compressed at the root of the neck by enlarged lymph nodes or may suffer damage at thyroidectomy.

7. Myxoedema causes hoarseness and should always be borne in mind when there is no apparent local cause.

Cyanosis

Cyanosis is dealt with in the section on cardiac disorders (see Ch. 7); it may result from any pulmonary condition that interferes sufficiently with oxygenation of the blood.

Finger clubbing

The term finger clubbing is used to describe an enlargement of the ends of the finger which occurs in certain disease processes. A typical example of finger clubbing is shown in Fig. 8.3. The first change is an increase in the soft tissues of the nail bed so that the angle between the base of the nail and the skin is lost. Later there is a diffuse increase in the soft tissues of the finger end which becomes

Fig. 8.3 Clubbing of the fingers.

thickened both anteroposteriorly and laterally. The precise mechanism of finger clubbing is not fully understood, but the main factor is probably alteration in the oxygenation of the peripheral tissues. In marked cases the toes may also be involved.

Pulmonary causes. Suppuration in the lungs as in cases of bronchiectasis, lung abscess, and empyema usually produces finger clubbing which may be of a marked degree. Carcinoma of the lung is an important cause.

Cardiac causes. The cyanotic group of congenital heart disease is associated with finger clubbing which is often marked. Subacute bacterial endocarditis often causes finger clubbing, but the degree is usually slight.

Cirrhosis of the liver is a less common cause of finger clubbing.

Halitosis

The causes of halitosis, or foul breath, may conveniently be described in four main groups.

1. *Sepsis or putrefaction in mouth and nasal sinuses.* The dentist will encounter many examples of halitosis due to carious teeth, pyorrhoea, sepsis under crowns, etc. Other causes to be mentioned include Vincent's infection, septic tonsillar infection, neoplasm of nasal sinuses or nasopharynx, and syphilitic or tuberculous ulceration. Careful local examination usually yields the diagnosis in these cases.

2. *Sepsis or putrefaction in lungs.* The most important causes are lung abscess, bronchiectasis, and tuberculous cavitation with secondary infection. In most of these cases the patient will give a history of cough and spit, and examination of the fingers may show clubbing.

3. *Drugs and foods.* Excessive tobacco smoking is a well-known cause of halitosis while onions and garlic are notorious for their effect on the breath. Paraldehyde is a drug that is used as a hypnotic in restless patients and its excretion in the breath gives a characteristic odour which may be smelt at some distance.

4. *Other causes.* In advanced renal failure the breath may have an unpleasant ammoniacal odour. In many alimentary disorders, ranging from simple gastric upsets to conditions like typhoid fever or peritonitis, the breath becomes foul.

Chest shapes

The principal medical terms for the common abnormalities of chest shape are as follows.

Kyphosis is the term used to describe increased curvature of the spine in the anteroposterior direction. This is seen commonly in the thoracic region giving rise to a hump-back. It occurs, in slight degree, as a more or less normal feature of ageing. It is seen in many cases of chronic bronchitis and emphysema. In some instances it is due to disease of the vertebrae, most often tuberculosis; this is the usual cause in severe hunch-back deformity.

Scoliosis signifies lateral curvature of the spine. Slight degrees are not uncommon and are usually due to faulty posture and development in childhood. Poliomyelitis may cause scoliosis if the vertebral muscles are unequally involved. Severe unilateral lung disease (e.g. tuberculosis, empyema) is an important cause of thoracic scoliosis. Unilateral hip joint disease frequently leads to lumbar scoliosis.

The term *barrel chest* is used where the anteroposterior diameter is greatly increased; there is increased curvature of the thoracic spine, the ribs

Fig. 8.4 Barrel-shaped chest.

are held more horizontally, and the sternum is usually more prominent (Fig. 8.4). Barrel chest is seen in some cases of chronic bronchitis and emphysema but its association with this form of lung disease is by no means constant. In chronic asthmatics barrel chest may develop but again the relationship is not constant. It is sometimes present in people with apparently healthy lungs.

CORYZA

Coryza, or the common cold, is an extremely frequent infection particularly in the winter months. The rhinovirus responsible has a high infectivity and there are many strains, hence recurrent attacks are frequent. The incubation period is short, in the majority of cases being two to three days.

Clinical features

These are so well known from personal experience that a description is hardly necessary. The individual has symptoms of a mild or moderate toxaemia which is followed by catarrhal inflammation of the nasal passages, i.e. rhinitis.

Treatment

No specific treatment is available. Rest, warmth, hot drinks and aspirin usually alleviate symptoms but it is doubtful if they shorten the course of the illness. Instillation of nasal drops containing a vasoconstrictor substance such as ephedrine may be employed to relieve nasal congestion.

Complications

Complications of the common cold are very frequent and are due to secondary bacterial infection, e.g. with staphylococci, streptococci, pneumococci and *Haemophilus influenzae*. There is an increase of general malaise, commonly with mild or moderate fever, and symptoms are indicated below.

1. Sinusitis — frontal headache or a dull ache over the maxillary sinus. In a severe case of maxillary or frontal sinusitis appropriate irrigation may be necessary in addition to antibiotic therapy.
2. Pharyngitis—sore throat, dry irritating cough.
3. Laryngitis — sore throat, hoarse voice, and cough.
4. Tracheitis — soreness or rawness behind the upper sternum increased by cough.
5. Bronchitis—cough and purulent sputum.
6. Bronchopneumonia—see details below.
7. Otitis media—Eustachian tube catarrh leads to deafness and when the middle ear is involved there is also pain in the ear.

Acute otitis media

Acute otitis media is almost exclusively a problem of childhood. It is often associated with infected lymphoid tissue of the nasopharynx and adenoid hypertrophy. This may be associated with nasal obstruction and mouth breathing. Adenoidectomy may minimize nasal difficulty and reduce the chances of chronic infection.

The most common bacteria involved in otitis media are *Streptococcus pneumoniae* and *Haemophilus influenzae*. Symptoms consist of early stuffiness of the ear followed by severe pain. If the tympanic membrane ruptures a serous or purulent discharge may present at the external ear. Treatment consists of systemic antibiotics (e.g. amoxycillin or erythromycin) continued for at least 10 days. If the infection does not respond readily an alternative drug should be substituted. Nasal and auditory tube decongestants in the form of nose drops or sprays may help. When the pain is especially severe and associated with bulging of the tympanic membrane, incision of the tympanic membrane (myringotomy) should be considered. This gives immediate and dramatic relief of pain.

Complications of acute suppurative otitis media are meningitis, facial paralysis, mastoiditis, and subdural or brain abscess.

Chronic otitis media characterized by persistent perforation of the tympanic membrane may necessitate mastoidectomy.

INFLUENZA

Aetiology

Three related viruses, termed A, B and C, may cause influenza. Virus A is responsible for most of the epidemics, virus B tends to cause more limited outbreaks, while infection with virus C is rare. Epidemics occur approximately every 10 years, due to antigenic change in the virus, which then spreads through the non-immune population. If the infection becomes particularly widespread the term *pandemic* is used — in the great pandemic of 1918–19 it is estimated that approximately 20 million people died, the majority of them from secondary bacterial pneumonia.

Clinical features

The incubation period is short, in most cases being 1–3 days.

The onset is abrupt with headache, aches and pains in the limbs and in the trunk, sweating, fever, and often vomiting. There is usually an associated catarrhal inflammation of the upper respiratory passages.

In most cases recovery takes place after a few days. In some, secondary bacterial infection leads to bronchitis or bronchopneumonia while in others, fortunately a minority of those infected, the illness takes an extremely rapid and fatal course.

Treatment

Bed rest, warmth, hot drinks and aspirin are sufficient to control symptoms in the majority of cases while the disease runs its course. Antibiotics should be given in full dosage if there is suspicion of secondary bacterial infection especially in the old, the very young, patients with chronic lung or heart disease, or the frail. Influenza virus vaccines, which give relatively short-lived protection, may be given annually or at times of epidemics.

ACUTE BRONCHITIS

Aetiology

Acute bronchitis is most often the sequel to a severe or neglected attack of the common cold; the common bacterial invaders are streptococci and pneumococci.

It should be remembered that when a child has an attack of what appears to be acute bronchitis he may be in the prodromal stages of one of the common infectious diseases such as measles or whooping cough.

Clinical features

The bronchial mucosa is red and congested and covered with an exudate which is first thin and later purulent. There is evidence of the constitutional upset that is usually associated with any bacterial infection — malaise, shivering, sweating, fever, tachycardia, and leucocytosis. The respiratory symptoms comprise cough and spit. The spit may be small in amount at first but later becomes purulent. Auscultation of the chest reveals abnormal sounds (rhonchi) produced by the secretion in the bronchi.

Prognosis

The prognosis is very good in otherwise healthy people but in infancy, old age, and in association with other illnesses, acute bronchitis can be a serious problem and may be followed by bronchopneumonia.

Treatment

The general measures used for the treatment of an infection, namely rest, warmth, and a light diet, are employed. Antibiotics are usually reserved for severe infections or at the extremes of life.

CHRONIC BRONCHITIS

Aetiology

Chronic bronchitis is an extremely common condition in Britain, especially in industrial districts. The most important aetiological factors are the contamination of the atmosphere in large towns with products from open fires and industrial processes, and vehicle exhaust fumes, the prevalence of cigarette smoking, and the unfavourable atmospheric conditions associated with certain occupations such as foundry workers and miners. Other factors that may be of importance in individual cases are faulty chest development, chronic foci of infection in the sinuses, and damage to the bronchial passages from repeated attacks of acute bronchitis. In many cases there is a combination of predisposing factors, e.g. a dusty occupation, excessive cigarette smoking, and residence in an area where 'smog' is or has been common.

Clinical features

The individual has a history of chronic cough and spit which is characteristically worse in the winter months when atmospheric conditions deteriorate. The spit may be relatively clear at times but is purulent when exacerbations of the bronchitis occur. Breathlessness on exertion occurs and may be very marked. In the majority of cases emphysema develops and this may be followed by right heart failure. There may be attacks of asthma superimposed particularly when the bronchitis undergoes an acute exacerbation.

Finger clubbing is not usually present unless there is a marked degree of suppuration in the bronchial tree; in such instances the presence of underlying bronchiectasis should be considered.

Treatment

In the majority of cases it is impossible to produce a cure but treatment may lead to considerable improvement. The principal measures are:

1. Reduction in cigarette consumption.
2. Antibiotic therapy when there is active infection present and, in some cases, over the winter months. A broad-spectrum antibiotic such as amoxycillin, which is active against *Haemophilus influenzae* as well as the pneumococcus, should be used.
3. Instruction in breathing exercises.
4. Change of occupation if this is an aetiological factor, if possible.

The public has great faith in cough mixtures but it is certain that many have little action other than a psychological one. A sedative cough mixture such as syrup of codeine phosphate is useful at night, however, while bronchospasm may be relieved by a bronchodilator such as salbutamol (see Ch. 16).

Patients suffering from chronic bronchitis tolerate anaesthesia badly and have a marked tendency to develop a postoperative bronchopneumonia. Patients should where possible be stopped from smoking for at least one week before operation and it has been shown that prophylactic antibiotics reduce the incidence of postoperative chest infection, especially for operations in the upper abdomen and involving the chest wall.

CHRONIC SINUSITIS

Recurrent or chronic attacks of sinusitis despite adequate antibiotic therapy should suggest some underlying disease such as dental infection, scarring from previous trauma with inadequate drainage, or perhaps diabetes. Medical or surgical attention to these underlying problems is essential in order to eliminate secondary infection.

The condition is important to the dentist and indeed pain in maxillary teeth with tenderness to percussion is not infrequent. Furthermore, the condition may be associated with meningitis, orbital cellulitis and abscess, or even with brain abscess. Surgical drainage procedures may be necessary as part of the treatment.

EMPHYSEMA

Emphysema is most commonly seen as a sequel to chronic bronchitis. Prolonged overdistension of the alveoli by the strain of repeated coughing leads to weakening and rupture of the alveolar walls with the formation of larger air-containing spaces or bullae. The lungs occupy a greater volume and usually cover the anterior surface of the heart. Emphysema has two important effects:

1. There is a reduction in the total alveolar surface available for gaseous exchange so that there is impaired oxygenation of the blood and a tendency to carbon dioxide retention.
2. There is interference with the blood flow through the lungs leading to hypertrophy and failure of the right ventricle (cor pulmonale).

Clinical features

Breathlessness on exertion is the dominant symptom. Physical examination is a notoriously poor guide to the presence of emphysema and it is now appreciated that the erstwhile textbook picture of a barrel-chested individual with increased resonance on percussion is by no means constant. Poor chest expansion is almost always present and the vital capacity is reduced. Cyanosis may be evident.

Chest X-ray usually shows the increased volume and increased translucency of the lungs.

If right heart failure supervenes, dyspnoea and cyanosis are intensified and oedema and hepatic engorgement develop.

Treatment of cor pulmonale

The measures outlined for chronic bronchitis are required in the majority of cases. Oxygen and diuretics are used when cardiac failure develops. Oxygen should be given in controlled, low doses (24% or 28%) using special masks in chronic bronchitis. Due to chronic carbon dioxide retention, these patients' ventilation is driven by hypoxia rather than hypercapnia; high concentrations of oxygen may cause hypoventilation and fatal respiratory failure.

LOBAR PNEUMONIA

Lobar pneumonia usually attacks young, previously healthy adults. The incubation period is short, often two to three days. The organism responsible is most frequently the pneumococcus. However in recent years infection with *Legionella pneumophilia* (legionnaire's disease) has been increasingly recognized. This bacterium lives in stagnant water, and epidemics may spread in ventilation systems, e.g. hospitals and hotels. *Staph. aureus* also causes lobar pneumonia, often with cavitation.

Pathology

As the name indicates, there is inflammation of part or all of a lobe or lobes of a lung. In the earliest stages the principal change is intense engorgement of the lung tissue which still contains air, but this is soon followed by the infected alveoli becoming packed with oedema fluid and cells and thus the lung tissue becomes airless or consolidated. Red cells predominate initially (the stage of red hepatization), and leucocytes and phagocytes later (the stage of grey hepatization). During the stage of resolution the alveolar contents are liquefied by proteolytic enzymes, and debris is removed by phagocytosis and by coughing.

Clinical picture

There is a sudden onset often with a rigor. The temperature rises quickly and may reach 40°C (104°F) or higher. The individual is breathless and has pain over the affected lobe due to involvement of the overlying pleura; the pain is increased by deep breathing or coughing and, in consequence, the patient takes quick, shallow breaths and tends to place the hand over the affected area when coughing. The cough produces sputum which is tenacious, small in amount at first, and tinged with blood giving it a rusty colour. The pulse is rapid, cyanosis is present, and there is a leucocytosis. Herpes labialis is often a feature (see Ch. 9).

The doctor can detect the consolidated lobe by percussion and ausculation. X-ray of the chest confirms the diagnosis.

Course and prognosis

Before antibiotics were produced the course of the illness was determined by a battle between the infecting organism and the patient's resistance. The usual picture was of a very severe illness with a high fever for 5–7 days, at the end of which time there was, in favourable cases, a rapid drop in temperature and a lessening of dyspnoea and other symptoms; this was termed the crisis. The aim of treatment was to sustain the patient's strength until by the production of antibodies he had overcome the infection.

The organisms were not always overcome in this favourable manner and peripheral circulatory failure (often fatal), spread of infection to the pleural cavity with suppuration (empyema), and lung abscess were important complications.

Treatment

Antibiotic treatment should be instituted promptly. Penicillin or amoxycillin is given for pneumococcal pneumonia. Erythromycin is added if Legionella is suspected, and flucloxacillin if staphylococci are suspected. Some guidance may be obtained from bacteriological examination of the sputum. Oxygen may be required initially. Pleuritic chest pain may require to be relieved by an analgesic.

Bronchopneumonia

Pathology and bacteriology

Bronchopneumonia, or lobular pneumonia, is characterized by a patchy infection of many lobules of lung tissue usually scattered through more than one lobe. The lung bases are most often involved. Normal, or relatively normal, areas of lung are seen between the airless, consolidated areas.

Bronchopneumonia is due to a descending infection from the upper respiratory passages by organisms that are often found normally in the respiratory tract, e.g. staphylococci, streptococci, *Haemophilus influenzae*, and pneumococci (group 4). It occurs as a complication of acute bronchitis, especially at the extremes of life, and is often the final mechanism of death in terminal illness: the 'old man's friend'. It also occurs after measles, whooping cough, severe influenza, or following inhalation of infected material into the respiratory passages. Importantly, bronchopneumonia occurs as a complication following anaesthesia and operations, especially if there have been collapsed areas of lung (atelectasis).

Clinical features

There is usually evidence of the predisposing cause. The symptoms and signs of any bacterial infection develop, namely malaise, fever, tachycardia and leucocytosis. Dyspnoea and cyanosis are present and may be of alarming degree in the infant. Cough and purulent spit may not be as prominent as in lobar pneumonia and this is particularly the case in young children who tend to swallow what sputum is produced. Discomfort or actual pain in the chest, worse on breathing or coughing, may be experienced but again it is not usually as marked as in lobar pneumonia.

The areas involved are revealed by the presence of crepitations; dullness on percussion is less striking than in lobar pneumonia.

Course and prognosis

As in the case of lobar pneumonia the prognosis has been immeasurably improved by the use of antibiotics but bronchopneumonia is still a serious condition at the extremes of life and in the frail or terminally ill.

Treatment

The measures described for lobar pneumonia apply. In inhalation bronchopneumonia the inhaled material may have to be sucked out. After operation the patient may be unable to cough effectively, so tracheostomy with assisted ventilation and suction toilet of the bronchial tree may be necessary to assist in clearing secretions.

Hypostatic pneumonia

This is the term given to the pneumonic change which occurs in the congested and oedematous lung bases of the bed-ridden individual in whom it is a common terminal event.

Pneumocystis carinii pneumonia

This is characteristic of severe immunodeficiency, especially HIV infection in which it is the commonest cause of death (see Ch. 2).

LUNG COLLAPSE

Collapse of a lung, or a portion of a lung, most frequently results from obstruction of the related bronchus. The air in the portion of lung supplied by the bronchus becomes absorbed and the lung becomes much reduced in volume or collapsed; this is often termed absorption collapse. Bronchial obstruction may result from:

1. *Inhalation of a foreign body*. The dentist is particularly concerned with the possible inhalation of a blood clot or portions of teeth in the anaesthetized patient. Children may inhale coins or other small objects placed in the mouth. If vomiting occurs in an unconscious patient there is considerable danger of the vomit being inhaled into the respiratory passages.

2. Bronchogenic carcinoma.

3. External pressure on bronchus, e.g. by enlarged tuberculous or neoplastic lymph nodes.

4. Postoperative collapse due to blockage of a bronchus by tenacious mucus or secretions.

Of these various causes the most important from a dental viewpoint is, of course, inhalation of foreign bodies, and the remarks which follow apply to this variety of lung collapse.

Clinical features

Following the inhalation of a foreign body into the lungs there is sudden breathlessness and cyanosis. Absorption collapse occurs distal to the site where the bronchus is obstructed. The affected lung is smaller in volume and there is a compensatory shift of the mediastinum to that side; clinically this may be detected by noting alteration in the position of the trachea and the apex beat. The doctor will be able to detect dullness on percussion and reduced breath sounds over the affected area. Infection is likely to supervene (see Fig. 4.2).

The inhalation of infected blood from a tooth socket or other operation site in the mouth or throat is more likely to result in a patchy bronchopneumonia than in lung collapse.

The principal complications which may later develop as a consequence of inhalation of foreign material in the respiratory tract are lung abscess and bronchiectasis (Fig. 8.5).

Treatment

Prophylaxis is extremely important. During any operation in the mouth or throat, precautions must be taken to guard against the possible entry of blood clot, etc. into the respiratory passages and this is particularly important in the anaesthetized patient. If a foreign body is inhaled then it is worth while, as a first-aid measure, leaning the patient forward and thumping him firmly on the back in the hope that this, plus coughing, will lead to the foreign body being dislodged. If this is not successful, or if there is any anxiety that there is residual material in the lungs, then medical advice should be sought immediately; bronchoscopic removal of the material is indicated in view of the complications outlined above.

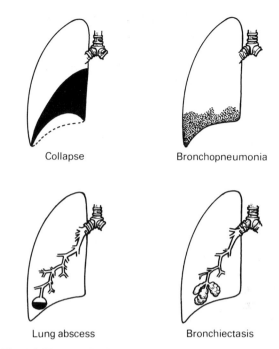

Fig. 8.5 The complications that may follow inhalation of foreign material into the respiratory passages.

LUNG ABSCESS

Aetiology

Lung abscess is a less common occurrence since the introduction of antibiotics but it may still be seen in the following circumstances:

1. Inhalation of infected material into the bronchial passages after operations on the mouth and throat conducted under general anaesthesia unless proper care has been taken.

2. Sepsis distal to obstruction of the bronchus by carcinoma.

3. The sequel to a severe pneumonia caused by antibiotic-resistant organisms.

Pathology

The organisms responsible are most commonly streptococci, staphylococci, and pneumococci. The abscess cavity is filled with pus, has fibrous tissue walls which, in chronic cases, may be very thick, and is surrounded by a zone of lung inflammation. If the abscess is near the surface of the lung there is likely to be a pleural reaction with pleural effusion and possible empyema.

Clinical features

A history suggesting a causative factor is usually obtained. A swinging temperature, sweats, rigors, tachycardia, and leucocytosis indicate the presence of sepsis. Finger clubbing occurs. A cough and purulent sputum are present if the abscess is in communication with a bronchus. The signs in the chest are usually those of consolidation or effusion. It may be possible to see a fluid level in the abscess cavity on X-ray film.

Treatment

Prevention is important, as emphasized in the preceding section of lung collapse. This is particularly so after inhalation of infected material into the respiratory passages. Bronchial obstruction due to carcinoma cannot always be relieved. Antibiotics are given preferably after determination of the sensitivity of the infecting organism. Drainage of the abscess cavity via the chest wall is sometimes necessary and if there is empyema then surgical drainage is mandatory.

BRONCHIECTASIS

Aetiology

In clinical practice there are two main types of onset. The more common variety is that which dates from a severe childhood attack of measles or whooping cough complicated by bronchopneumonia and bronchial obstruction due to viscid plugs of mucus. The other variety, which is of direct dental interest, is that following bronchial obstruction by an inhaled foreign body. In both instances the bronchiectasis results from the combined effects of bronchial obstruction and infection. Obstruction leads to absorption collapse with outward tension on the bronchial walls while the infection weakens the walls.

Pathology

There is a dilation, which may be saccular or cylindrical, of the terminal portions of the bronchi especially at the lung bases. Chronic sepsis develops in these dilated portions and may spread to adjacent lung tissue or even to distant parts via the bloodstream, e.g. to produce brain abscess.

Clinical features

Cough and spit, worse in the mornings, are the dominant symptoms. The sputum is copious, purulent, and sometimes blood-streaked. Halitosis is common and the dentist is likely to be made unpleasantly aware of this sign in a bronchiectatic patient. Clubbing of the fingers is a typical feature. If the degree of suppuration in the chest is marked then the general health will suffer and the individual is likely to be underweight and have a poor appetite.

On auscultation of the chest the doctor may be able to hear adventitious sounds at the lung bases. Confirmation of the diagnosis is usually obtained by means of a bronchogram. This comprises an X-ray picture of the bronchial tree after it has been delineated by a radio-opaque material (Figs. 8.6, 8.7 and 8.8). The bronchiectatic areas are sometimes likened to a bunch of grapes.

Prognosis

The prognosis has been much improved by antibiotics. The infection can be more readily controlled so that the dangers of secondary pneumonia or metastatic abscess are lessened.

Fig. 8.6 Normal right lower lobe bronchogram.

Fig. 8.7 Bilateral cylindrical bronchiectasis.

Fig. 8.8 Saccular left lower lobe bronchiectasis (lateral view).

Treatment

This may be either medical or surgical. The aim of medical treatment is to keep the dilated portions empty and free from infection by the use of postural drainage and antibiotics. Successful postural drainage necessitates careful localization of the affected areas so that the optimum position for drainage may be adopted. The procedure must be carried out regularly.

Surgical treatment is possible only where the bronchiectasis is localized to one lung and preferably to one lobe of that lung. In such cases lobectomy may give a permanent cure.

CYSTIC FIBROSIS

This is a genetic disorder with autosomal recessive inheritance. Affected children have malabsorption (see Ch. 9) due to pancreatic fibrosis, while chronic pulmonary infection and fibrosis occur due to abnormally viscid secretions blocking the bronchi. Treatment is with daily physiotherapy and antibiotics, but early death is usual. Antenatal diagnosis is now available, which allows parents the option of selective termination of affected pregnancies.

MALIGNANCY OF THE RESPIRATORY SYSTEM

Laryngeal neoplasms

Cancer of the larynx is much more common in people who smoke and drink heavily. As in the mouth, such neoplasms may arise from areas of leukoplakia. Squamous cell carcinoma is the most common tumour of the larynx. It has significantly different clinical behaviour in different locations. Vocal cord cancers have a favourable prognosis because early presentation with hoarseness leads to early detection and therapy. In addition the vocal cord is especially devoid of lymphoid tissue and drainage and therefore cervical spread does not generally occur early. Radiotherapy is the treatment of choice for early vocal cord cancer.

Cancer of the supraglottic and subglottic larynx on the other hand tends to metastasize early to the cervical lymph nodes because of the rich lymphatic drainage. Clinical presentation is generally later than in a case of vocal cord tumour. The most common early symptom is pain, particularly on swallowing, with referred pain to the ear. Palpable lymph node metastases may also be one of the presenting signs. Since these tumours are generally more advanced when first detected, they are usually best treated with combination surgery and X-ray treatment.

Carcinoma of the maxillary antrum

A cancer may arise from the lining of the maxillary antrum. This may present as sinusitis, as unilateral facial swelling, or with erosion into the oral cavity presenting with loosening of the upper teeth, or of a previously well-fitting denture. The diagnosis is confirmed by appropriate biopsy. Treatment is by a combination of surgery which involves complete maxillectomy and radiotherapy. The resultant defect must be repaired and the dentist is often required to fix an appropriate obturator.

Bronchogenic carcinoma

Bronchogenic carcinoma is the most common variety of malignant tumour seen in the medical wards of hospitals. This is because of a real increase in the incidence of the disorder (see Fig. 1.2) due to cigarette smoking. It is seen more frequently in men and the majority of cases occur over the age of 40 years. However it is increasing in women following their increasing tendency to smoke.

Aetiology

The basic cause is cigarette smoking. Men who regularly smoke more than 20 cigarettes a day are more than 20 times more liable to develop carcinoma of the bronchus than non-smokers. Pipe smoking or cigar smoking is much less harmful in this respect. Atmospheric pollution may be an additional aetiological factor in large towns. Some cases are due to asbestosis.

Pathology

The growth starts in the wall of a bronchus usually near the lung hilum although a few are peripheral and a few apical. There are three histological types — the round cell tumour which is most malignant, the columnar cell adenocarcinoma which is intermediate in malignancy, and squamous cell adenocarcinoma which has the slowest rate of growth.

The tumour spreads to the lymphatic glands in the mediastinum and neck, to the pleura, and by the bloodstream to bones, brain and liver.

Clinical features

Bronchogenic carcinoma may present in many ways and a high level of clinical skill is necessary if the diagnosis is to be made at a time when surgical treatment is possible. Cough and haemoptysis may occur early or late; their presence is always an indication for a detailed examination of the lungs. When the growth is large enough to cause bronchial obstruction, infection in the retained secretions distal to the block is likely to occur and the patient may develop a febrile illness which is taken for pneumonia; only when the 'pneumonia' does not clear up may the underlying neoplasm be suspected. Spread of the tumour to the pleura results in chest pain, which is worse on breathing, and a blood-stained pleural effusion develops. Spread of the growth to the glands in the mediastinum is likely to produce congestion of the neck veins, fullness of the neck, and hoarseness due to pressure on the recurrent largyneal nerve. In some patients the first indication of the presence of the tumour is symptoms arising from secondary deposits in the bones, brain, or liver. Loss of appetite, energy, and weight, which are features common to the cachexia of any malignant neoplasm, may occur before, or together with, any of the above symptoms.

Diagnosis

It is important that the doctor thinks of bronchogenic carcinoma if an adult presents with any of the symptoms or signs mentioned above. Chest X-ray and sputum cytology may establish the diagnosis, while bronchoscopy is a further valuable step as it enables visualization of the tumour and biopsy. In some patients lymph node biopsy is required for diagnosis.

Treatment

The only curative treatment possible is surgical removal of the growth by lobectomy or pneumonectomy but, unfortunately, this is not a feasible step in the majority of patients as, by the time symptoms bring them for medical attention, the condition is too far advanced. Deep X-ray therapy may slow the progress of the disorder and relieve, to some extent, troublesome symptoms, e.g. mediastinal compression or painful bony metastases. Morphine is the most useful drug in the latter stages of the disease.

Other tumours of the respiratory system

Adenoma of the bronchus is an infrequent cause of cough and haemoptysis. Bronchoscopy and biopsy are required in diagnosis.

Secondary deposits in the lung occur commonly; the most important primary sites are the breast, thyroid, prostate, kidney, stomach, colon, and bone.

LUNG DISEASE DUE TO DUST

Those lung diseases that are caused by the inhalation of dust are known collectively as the pneumoconioses. There are many varieties, but *silicosis* and *asbestosis* are the most important.

Silicosis

Aetiology

The disease is due to the inhalation over long periods of fine particles of silica; this is an occupational hazard of miners, stone masons, sand blasters, etc. The tiny particles of silica pass to the alveoli, where they are taken up by macrophages and deposited in lymph nodes throughout the lungs. The silica slowly goes into solution and sets up an irritative fibrotic reaction.

Clinical features

The individual gives a history of having been in an occupation involving exposure to silica dust for many years. A latent period of several years is usually present before symptoms arise. The main symptoms are cough, spit, and dyspnoea which is progressive and eventually incapacitating. The diagnosis may be confirmed by chest X-ray which shows diffuse shadows.

Complications

Patients with silicosis have a greatly increased liability to develop pulmonary tuberculosis. The other main complication is right heart failure secondary to the fibrotic changes in the lungs.

Treatment

There is no curative treatment for the condition and preventive measures are all-important. The dust in the atmosphere should be kept down as far as possible by various mechanical means, and if this is not sufficient respirators should be worn. Those at risk should be examined at regular intervals and at the earliest sign of the disease should be removed from that occupation. Silicosis is one of the industrial diseases prescribed by the DHSS for which disablement benefit may be paid.

Asbestosis

This follows exposure to high concentrations of asbestos dust, e.g. from insulation materials. Its features include lung fibrosis, bronchial carcinoma, and pleural malignancy (mesothelioma). Asbestosis is also a prescribed industrial disease.

PNEUMOTHORAX

Aetiology

Pneumothorax, which means air in the pleural space, may be due to a penetrating wound of the chest wall, rupture of a tuberculous focus near the surface of a lung, escape of air through a weakened portion of the visceral pleura (the spontaneous variety), or it may be induced as a therapeutic measure in tuberculosis.

Features of spontaneous pneumothorax

The patient is usually a young adult who suddenly develops pain in the affected side of the chest and becomes breathless and cyanosed. Examination shows that the mediastinum is shifted to the opposite side and the percussion note on the affected side is more resonant than usual (Fig. 8.9). Chest X-ray shows the air-containing pleural space and the collapsed lung.

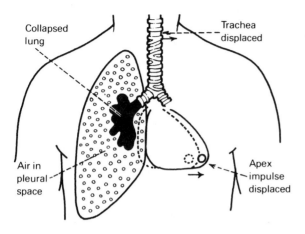

Fig. 8.9 The changes in a right sided pneumothorax.

In some cases there is no continued leak, the air in the pleural cavity is absorbed in two or three weeks, and the lung re-expands. All that is required is analgesia to relieve the initial pain and a period of rest. In the valvular type air passes into the pleural cavity with inspiration but none escapes during expiration; in such cases the tension in the chest must be relieved via a needle passed through an intercostal space. The pneumothorax which follows penetrating wounds is often accompanied by bleeding into the pleural cavity (haemo-pneumothorax). There is frequently a valvular mechanism with a build-up of air in the pleural cavity (tension pneumothorax). In such cases the air must be relieved by the passage of one or more large intercostal drains connected to an underwater drainage system and suction may be necessary to keep the lung expanded. Continuing leakage of air or bleeding may necessitate operation on the chest (thoracotomy) to seal the air leak and control bleeding.

In some cases of pneumothorax air may escape from a punctured lung via the pleural cavity into the muscle planes and subcutaneous tissues (surgical emphysema). This is usually a harmless condition and is diagnosed by a subcutaneous crackling on palpation. Occasionally large quantities of air escape and track upwards into the neck where they may cause respiratory embarrassment.

PLEURISY

Aetiology

The principal causes of pleurisy are as follows:

1. Trauma, e.g. fractured rib, pneumothorax.
2. Viral infection, e.g. Coxsackie.
3. Pulmonary infarction due to pulmonary embolism.
4. Lobar pneumonia.
5. Bronchial carcinoma or secondary tumour deposits in the lungs.
6. Tuberculosis, primary or secondary (see Ch. 1).

The last four causes may also cause a pleural effusion.

Pathology

The term *dry pleurisy* is often used to describe the early stages when the pleura is inflamed but there is little in the way of exudate. When fluid accumulates in the pleural cavity the terms *wet pleurisy* or *pleural effusion* are used.

The nature of the effusion varies with the cause. In the primary tuberculous variety it is straw-coloured, contains lymphocytes, is sterile on culture, and tubercle bacilli are usually demonstrable only after guinea-pig inoculation; in pleurisy following pneumonia pus cells are present in the fluid and all stages from a slightly hazy fluid to frank empyema may be seen; pleural effusion due to pulmonary infarction or carcinoma is usually blood-stained.

Clinical features

Pleuritic chest pain, which is characteristically sharp and increased by breathing or coughing, is most likely to be present before effusion develops. At this stage also the doctor may hear with the stethoscope pleural friction caused by the movement of the inflamed pleural layers. Breathlessness becomes progressively more marked as fluid accumulates in the pleural cavity. The effusion produces impaired movement, dullness of percussion note, impaired or absent breath sounds on the affected side, and a shift of the mediastinum to the opposite side (Fig. 8.10). Chest X-ray shows an opacity due to the fluid.

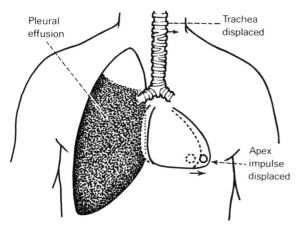

Fig. 8.10 The changes in a right sided pleural effusion.

It is relatively simple matter to remove the fluid, either for diagnostic purposes or for relief of breathlessness, through a hollow needle passed under local anaesthesia through an intercostal space. Treatment depends upon the basic cause.

EMPYEMA

The term empyema is employed where there is pus formation in the pleural cavity. It used to be a relatively frequent complication of severe pneumonia or lung abscess but is now uncommon.

The patient shows all the features of a severe bacterial infection with a swinging temperature, rigors, leucocytosis, etc., while examination of the chest shows evidence of fluid in the pleural cavity. Diagnosis is confirmed by paracentesis of the chest.

The main points in treatment are the intensive use of antibiotics and the aspiration of pus from the pleural cavity. Formal surgical drainage with a removal of a rib to gain access may be necessary.

OTHER RESPIRATORY DISORDERS

These include tuberculosis (see Ch. 1), pulmonary embolism (see Ch. 4), and hay fever and asthma (see Ch. 16).

SMOKING AND HEALTH

The annual Report of the Chief Medical Officer of the Ministry of Health for the year 1967 contains the following statement: '. . . the abolition of cigarette smoking would be the greatest single contribution to the improvement of the public health still open to us'.

The principal reasons for such a view may be summarized as follows:

1. Deaths from cancer of the lung continue to increase and there is a greatly increased incidence in those who are heavy cigarette smokers.

2. Chronic bronchitis is a widespread condition, with a considerable morbidity and significant mortality, and it is very much more common in heavy cigarette smokers.

3. Morbidity and mortality from coronary heart disease, stroke, and peripheral vascular disease (e.g. of the lower limb) continue to rise and are greater in the heavy cigarette smoker.

In addition to these major causes of morbidity and mortality it should be remembered that the heavy cigarette smoker is usually a greater anaesthetic risk.

Abolition of cigarettes appears an impracticable dream but health education in regard to the hazards of cigarette smoking should nevertheless be pursued. Young people should be advised to stop, to reduce, or to change to a pipe or cigars. Some patients find nicotine chewing gum useful in giving up cigarettes, since nicotine is the major addictive agent.

9

Disorders of the alimentary tract

THE BUCCAL CAVITY

General considerations

The buccal cavity is referred to by Sir William Osler as a mirror of the rest of the body and it is essential that the dentist should have a clear understanding of the oral changes produced by systemic disorders. He should also appreciate the possible effects of dental abnormalities on the body generally.

For the efficient mastication of food, it is necessary that a sufficient number of teeth are present and that the soft tissues of the mouth be healthy. Thorough mastication of food is a very important first step in the complex process of digestion. While it is probably true that no specific alimentary disease is actually due to inadequate mastication, it must be accepted that insufficient teeth, extensive dental caries, and poor oral hygiene are wholly undesirable in any person and that they may well have a positively adverse influence in those with gastritis, peptic ulceration or disordered bowel function. Lack of teeth is likely to be more important in older people in whom the digestive powers of the stomach may be diminished.

A patient suffering from illness of a medical nature may initially consult his dentist because of oral symptoms. As an example of this, we may recall the bleeding gums of acute leukaemia. One of the authors well remembers a case of acute monocytic leukaemia occurring in a middle-aged man in whom the bleeding gums led him to seek dental advice. Unfortunately, the dentist's suspicions were not aroused by the obvious pallor and ill-health of the man and he proceeded to extract several teeth in the mistaken belief that he was dealing with an advanced case of periodontal disease.

Similarly, scurvy due to vitamin C deficiency may present with bleeding gums.

In other instances, the dentist may observe during the course of routine work some oral abnormality which gives a clue to the fact that a general medical disorder is developing. In this connection, one may note that the dentist often sees patients at regular intervals for a 'check-up' on the state of the teeth, whereas the doctor is seldom consulted until the patient feels positively ill. The classically quoted, but seldom seen, buccal pigmentation of Addison's disease is an example of an early oral manifestation of systemic disease. Similarly, infectious mononucleosis may present with oral signs of oedema of the fauces, enlarged cervical lymph nodes, and occasionally with oral petechial haemorrhages seen in the palate.

The dentist should have an awareness of the various systemic infections that may produce local lesions in the mouth. This is partly for reasons of his own safety as in syphilis but also so that he may not continue with local measures alone in circumstances where general measures are urgently required. Perhaps the most striking example of this is the folly of attempting to deal locally with the oral lesions of syphilis or tuberculosis.

There has been much speculation regarding the role of dental sepsis in the aetiology of disorders of the alimentary tract. At one time some held that the swallowing of septic material from diseased periodontal tissues might predispose to peptic ulceration but support for this view is now very scanty. Haematogenous spread of organisms from the buccal cavity to the gall-bladder to produce cholecystitis is, however, still actively considered by some to be of importance.

In subacute bacterial endocarditis there is no

doubt that the buccal cavity is the source of infection in the majority of cases.

Examination of the buccal cavity

A dentist, by the nature of his training and profession, should be extremely proficient at examining the buccal cavity, but there may be a tendency, particularly if he has a very full schedule, for him to devote his attention to the teeth and gums to the exclusion of the other structures in the mouth. This is obviously undesirable and when one considers the number of disorders that may have local manifestations in the buccal cavity it is apparent that the dentist should include at least a brief examination of all the structures in the mouth in his initial appraisal of the patient.

The essentials for a proper examination are good illumination, a comfortable relaxed patient, and a well-practised routine on the part of the dentist. It does not matter in what order the various structures are examined provided they are all included. The lips, the gums, the mucosal lining of the cheeks, the palate, the tongue and the throat should all be inspected. Regarding the tongue, it may be noted that while it is seldom examined nowadays with the detail and reverence accorded it by the physicians of Victorian times, it is an important mirror of disease and should never be ignored. The dorsum of the tongue, the sides and the under surface should all be inspected and this should be followed by observations of the movements of the tongue and soft palate. Palpation of the tongue is necessary to detect any lesion or abnormality within the substance of the organ such as a lingual thyroid. In health, the tongue is moist, pinkish in colour, has a slight fur on the surface, and the papillae are easily seen.

THE LIPS

Colour

Cyanosis is often most evident in the lips; it is more prominent after exertion or in cold weather. Pallor of the lips may be due to shock (e.g. after haemorrhage or myocardial infarction) or due to anaemia. With regard to pallor of the lips it must be remembered that examination of the skin and mucous membranes affords only a rough guide to the haemoglobin level. Lipstick may, of course, mask the true colour of the lips.

Herpes and other viral infections (see also Ch. 1)

Many viruses can affect the oral tissues but the herpes viruses in particular seem to result in significant oral disease. Primary herpetic gingivostomatitis is common as the result of infection with the herpes simplex virus. The infection is characterized by small painful blisters or vesicles situated near the mucocutaneous junction of the lips. These may enlarge and coalesce and cervical lymph node enlargement is common. The lesions may become severe in eczema herpeticum or in immunologically suppressed patients. The virus is probably a normal inhabitant of the buccal cavity, capable of producing inflammatory changes only when the resistance is lowered (e.g. during an attack of coryza, influenza or pneumonia). Acyclovir cream or tablets may be prescribed by dentists for oral herpes of the lips or mouth respectively, and should be started as early as possible.

Recurrent herpes simplex infections are common and a recurrence may be precipitated by a minor cause such as exposure to sunlight or menstruation. Most recurrences are manifest on the lips (herpes labialis).

Herpes zoster of the maxillary or mandibular division of the trigeminal nerve produces a unilateral facial rash limited to the affected dermatome and in association with unilateral oral ulceration. The pain is severe and may simulate toothache; this is important since the pain may precede the appearance of the characteristic rash. In some rare cases the facial nerve is affected, causing a unilateral lower motor neurone facial nerve palsy in association with skin lesions in the external ear and oral ulcers on the palate (Ramsay Hunt syndrome). Once the rash has disappeared there may be postherpetic neuralgic pain. Treatment is with oral acyclovir or topical idoxuridine, started as early as possible.

In infection due to *measles*, spots resembling grains of salt on a red erythematous mucosa may develop in the buccal cavity (Koplik's spots). The oropharynx is also inflamed and the characteristic macular skin rash appears soon after.

Other abnormalities

The effects of vitamin deficiency and of syphilis on the lips are considered later in this chapter along with the effects of these disorders on the buccal cavity generally. Carcinoma of the lip is discussed with other tumours in Chapter 6.

CLEFT LIP AND PALATE

Approximately 1 in 800 babies is born with either a cleft lip, a cleft palate, or both. The deformity is a major challenge to plastic surgeons and requires in addition the help of a speech therapist and frequently other specialist care, including expert counselling of the parents.

The condition is classified as to whether the primary palate (that is, the lip and alveolar ridge) or the secondary palate (that is, the hard and soft palate) or both are involved. Clefts of the lip may be minor but may extend well up into the nostril and the condition may be bilateral, extending back through the primary palate on both sides and involving the central area of the secondary palate.

Management of the condition is best undertaken by early consultation between the surgeon and orthodontist. The case is evaluated and it may be advisable to insert a dental obturator very early on in the neonatal period in order to prevent later arch deformity.

Surgical repair is carried out for cleft lip at an early stage, usually the first three months of life, but in cleft palate surgical treatment is best delayed for some time. However it should be performed somewhere between one year and eighteen months of birth.

GINGIVAL HYPERTROPHY

Hypertrophy of the gingival tissues is most frequently the result of local causes (e.g. chronic sepsis and irritation) and the dentist, who will be familiar with such conditions, should always consider such local aetiological factors before turning to the less common systemic causes of gum hypertrophy described below.

1. In scurvy the gums are swollen and haemorrhagic.

2. In acute leukaemia, especially the monocytic variety, bleeding swollen gums are often present.

3. The drug phenytoin (Epanutin®), which is used in the control of epilepsy, may lead to gingival hyperplasia. In severe cases alternative anticonvulsant therapy may have to be employed.

4. Gum hypertrophy develops in some women during pregnancy and may be sufficiently marked as to cause prominent gingival swellings or 'pregnancy tumours'. Similar, but less prominent, changes may be seen at menstruation. In many of these cases the gum changes are probably hormonally induced exaggerations of pre-existing minor gingival hypertrophy caused by local infection.

STOMATITIS AND GINGIVITIS

Stomatitis simply means inflammation of the mouth and gingivitis a more localized inflammation of the gums adjacent to the teeth. The changes may occur on the tongue or on the buccal mucosa.

A generalized form of stomatitis may be found within the mouth and may occur in infants where the hygiene is poor, or in any ill person where care of the mouth is neglected. It may be seen after excess smoking or alcohol consumption or, in some cases, after the prolonged use of penicillin or other antibiotic lozenges. The mucosa of the mouth is red and dry, the tongue swollen and covered with a brownish fur, and the breath foul. Care of the mouth is extremely important in any severe or prolonged illness and in hospitals it is standard practice to pay careful attention to maintaining a healthy state of the buccal cavity. Mouth washes, e.g. with hydrogen peroxide, followed by swabbing of the tongue with a preparation such as Compound Glycerin of Thymol BPC is carried out at frequent intervals.

Aphthous stomatitis

Aphthous stomatitis is characterized by the appearance of small, painful, superficial ulcers in the mouth (dyspeptic ulcers). Excess salivation is usually associated. Sometimes these ulcers occur for no particular reason while in other instances they occur following some gastrointestinal upset or a febrile illness. Mild cases often clear up spontaneously although recurrence is common. Mouth washes containing hydrogen peroxide, or the local application of a 1 per cent solution of gentian violet or of a paste containing triamcinolone acetonide (a steroid preparation) are often helpful.

Yeast infections (see also Ch. 1)

Stomatitis due to infection of the buccal cavity with yeasts is common. The most frequent cause in Britain is by the yeast *Candida albicans*. This is known as thrush. Many normal people harbour *Candida albicans* in the oral cavity but infection becomes clinically apparent when the resistance is lowered. Candidiasis thus provides a reflection of health and tends to become rampant where there is general debility and especially after the use of broad-spectrum antibiotics in the treatment of general infection.

It tends to manifest at the extremes of age, and is common in pregnancy and in bottle-fed infants if hygiene is imperfect. It is frequent also in the elderly, especially where there is associated generalized debility. A variety of immunological disorders predispose to candidiasis, especially HIV infection (see Ch. 2), leukaemia (see Ch. 12) and diabetes mellitus (see Ch. 15). It is a frequent finding in the dehydrated ill patient. White or yellow patches appear in the buccal mucosa and on the throat and may lead to considerable discomfort and interference with eating. The disorder frequently responds to the local application of 1% aqueous solution of gentian violet but a more efficacious form of treatment is with the antibiotic nystatin and this is usually given by topical administration (lozenges or paint). Amphotericin lozenges are an alternative. In some patients a form of chronic candidiasis develops in association with the wearing of dentures (denture stomatitis). This affects the palate only but is sometimes associated with cracks and inflammation at the corners of the mouth (angular cheilitis).

Ulceromembranous stomatitis

Ulceromembranous stomatitis (Trench mouth, or Vincent's infection) is due to the combined effects of a fusiform bacillus and an anaerobic spirochaete. A healthy mouth has a considerable degree of natural resistance to these organisms, but again this may be lessened by systemic illness, fatigue, or local factors.

The infection usually commences and is most severe at the gum margins and in the interdental papillae which are quickly affected, but it also may spread to the rest of the buccal cavity and to the throat. Vincent's infection is rare in the edentulous mouth. The characteristic lesion is a superficial ulcer of a rather irregular shape. It is usually covered with a greyish membrane. The adjacent mucosa is markedly inflamed. Excess salivation is present and the breath is offensive with a characteristic odour. The submandibular lymph nodes are usually tender and enlarged.

The drug of choice is metronidazole, and mouthwashes containing hydrogen peroxide often lead to rapid improvement. It is important to ensure that the infection has been completely eradicated, especially from the interdental areas. In chronic or recurrent cases, attention must be paid to the general health of the individual and a search made for local factors which may predispose to persistence of the infection.

Diabetes mellitus

Patients with diabetes mellitus are prone to infection and the oral cavity is no exception. It should be noted that the forms of stomatitis referred to above are more likely to develop in the diabetic patient and meticulous dental care and careful stabilization of diabetes are indicated.

Gangrenous stomatitis

Gangrenous stomatitis, noma, or cancrum oris is now uncommon. It used to be seen as a complication of severe illnesses in debilitated children with very poor resistance. The gangrenous changes were usually maximal in the tissues of the cheeks and sometimes caused penetration to the exterior.

DRUGS AND THE BUCCAL CAVITY

Several drugs may produce symptomatic or objective changes in the buccal cavity and it is important that the dentist has an awareness of them. Some of these are mentioned in other chapters but it will be of value to summarize them here. Mouthwashes and other local remedies are not included.

Iron

Fluid preparations of iron, used in the treatment of hypochromic anaemia, produce blackening of the tongue and teeth unless taken through a straw. The same effect, though usually in lesser degree, observed with iron tablets if the patient does not swallow them promptly.

Liquorice

Mixtures containing liquorice produce blackening of the tongue; their use is now much less common.

Phenytoin

Gum hypertrophy may follow the use of the anti-convulsant drug phenytoin (Epanutin®).

Atropine

Dryness of the mouth is an important side-effect of treatment with atropine, which is used to treat sinus bradycardia (see Ch. 7).

Heavy metals

The long continued administration of bismuth, lead, and mercury leads to a blue line on the gum margin around the natural teeth due to a deposit of the sulphide salt of the metal in the presence of local infection. Stomatitis, excess salivation, and foul breath are usually also present. Lead poisoning may occur as an industrial disease or be due to contaminated drinking water.

Antibiotics

Stomatitis may occur as a complication of antibiotic therapy due to alterations in the bowel flora causing deficient synthesis of the vitamin B complex. A brownish-yellow discoloration of the teeth may result from administration of tetracycline in childhood.

Drug allergy

Oedema of the throat and glottis may occur as an allergic response to certain drugs in susceptible individuals. Some patients develop stomatitis, excess salivation, rhinitis, and conjunctivitis if they are given iodides or bromides (iodism, bromism); a skin eruption may also be present.

Aspirin burn

Painful burns are seen commonly in the buccal cavity due to the local irritative effect of an aspirin tablet held in the mucobuccal fold near a painful tooth in the mistaken belief that proximity to the site of pain enhances the analgesic effect of the drug.

THE BUCCAL CAVITY AND SYSTEMIC DISORDERS

The principal systemic disorders which may produce changes in the buccal cavity are summarized below. The student is referred to the appropriate chapter for an account of the various diseases.

Blood diseases

The principal changes to be remembered are the glossitis of hypochromic anaemia and pernicious anaemia, and the tendency to haemorrhage and infection in acute leukaemia, thrombocytopenia, and agranulocytosis.

Vitamin deficiency

The gum changes of scurvy, the tongue and lip changes of vitamin B deficiency, and the dental consequences of vitamin D deficiency are the important oral manifestations.

Endocrine disorders

The pigmentation of Addison's disease, the tongue enlargement of cretinism, and the enlargement of the jaw and tongue of acromegaly are the main points to be remembered.

Infectious diseases

The principal buccal changes to recall in the common infectious disorders of childhood are the Koplik's spots of measles, the vesicles of chickenpox, the difficulty in mastication and swelling of the parotid duct orifice in mumps, the tongue changes in scarlet fever, and ulceration of the fraenum of the tongue in whooping cough. Buccal lesions may occur in congenital, primary, secondary and tertiary syphilis. Superficial ulceration may be present in chronic pulmonary tuberculosis. In the United States actinomycosis, blastomycosis, histoplasmosis, and coccidioidomycosis are important causes of chronic, indurated, suppurative lesions of the buccal cavity and jaws.

Neurological disorders

The main changes are the paralysis of tongue associated with bulbar and pseudobulbar palsy, hypoglossal paralysis, scars of the tongue in epilepsy, tremors of the tongue in various diseases, and the jack-in-the-box movements in chorea.

Gastrointestinal disorders

Halitosis, whilst often a symptom of oral disease or dental caries, also occurs in association with fungating infected carcinomata of the stomach or oesophagus. Crohn's disease, a chronic inflammatory disease of the bowel, may also present with oral ulceration, mucous tags, or areas of induration within the oral cavity. Peutz-Jeghers syndrome consists of intestinal polyposis affecting predominantly the small bowel associated with pigmented areas on the lips within the buccal cavity and on the dorsum of the hand. It may present with small bowel obstruction.

MISCELLANEOUS CHANGES IN THE TONGUE

Leukoplakia

This is an uncommon condition, the causation of which is poorly understood. The main aetiological factors usually considered are irritation of the tongue from roughened edges of teeth or dentures, irritation from chronic smoking, and syphilis. It should be noted that dysplastic degeneration of the mucous membranes occurs most commonly in those who smoke and drink alcohol to excess.

White, firm, smooth patches develop on the surface of the tongue particularly on the lateral aspects, and also on the undersurface of the tongue and the adjacent floor of the mouth. This area is often overlooked in routine oral and pharyngeal examination and should be given special attention. In chronic cases, fissures appear and may cause considerable pain and discomfort. In severe cases, the process may also involve other parts. Good oral hygiene is essential and any possible aetiological factors such as carious or roughened teeth should be dealt with. Leukoplakia may be associated with syphilis (see Ch. 1), and hairy leukoplakia with HIV infection (see Ch. 2). If suspected, such patients should be referred to a doctor for consideration of testing for syphilis or HIV infection.

Leukoplakia is a precancerous condition, so patients with leukoplakia should be kept under careful observation. The development of nodules or ulcers indicates that a biopsy should be performed. If the histological changes reveal incipient neoplasia then excision of the affected mucosa with skin grafting can be performed. If frank neoplastic change is confirmed, surgical resection and radiotherapy are employed as described in Chapter 6.

Lichen planus

This is a skin disorder which may produce lesions in the mouth resembling leukoplakia to some extent. It never, however, produces a uniform white patch but rather a framework of whitish lines, often radiating from a central area. It may also present as a silvery or violaceous patch on a mucosal surface and this may be associated with some burning pain. Topical corticosteroids may be helpful in some cases.

Dryness of the tongue

Dryness of the tongue occurs in people who habitually breathe through the mouth as a result of nasal obstruction; this may be caused by hypertrophy of adenoidal tissue or be due to deviation of the nasal septum. Dryness of the tongue is an important manifestation of dehydration (e.g. in diabetic coma) and is a useful clinical guide in assessing the fluid balance of the patient. Dryness of the mouth due to drugs is discussed above. Deficient secretion from the parotid glands results in dryness of the mouth; this is considered below.

Furring on the tongue

Some individuals become very alarmed if they notice that the tongue is furred and they may seek medical advice regarding this. The majority of them believe that fur on the tongue is a sign of disorder of the bowels or stomach, but in many instances it does not have any serious significance. It is seen after excess smoking, on 'the morning after the night before', after milk drinking if the hygiene of the mouth is poor, and in any febrile illness. It also occurs in many alimentary disorders ranging from simple gastric upsets to serious conditions such as peritonitis and typhoid fever. In severe renal failure a brownish fur on the tongue is common, especially if the hygiene of the mouth has been neglected. The characteristic fur on the tongue in scarlet fever has already been noted. Lastly it should be noted that some apparently perfectly healthy individuals have a rather prominent fur on the tongue.

Fissured or scrotal tongue

In this condition the fissures on the tongue are abnormally deep. The fissures may run longitudinally, transversely, irregularly, or radiate out in a herring-bone pattern from the centre. The disorder is congenital in origin and does not signify any disease.

Geographical tongue

Geographical tongue, or wandering rash of the tongue, is the descriptive term employed for a condition characterized by patchy desquamation of the superficial epithelium after initial local overgrowth. The patch is slightly raised and has a yellowish-white or greyish colour; where desquamation has occurred there is a red, raw-looking area. The patches gradually change in shape, often forming circles which may touch. Healing occurs slowly but fresh patches may form over several months until

the condition finally clears up. Pain is not usually present but the disorder often produces considerable anxiety to the patient until he is reassured that it is not of serious import. The cause of the disorder is unknown. There is no specific treatment but it is worth while trying the effect of simple mouthwashes.

Black hairy tongue

This is an unusual condition which usually occasions considerable alarm on the part of the sufferer. It is due to infection with a fungus which produces a dark pigment and causes proliferation of the filiform papillae. The infection may occur without apparent antecedent cause or it may follow systemic or local antibiotic therapy due to an upset of the normal mouth or bowel flora. The disorder improves following the use of hydrogen peroxide mouthwashes or alternatively the use of 10% salicylic acid.

The burning tongue

Sometimes the dentist is consulted by patients whose principal symptom is a burning sensation in the tongue and in whom examination of the organ is either negative or reveals nothing more than a little redness. The symptom is usually more pronounced after taking hot, well-seasoned, or rough items of food and drink.

In these circumstances the main considerations which the dentist should bear in mind are set out below. It will be readily seen that in many cases both dental and medical advice may be necessary.

1. Is there any occult source of irritation in the mouth such as rough edges of teeth, ill-fitting dentures, etc.?

2. Sometimes a burning tongue may be associated with denture stomatitis (see above) and in such cases a stainless steel denture which does not cover a wide area of the palate is a useful alternative.

3. Are there dental fillings of different metallic composition which when in contact produce a minor electric current in the buccal cavity?

4. Is the patient anaemic?

5. Is there deficiency of the vitamin B complex?

6. Has the patient been taking any medicines which could directly irritate the mucous

membranes of the mouth (e.g. too strong mouth-washes) or upset the normal buccal or bowel flora (e.g. antibiotics)?

7. Is coronary artery disease present? The pain of myocardial ischaemia is usually experienced in the chest and may be referred to the shoulders, arms, and jaws and gums; occasionally it may be maximal in one of the referred sites.

8. In some instances the symptom occurs in women at the time of the menopause and it is generally believed that hormonal imbalance is responsible, although the mechanism is obscure. A chronic desquamative gingivitis may also be seen at the menopause.

9. Traumatic ulcer of the tongue: chronic ulceration of the tongue which can be difficult to differentiate from carcinoma may develop as a result of chronic trauma from a roughened tooth or dental appliance. Such ulcers heal rapidly after elimination of the cause of irritation and failure to do so is an indication for biopsy.

Oral antral fistula

Occasionally an oral antral fistula develops after extraction of an upper molar tooth, the roots of which often protrude into the maxillary sinus. Such a fistula is easily closed by rotating a small flap of oral mucosa across the defect. Oral antral fistulae may also develop as a result of tumours, but this is a much more rare event and, if suspected, biopsy is essential.

THE SALIVARY GLANDS

The principal diseases of the salivary glands are considered below, although epidemic parotitis, or mumps, is described in Chapter 1.

Ptyalism

Excess secretion of saliva is a distressing symptom. It may occur in any irritative or inflammatory lesion of the buccal cavity, in parkinsonism (see Ch. 18), as a result of the administration of iodides or heavy metals, and in anxiety states. Ptyalism may also occur in some instances of carcinoma of the oesophagus. Management consists in correction of

any causal factor and the symptomatic use of atropine preparations.

Xerostomia

The term means a dry mouth. It occurs in habitual mouth breathers and where there is a deficient secretion of saliva. The latter occurs in dehydration from any cause, in Sjögren's disease (see Ch. 17), and from excessive use of atropine.

Inflammatory parotitis

Associated with salivary calculus

Calculus formation is common in the submandibular gland, unusual in the parotid gland, and unknown in the sublingual gland. The submandibular gland secretes a highly mucous saliva and the duct has a long course. The calculi are composed of calcium phosphate and carbonates. Their clinical features consist of swelling below the angle of the jaw which develops at meal times and is accompanied by mild discomfort and sometimes severe pain. There is oedema and swelling of the floor of the mouth and frequently a discharge of purulent saliva from the duct. There is sometimes an unpleasant taste present. In a proportion of patients the stone can be palpated bimanually and X-ray shows the calculus. If the stones are in the floor of the mouth they can be removed through an intra-oral incision but if in the submandibular gland then the gland itself must be removed since it is fibrosed and chronically damaged. Calculi within the parotid gland or duct are uncommon, the stones being usually translucent and seen as filling defects on a sialogram.

Acute suppurative parotitis

Suppurative parotitis (Fig. 9.1) is seen as a complication of debilitating illness or in postoperative patients in whom the hygiene of the mouth has been neglected; dehydration is an important predisposing factor. There is a spread of bacteria, usually staphylococci or streptococci, up the duct of the gland. The gland becomes swollen, very tender, and pus may be seen extruding from the ductal orifice within the mouth. Pyrexia and leucocytosis, together with generalized illness, develop.

Fig. 9.1 Acute parotitis. Affected left parotid gland in a debilitated patient. Appearance of mixed parotid tumour is very similar.

Prevention by strict oral hygiene is very important. In established cases antibiotics are employed and surgical drainage may be required in staphylococcal infection.

Chronic recurrent (non-calculus) parotitis

In a minority of cases this condition may be due to main duct obstruction, e.g. stenosing papillitis as a result of operative trauma or ill-fitting dentures. In such cases dilation may be successful. The remainder of patients have no such stricture, the disease being of unknown aetiology. It is frequently seen in children, the individuals suffering from periodic pain and swelling of one or both parotid glands, often for many years. Radiological studies may show sialectasis (dilatation of the duct system). Treatment is by the establishment of drainage, by massage of the gland, and sialogogues and parotidectomy may be required in severe cases. Division of the auriculo-temporal nerve in the middle ear has been successfully employed.

Mikulicz's disease and syndrome

The term Mikulicz's disease should be reserved for cases of benign enlargement of the salivary and lacrimal glands of unknown cause. Histological examination shows atrophy of the gland acini and an increase of lymphoid tissue. When the glandular enlargement is due to some recognizable pathological process such as lymphatic leukaemia or lymphoma the term Mikulicz's syndrome is used.

Sjögren's disease

This comprises an affection of the salivary and lacrimal glands producing troublesome xerostomia and a sense of grittiness in the eyes. The majority of patients are women and they may also suffer from rheumatoid arthritis. It is thought to be due to an autoimmune process (see Ch. 17).

Uveoparotitis (Heerfordt's disease)

This is a local expression of sarcoidosis which is an uncommon disorder characterized by histological changes similar to those seen in tuberculosis except that caseation does not occur and tubercle bacilli are not present. The Mantoux reaction is negative. There is a concomitant swelling of the parotid glands and inflammatory changes in the uveal tract of the eyes. Other manifestations of sarcoidosis may be extremely varied and include enlargement of the mediastinal lymph nodes, lesions of the lung tissue, enlargement of the spleen, and skin lesions.

Salivary tumours

Simple adenomata and cysts of the salivary gland may occur but are extremely uncommon. Similarly lipomata and neurofibromata of the facial nerve may present as swellings within the parotid gland, and bony tumours such as adamantinoma of the mandible may be mistaken for true lesions arising within the parotid.

Mixed salivary tumour (pleomorphic adenoma)

This is a slow growing tumour usually found in patients over 30 years old. 90% in the parotid gland and 5% in the submandibular gland and the remainder are found in the palate, cheek or lip. The tumour is lobulated and has a false capsule. On cutting it has a translucent appearance and histologically is composed of cellular elements which are epithelial and a myxomatous matrix which may have the consistency of cartilage. Treatment is by removal of the tumour with the surrounding parotid gland (superficial parotidectomy) and care must be taken to preserve the facial nerve. In the submandibular gland and in other areas such as the lip or palate complete excision is practised.

Adenocarcinoma

This presents as a hard, ill-defined swelling steadily enlarging and infiltrating the surrounding skin. If involving the parotid gland there is, unlike the pleomorphic adenoma, involvement of the facial nerve with facial palsy and subsequently, as the base of the skull is involved, other cranial nerves become affected. Glandular metastases may occur in the neck and more rarely distant metastases in liver or lung. Treatment is by wide excision and skin grafting and by deep X-ray therapy.

Adenoid cystic carcinoma (cylindroma)

This is a malignant tumour arising usually in the submandibular gland or in the palate. It metastasizes along nerve sheaths or tissue planes rather than to regional nodes. The tumour is radioresistant and requires very wide excision.

Adenolymphoma (Warthin's tumour)

This accounts for approximately 10% of all parotid swellings. It is a round or ovoid cystic tumour with a smooth surface and is filled with brownish material. Histologically it consists of columnar epithelium with lymphoid stroma probably arising from salivary duct epithelium and lymphoid tissue within the gland. Local enucleation is curative.

SORE THROAT

Sore throat is a very common complaint. The majority of cases are due to simple upper respiratory tract infections, which are self-limiting, but it is important to remember that there are more serious causes.

Soreness of the throat due to local infection. The more important of the local infections of the throat are the pharyngitis of the common cold, adenoviruses, streptococcal sore throat, Vincent's infection spreading from the buccal cavity, and extension of thrush from the buccal cavity. There is seldom any diagnostic problem in these cases but, if in doubt, the diagnosis can be quickly established by microscopic examination of a stained smear from the throat.

Soreness of throat in association with the infectious fevers. The infectious fevers are discussed elsewhere, but it may be recalled here that sore throat is a feature of the early stages of measles, meningitis, and whooping cough, and is a cardinal part of the clinical picture of diphtheria and scarlet fever.

Secondary syphilis. Soreness of the throat may be present in secondary syphilis if the mucosal lesions, which are characteristic of this stage of the infection, spread from the buccal cavity to the throat.

Sore throat associated with blood disorders. The principal disorders of the blood that may be associated with sore throat are acute leukaemia, agranulocytosis, and infectious mononucleosis.

Investigation of sore throat

A careful history often reveals helpful information, e.g. contact with cases of infectious disease, presence of a recent tendency to haemorrhage, or skin rashes. On general examination attention should be paid to the presence of pallor, skin rashes, enlarged lymph glands, enlarged spleen, evidence of bruising, and purpura. The appearance of the mouth and throat may give diagnostic help (e.g. the difference between the streptococcal throat and the throat of diphtheria, or the presence of Koplik's spots). A swab of the throat for bacteriological study yields diagnostic information in many instances and, in addition, gives valuable therapeutic help by indicating the sensitivity of the organisms to the various antibiotics. Examination of the blood is necessary to establish the diagnosis in cases of leukaemia, agranulocytosis, and infectious mononucleosis. Serology is useful for diagnosis of infectious mononucleosis and syphilis.

DISORDERS OF THE OESOPHAGUS

Anatomical considerations

The oesophagus is a hollow tube, about 25 cm long,

which extends from the lower border of the cricoid cartilage to the cardiac orifice of the stomach which is at the level of the eleventh thoracic vertebra. The distance from the incisor teeth to the lower end of the oesophagus is about 40 cm.

The oesophagus lies in a loose bed of areolar tissue in the posterior mediastinum. The principal relations are the trachea, the thyroid, the aortic arch, and the left main bronchus anteriorly, while the vertebral column lies posteriorly. The left recurrent laryngeal nerve lies between the aortic arch and the oesophagus.

The oesophagus has an outer longitudinal and an inner circular muscle layer with connective tissue containing nerves (Auerbach's plexus) and the blood vessels between. The mucous membrane consists of stratified squamous epithelium which changes abruptly to gastric mucosa at the cardia.

The upper end of the oesophagus is kept closed, except on swallowing, by a sphincter formed by the cricopharyngeus muscle. Reflux of gastric contents into the lower end of the oesophagus is prevented by the cardiac sphincter of the stomach, the muscles of the diaphragm around the oesophageal opening, and the difference between the thoracic and intra-abdominal pressure. Ordinarily it takes about five seconds for a bolus of food to traverse the oesophagus. The parasympathetic fibres to the oesophagus are carried in the vagus nerves. Should oesophageal obstruction exist then the level of obstruction can often be precisely located by the patient. Oesophageal pain is felt in the retrosternal area and at the root of the neck and may mimic angina pectoris.

Dysphagia

The commonest symptom in disorders of the oesophagus is difficulty in swallowing, or dysphagia, and a description of the main causes of dysphagia will, in fact, be an account of the principal oesophageal lesions. In addition it should be remembered that dysphagia may result from painful conditions of the throat which have already been described. The causes of dysphagia are shown diagrammatically in Figure 9.2.

Dysphagia may result from lesions in the posterior one-third of the tongue or in the oral or the laryngo-pharynx but it more commonly results from disorders affecting the oesophagus.

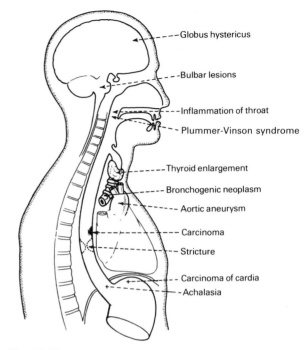

Fig. 9.2 The causes of dysphagia.

Dysphagia due to pressure on the oesophagus

Enlarged lymph glands in the mediastinum are a common cause of dysphagia. The enlargement may be due to lymphomas, tuberculosis, or metastatic carcinoma particularly from the bronchi.

Thyroid enlargement must be of considerable degree before it causes difficulty in swallowing if the thyroid is in its usual position but if the thyroid is retrosternal then relatively slight enlargement may be sufficient to cause dysphagia as the gland cannot readily be enlarged in an anterior direction. Dysphagia due to thyroid enlargement may be accompanied by tracheal deviation and compression.

Bronchial carcinoma. Carcinoma of the bronchus near the carina or involving mediastinal glands close to the oesophagus may directly invade the oesophageal wall.

Abnormalities of the great vessels. Aneurysms of the aortic arch or of the great vessels at the root of the neck or abnormalities in their origin and anatomical course are rare causes of dysphagia.

A pharyngeal diverticulum may develop from a weak area between the inferior constrictors of the pharynx and the cricopharyngeus. The dysphagia is accompanied by a gurgling in the neck when the diverticulum empties and there may be halitosis and attacks of coughing. An oesophageal diverticulum is more likely to result from traction on the oesophagus by a localized area of postinflammatory fibrosis, e.g. infected lymph glands. Either form may exert pressure on the oesophagus and cause dysphagia. Barium swallow is usually diagnostic.

Dysphagia due to intrinsic oesophageal lesions

Carcinoma of the oesophagus is a very important cause of dysphagia which progresses until the patient cannot swallow even his own saliva. The disease is discussed in detail in Chapter 6.

Simple fibrous stricture of the oesophagus may result from trauma caused by swallowing a foreign body, a corrosive substance, or extremely hot fluids. The most common cause of stricture, however, results from long-standing oesophagitis consequent on reflux of acid gastric contents and bile into the oesophagus. This may be accompanied by a hiatus hernia. The dysphagia which results may cause considerable loss of weight as a result of impaired nutrition but is not associated with the cachexia of malignant growth. The treatment in most cases is by periodic dilatation of the stricture by oesophageal bougies. If a hiatus hernia is present and reflux can be demonstrated then repair of the hernia and prevention of reflux can result in cure. Occasionally, it is necessary to resect a very tight stricture and reconstruct the defect by an oesophagogastric anastomosis.

The dysphagia of the Plummer–Vinson or Kelly–Paterson syndrome is due to degenerative changes occurring in the upper part of the alimentary canal, particularly the pharynx. In severe cases webs of tissue form in the pharynx and upper oesophagus. The syndrome comprises chronic iron deficiency anaemia, glossitis, dysphagia, and koilonychia. The term 'sideropenic dysphagia' is sometimes employed (see Ch. 12).

Dysphagia due to neuromuscular or functional causes

Difficulty in swallowing is a common symptom in anxious individuals. The usual description is of a constant lump in the throat as though something was lodged there. The main points of diagnostic value are the absence of evidence of any organic lesion and the personality of the patient. The condition is termed *globus hystericus*.

Difficulty in swallowing is an important feature of lesions of the lower brainstem nuclei (*bulbar palsy*) or of the pyramidal fibres which supply these nuclei (*pseudobulbar palsy*). Vascular lesions and degenerative processes account for the majority of cases. Impaired function of the tongue and larynx causing difficulty in eating and speaking are associated symptoms (see Ch. 18).

Dysphagia may be due to disturbed function of the sphincter at the lower end of the oesophagus, which does not open in the usual reflex manner in response to swallowing. *Achalasia*, which means failure to relax, is a better term than cardiospasm which was used when it was thought that there was active spasm of the sphincter. It occurs more often in women and the aetiology is poorly understood. Diagnosis is by oesophageal manometry.

The dysphagia is often intermittent at first. In severe cases there may be considerable weight loss because of impaired nutrition. An attempt may be made to improve the faulty mechanism of the cardiac sphincter by forceful pneumatic or hydrostatic dilatation. This is sufficient in many cases but, if it fails to give relief, recourse may be made to surgical division of the muscle fibres at the lower end of the oesophagus (Heller's operation). In long-standing achalasia there is an increased risk of carcinoma of the oesophagus and this possibility should be borne in mind during investigation.

Investigation of a case of dysphagia

A careful history may reveal some causal factor such as swallowing a foreign body or a corrosive substance, or there may be associated symptoms of the cause such as cough or haemoptysis in bronchogenic carcinoma. It should be ascertained whether the dysphagia is progressive as in carcinoma or intermittent as in achalasia. Often the patient will indicate the level of obstruction accurately.

The clinical examination should pay particular attention to the presence of anaemia, koilonychia, weight loss, thyroid gland enlargement, and cervical lymphadenopathy. In the mouth the tongue should be inspected carefully for glossitis and the throat should be thoroughly examined. Blood examination is required if anaemia is suspected.

The next step in investigation is usually recourse to radiology. An X-ray of the chest will reveal evidence of most of the causes of external pressure on the oesophagus. An X-ray of the oesophagus, taken after the patient has swallowed a thick paste of barium, will reveal the level of hold-up and, in many cases, gives a clue to the nature of the obstruction. In carcinoma the characteristic finding is an irregular filling defect, in simple stricture the narrowing is usually symmetrical, while in achalasia there is smooth uniform enlargement of the lower part of the oesophagus above the closed sphincter.

A further diagnostic step is oesophagoscopy — this is essential and can be carried out with either a flexible or a rigid oesophagoscope and is of particular value in differentiating carcinomata from benign strictures as the lesion can be visualized and a biopsy taken for histological examination.

Other oesophageal conditions

Oesophageal varices

Dilation of the veins at the lower end of the oesophagus results from a rise in pressure in the portal circulation most commonly as a consequence of cirrhosis of the liver. These oesophageal varices are prone to bleed, giving rise to copious haematemesis. They may be visualized as small filling defects on barium swallow X-ray examination, or be directly observed at endoscopy.

Reflux oesophagitis

This is an important cause of indigestion and heartburn, especially in women of middle age and over. It may also cause chronic blood loss and iron deficiency anaemia. Causal factors include obesity, corsets, alcohol, smoking, hyperacidity and hiatus hernia. In hiatus hernia, due to widening of the opening in the diaphragm through which the oesophagus passes, a portion of the upper part of the stomach passes through into the thorax (Fig. 9.3). This is associated with inefficiency of the cardiac sphincter and a reflux of acid gastric contents resulting in oesophagitis. The symptoms in reflux oesophagitis are characteristically worse on stooping or lying flat since in these positions oesophageal reflux is more

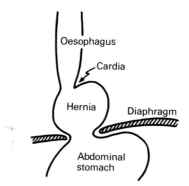

Fig. 9.3 Relationship of a hiatus hernia to the diaphragm.

likely to occur. Treatment is by weight-reducing diet and the avoidance of stooping. The patients are encouraged to sleep in a semi-upright position and to avoid precipitating factors such as corsets, alcohol and smoking. Drug treatment includes antacids, alginate foams (e.g. Gaviscon®), or H_2 receptor antagonists (e.g. cimetidine, ranitidine). Should these simple measures fail then surgery may be necessary for severe symptoms or for stricture.

DISORDERS OF THE STOMACH AND DUODENUM

Anatomical and physiological considerations

The shape and form of the stomach (Fig. 9.4) varies widely in different individuals and according to whether it is full or empty. The body of the stomach secretes most of the gastric juice, which contains hydrochloric acid, pepsin, mucus, and intrinsic factor. The secretion is initiated by a psychic flow produced by the taste, sight, smell or thought of food and completed by a reflex and humoral response to the presence of food, especially meat extracts, in the antrum of the stomach. The antrum mixes the food and propels it through the pylorus into the duodenum. The arterial blood supply, which is derived from several vessels arising indirectly from the abdominal aorta, is abundant.

The stomach is not an essential part of the alimentary tract but it has the following important functions.

Motor. It acts as a reservoir for the food enabling humans to take large meals relatively infrequently. The food mass lies initially in the body of the stomach where it is softened by admixture with the

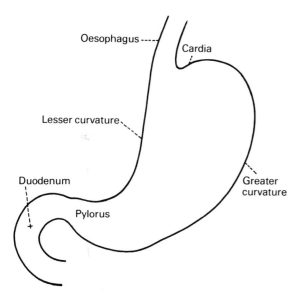

Fig. 9.4 The configuration of the normal stomach.

gastric juice. It then passes into the antrum where active peristaltic movements, plus gastric digestion, complete the transition of food to a semi-liquid consistency for delivery in small quantities to the duodenum over a period of two to six hours depending on the nature of the meal.

Digestive. If the presence of free hydrochloric acid, pepsin begins the digestion of proteins by breaking them down into proteoses and peptones, but the main digestive processes do not take place until the semi-liquid food reaches the small intestine.

Protective. The stomach protects the more delicate small intestine in several ways. Very hot or very cold foods are brought to body temperature, chemical irritants such as alcohol are diluted, many bacteria are destroyed by hydrochloric acid, grossly irritant material is rejected by vomiting, and improperly masticated food is softened and broken up by gastric peristalsis and digestion.

Haemopoietic. The cells of the gastric mucosa secrete a substance called *intrinsic factor* which is essential for the absorption of vitamin B_{12} (*extrinsic factor*). Deficiency of vitamin B_{12} is a very important cause of anaemia (see Ch. 12).

Investigation of gastric and duodenal disorders

A careful history is essential. Special tests include the employment of a barium meal examination and the performance of gastroduodenoscopy. This is carried out with the flexible fibre-optic instrument and allows confirmation of X-ray findings and biopsy of tissues for histological examination. Resting gastric juice or the secretion of gastric juice stimulated by the administration of a drug such as pentagastrin can be used to assess the acid-secreting ability of the stomach.

Other special investigations include the assessment of the speed of gastric emptying and of the integrity of its nerve supply.

It is important to realize that a proportion of barium meal X-ray examinations reveal no abnormality despite the presence of disease so that endoscopy is essential should symptoms continue.

Dyspepsia

One of the principal ways in which disorders of the stomach and duodenum may present is by indigestion, or dyspepsia. The main causes of this common symptom are as follows.

1. *Simple or functional dyspepsia.* This term is used to describe recurrent dyspepsia without any detectable lesion in the stomach or duodenum and in the absence of disordered function of other organs such as the liver and kidneys. It is most often seen in nervous, tense people especially when they are overworked or otherwise keyed-up. The reason for the dyspepsia is not known with certainty, but hypermotility and spasm of the pylorus and duodenum are likely factors. Symptomatic relief is often obtained with alkalis and sedation.

2. *Gastritis.* Acute inflammatory change in the gastric mucosa is most often due to dietary and alcoholic indiscretion. Abdominal discomfort, nausea, and vomiting are present and there may be haematemesis in severe cases. Atrophic and hypertrophic forms of chronic gastritis have been described largely on the basis of gastroscopic appearances. The aetiology of the condition is obscure. Dyspepsia, which does not usually have the periodicity characteristic of peptic ulceration, is the main symptom.

3. Peptic ulcer.

4. Carcinoma of stomach.

5. Reflux oesophagitis.

6. *Secondary dyspepsia.* Dyspepsia is frequently due to disordered function of the stomach

secondary to defects of other organs or systems. Important examples are gall-bladder disease, hepatic dysfunction (e.g. cirrhosis of liver), anaemia, congestive cardiac failure, and chronic renal disease.

Peptic ulceration

The term peptic ulcer includes duodenal ulcer, gastric ulcer, and the less frequent ulcers that may occasionally be seen at the lower end of the oesophagus or at the junction of a gastroenterostomy (stomal ulcer). Duodenal ulcer is the most common variety.

Incidence

Peptic ulceration is a common disorder which affects 10% of all adults at some time during their life. Duodenal ulceration is more common in men while the sex incidence of gastric ulcer is about equal. Duodenal ulcers usually start in early adult life whereas most gastric ulcers develop in middle age or later; either variety, however, may develop at practically any age. A family history of peptic ulceration is often present.

Aetiology

The causation of peptic ulceration is not fully understood although two facts seem reasonably clear:

1. The lesion occurs only in those parts of the alimentary canal in contact with the gastric juices, i.e. the stomach and duodenum, and the small intestine after short-circuit operations.

2. The actual ulceration is apparently caused by proteolysis of the mucosa and it is probable that pepsin and hydrochloric acid are the important constitutents of the gastric juice in this respect.

Many attempts have been made to define local predisposing factors in the upper alimentary tract. Inadequate blood supply to certain portions of the mucosa, deficiency of some protective enzyme rendering the mucosa vulnerable to the action of gastric juice, and focal sepsis causing mucosal damage have all been considered as possible aetiological factors but none has been proven. There is an increased incidence in patients with hepatic cirrhosis (see Ch. 10).

Pathology

The majority of duodenal ulcers occur in the first part of the duodenum. The most common site for a gastric ulcer is on the posterior wall of the lesser curvature. The ulcer is at first superficial, involving only the mucosa, but chronic ulcers may penetrate deeply into the wall of the stomach or duodenum and be surrounded by much fibrosis. Ulcers usually measure about $\frac{1}{4} - \frac{1}{2}$ inch in diameter but larger lesions may develop. In some cases more than one ulcer may be present. Malignancy may develop within the wall of a gastric ulcer.

Clinical features

The characteristic symptom of peptic ulceration is indigestion or dyspepsia. In a typical case of duodenal ulceration the patient usually states that about one to three hours after a meal, or just before a meal, he experiences discomfort in the upper part of the abdomen. This may be a vague, 'blown-up' feeling of distension, while at other times a gnawing pain may be experienced. The discomfort usually settles temporarily if food or an alkali is taken. Flatulence, a burning sensation behind the sternum (heartburn), and the eructation of mouthfuls of sour liquid (waterbrash), are often associated. When the dyspepsia is severe, vomiting is likely to be frequent. These symptoms may also waken the patient from sleep in the early hours of the morning.

In duodenal ulceration the dyspeptic symptoms are characteristically intermittent. A common pattern is dyspepsia for a few days to a few weeks, followed by a period of freedom from symptoms lasting for a few weeks or months. Recurrence of symptoms is frequently associated with worry or overwork. More severe symptoms include vomiting and the development of pain in the back.

The symptomatology in gastric ulceration is similar to that in duodenal ulceration with the exception that the discomfort usually comes on much sooner after meals and may be less intermittent.

Clinical examination of the patient is often not helpful in establishing the diagnosis. Weight loss may occur if the ulcer is very active and vomiting is pronounced, but it is not a feature in uncomplicated cases. Examination of the abdomen may reveal tenderness in the epigastrium.

Investigations

Should barium meal X-ray examination reveal a duodenal ulcer then endoscopy is unnecessary. However, in cases of gastric ulceration endoscopy is essential to visualize the lesion, obtain biopsy, and observe progress.

In duodenal ulceration there is characteristically a hypersecretion of acid gastric juice (hyperchlorhydria) although in gastric ulceration there is very seldom excess acid secretion.

Prognosis and course

An acute peptic ulcer may heal with or without treatment and remain healed. In many individuals, however, the lesion becomes chronic while, in others, the ulcer may heal but a further ulcer develops some time later. Many patients learn to 'live with their ulcer' and suffer only occasional discomfort. Others, however, find it a severe disability and economic handicap. Various complications (Fig. 9.5) may develop especially in the case of chronic ulcers.

1. Haemorrhage may occur from the ulcer producing haematemesis and/or melaena (see Ch. 5).

2. The ulcer may penetrate through the wall of the stomach or duodenum leading to perforation and acute peritonitis. There is a sudden onset of severe abdominal pain, rigidity of the abdominal muscles, and free gas under the diaphragm is shown on X-ray of the abdomen. Emergency surgery is performed to close the perforation and irrigate the peritoneal cavity, after resuscitation from shock.

3. Excessive fibrosis may develop around the ulcer which, if situated at the pylorus, produces pyloric stenosis. This causes profuse vomiting, often of old food. Treatment is usually surgical. A less common site for fibrotic narrowing is in the body of the stomach producing hour-glass deformity.

4. Malignant change may be found in a segment of the wall of an otherwise simple gastric ulcer. This is most important to recognize. Although there has been some debate as to whether the neoplasm is in fact a complication of gastric ulceration the argument is of no great clinical importance.

Treatment

Tea and coffee should preferably be taken rather weak with plenty of milk, and alcohol only in moderation after meals. Tobacco smoking is best avoided altogether and it has been shown that abstinence from smoking may be associated with an increased incidence of healing of duodenal ulceration.

Most patients find quick, albeit temporary, relief from dyspepsia with an alkali and in consequence there is great variety of proprietary preparations available for self-medication. Sodium bicarbonate, or baking soda, is one of the most commonly used drugs but, although reasonably effective, it is far from ideal as it causes liberation of carbon dioxide in the stomach producing flatulence, stimulates further secretion of hydrochloric acid, and may lead to an upset in the acid–base balance of the body (alkalosis) because it is so readily absorbed. Two widely prescribed substances which are efficient and safe are aluminium hydroxide and magnesium trisilicate. The symptomatic benefit obtained from the use of alkali drugs is without doubt but it is less certain that their longterm use promotes healing of the ulcer.

Recent years have seen remarkable changes in the management of peptic ulceration and in particular duodenal ulceration by the development of the drugs cimetidine and ranitidine. These drugs act by inhibiting histamine receptors in the stomach (H_2 receptors) and so inhibiting secretion of an acid gastric juice. These drugs have been shown to heal peptic ulcers and may be taken for prolonged

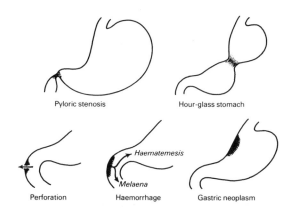

Pyloric stenosis   Hour-glass stomach

Perforation   Haematemesis   Melaena   Haemorrhage   Gastric neoplasm

Fig. 9.5 The complications of peptic ulceration. See text for discussion regarding gastric neoplasm.

periods as a maintenance therapy to prevent relapse. Alternative ulcer-healing drugs include bismuth chelate (De-Nol®), sucralfate, liquorice (Caved-S®, Rabro®), and carbenoxolone which is a liquorice constituent.

Indications for surgery in peptic ulcer

In gastric ulceration surgical treatment is clearly indicated in the presence of perforation or excessive fibrosis leading to hour-glass deformity. If there is doubt after observation as to the healing of a gastric ulcer or doubt as to whether an ulcer is simple or malignant, surgery is likewise required.

In chronic duodenal ulceration where the symptoms are persistent and intolerable, surgery is likewise required as it is in cases of perforation and pyloric stenosis.

Many patients with peptic ulceration bleed (haematemesis and/or melaena) and surgery may be required where bleeding is persistent or recurrent.

The results of surgery for gastric ulcer and duodenal ulcer are in general good but cure cannot be guaranteed and, especially in duodenal ulcer, recurrent ulceration or complications of operation develop in approximately 7−10% of patients.

Carcinoma of stomach

The stomach, especially the pyloric region, is a common site for cancer. The tumour is usually an adenocarcinoma. It may present as an ulcer and be difficult to distinguish from a simple peptic ulcer. Endoscopy and biopsy are essential in this differentiation.

Clinical features

The clinical features may be considered conveniently in three groups. Firstly, there may be symptoms specifically related to the stomach, the most important being a vague form of indigestion occurring for the first time often in late middle life in an individual with a previously good appetite. Dyspepsia is progressive and not subject to relapses and remissions as in peptic ulceration and is poorly relieved by alkalis. Abdominal pain and vomiting usually develop later. Secondly, there are the symptoms that are common to many malignant neoplasms, namely loss of appetite, loss of energy and loss of weight, and in addition there may be anaemia which often develops early and results from persistent slight bleeding. Thirdly, the tumour may present with secondary deposits in the liver, bones or abdominal lymph nodes and very occasionally there is a tumour deposit in the lymph nodes at the root of the neck, especially on the left side.

Diagnosis

Gastric neoplasm should be suspected in any middle-aged or elderly individual who loses their appetite and develops vague indigestion. Clinical examination in the early stages is often negative but later will show evidence of weight loss and an abdominal mass or an enlarged liver. A barium meal usually shows a filling defect while gastroscopy may permit visualization and biopsy of the growth. Specimens may be obtained for exfoliative cytology. The gastric juice commonly contains blood and has an offensive odour.

Treatment

The only curative treatment is surgical resection of the stomach (gastrectomy) but, unfortunately, the lesion is inoperable in many cases by the time a diagnosis is established.

Haematemesis and melaena

Causes

The main alimentary causes of haematemesis and melaena are acute erosive gastritis, acute or chronic peptic ulceration, ruptured oesophageal varices, and rarely gastric or oesophageal neoplasm. Other causes include vomiting of swallowed blood, e.g. after epistaxis, and the haemorrhagic blood disorders. Aspirin, which is irritant to the gastric mucosa, may precipitate alimentary bleeding, especially in those with peptic ulceration. Excess alcohol intake is a common precipitating factor in many instances.

Clinical features

If much blood is lost the patient is shocked (see Ch. 5). If the blood is vomited immediately after haemorrhage occurs it will be red in colour but more frequently it is retained in the stomach for some time and owing to the action of the gastric juice it becomes progressively darker and may come to resemble coffee grounds. The melaena stool is black, shiny and offensive in odour and is sometimes described as a tarry stool. In contrast to the appearance of the blood in haematemesis the blood in haemoptysis is usually bright red in colour and frothy due to admixture with air.

Treatment

The main points in treatment are hospital admission, intravenous fluids to replace blood volume, and adequate blood transfusion in severe cases. Patients are managed by a physician and surgeon acting together and early diagnosis of the site of bleeding, particularly by endoscopy, is important. Recently, there have been some successful results by coagulation of bleeding points using a laser beam directed endoscopically. Surgery is indicated for persistent or recurrent bleeding. The fibrinolytic inhibitor drug, tranexamic acid, reduces recurrent bleeding (see Ch. 12).

After the emergency is over diagnostic measures are necessary to establish the source of bleeding and the patient should receive iron to enable replacement of lost blood.

DISORDERS OF THE BOWEL

It is proposed to deal quite briefly with the various bowel disorders. In the majority of cases the main symptomatology is disordered bowel rhythm, i.e. diarrhoea and constipation. An account will be given of the principal causes of these two common symptoms, together with an explanatory note where desirable.

Diarrhoea

Diarrhoea may be defined as the abnormally rapid passage through the gut of the intestinal contents leading to frequent, loose stools. Colicky abdominal pain may occur. Considerable quantities of fluid and electrolytes may be lost in severe cases of diarrhoea and their replacement is an essential part of treatment (e.g. in bacillary dysentery, cholera, etc.). The presence of blood in the stools indicates ulceration of the colon.

Transient diarrhoea may result from many *simple causes*, e.g. the eating of indigestible food such as green apples, emotional upset, or a change in climate.

Infection of the bowel (see Ch. 1) is a very important cause of diarrhoea; in this group are bacterial food poisoning, bacillary dysentery, amoebic dysentery, typhoid and paratyphoid fever, cholera, and tuberculosis of the intestine. Bacterial food poisoning is most frequently due to Salmonella and Campylobacter bacteria, often acquired from meat and poultry. Other important agents are certain strains of staphylococci and *Clostridium botulinum* (botulism). The principal clinical features are an abrupt onset, nausea, vomiting, and diarrhoea. HIV infection (see Ch. 2) commonly causes chronic diarrhoea from several organisms, including Salmonellae and the protozoon *Cryptosporidium*.

Malignant tumour of the bowel is very common in the colon or rectum but much less so in the duodenum and small bowel. Adenocarcinoma is the common variety and this grows to form a circumferential lesion which causes stricturing and ulcerates. The symptoms are initially of intermittent diarrhoea alternating with constipation. For tumours on the left side of the colon or in the rectum bleeding is a common accompaniment whereas lesions in the ascending colon and in the caecum more often present with loss of weight, loss of appetite, and loss of energy. There is often a palpable mass and in rectal lesions the tumour can be felt by digital examination. The liver may be palpable due to the presence of secondary deposits. In some patients the stricture becomes so tight as to cause complete intestinal obstruction and the patient presents with a distended abdomen, colicky abdominal pain, and vomiting.

Diagnosis is by means of barium enema X-ray examination and by sigmoidoscopy or fibre-optic colonoscopic examination and biopsy. The treatment is surgical and involves excision of the primary tumour with either end-to-end anastomosis or the formation of a colostomy. Should there be secondary deposits in the liver then usually a palliative resection is carried out or the tumour is bypassed to avoid the complication of obstruction.

Crohn's disease. This is a relatively uncommon non-specific chronic inflammatory condition of the bowel of unknown cause. The most common area affected is the terminal ileum but the disease can affect any part of the gastrointestinal tract including the mouth. The presentation may be with pain in the right iliac fossa with diarrhoea, weight loss and anaemia, and with loss of energy but occasionally a more acute onset with fistula formation occurs.

Treatment is supportive by means of adequate nutrition and blood transfusion if anaemic. Effective drugs include corticosteroids and sulphasalazine. Surgical resection may prove necessary for obstruction, fistula formation, or other complications. Unfortunately resection is followed by recurrence of the disease in up to 50% or more of patients.

Ulcerative colitis is a relatively uncommon but very important cause of diarrhoea. The condition, which is of uncertain aetiology, affects young adults and is more common in females. The individual has recurrent bouts of diarrhoea, the stools containing blood and excess mucus. Progressive weight loss and anaemia occur. The disease is a serious one and may prove fatal. Some patients respond to a low residue diet, steroids (given rectally or systemically) and blood transfusion while in others surgery is necessary. It has been shown that the best results are obtained by total removal of the colon and rectum although some surgeons still practise partial colectomy. Removal of the colon and rectum (proctocolectomy) necessitates the creation of a permanent ileostomy.

It is important to know that long-standing ulcerative colitis involving the whole colon is a predisposing cause of cancer of the colon and this is an added reason to consider colectomy in severe disease.

Impaired absorption of fat from the small intestine (malabsorption) leads to the passage of pale, bulky, offensive stools containing excess fat. The disorder is termed *steatorrhoea; coeliac disease* is the most common variety. The absorption defect is seldom limited to fat, however: there is commonly associated a deficiency of iron, calcium and vitamins (especially folic acid, D and B) so that anaemia, glossitis, and rickets or osteomalacia, are usually present in addition to loss of weight.

Many cases improve on a diet free from gluten, which is a constituent of ordinary flour and which damages the small bowel mucosa (gluten enteropathy). Steatorrhoea may also be due to cystic fibrosis (see Ch. 8) or to chronic pancreatitis (see Ch. 10).

Diarrhoea may also result from *poisoning* with various substances. In medicolegal circles the most important is arsenic.

Self-medication with *purgatives* is a common cause of intermittent diarrhoea in introspective individuals with a 'bowel complex'. This is discussed further in the section below.

Constipation

Constipation may arise either from delay in the passage of faeces through the intestine or delay in the evacuation of faeces from the rectum. From a practical viewpoint, patients with constipation may be divided into two main groups, namely those in whom there is no organic cause, and those in whom there is some underlying pathology. It should be emphasized that the first group is by far the larger.

No organic lesion. A large number of individuals complain that they suffer from constipation. There are usually two main factors which have contributed to this state of affairs. The first is that in many there has been, in the early years of life, a tendency to neglect to empty the bowel when the reflex mechanism of the rectum has indicated that it is full, owing to social inconvenience or laziness. After a time there is blunting of the reflex mechanism and the individual, who now has a 'lazy bowel', begins to use purgatives at first intermittently but later regularly. The other factor is that many people have the erroneous idea that a variety of ill-defined diseases will overtake them if evacuation of the bowel is not frequent and regular. Advertisements in the press and elsewhere encourage this misconception and serve to focus still more the attention of the rather hypochondriacal individual on the bowel function. It should be realized that for some individuals it is perfectly natural for the bowels to move on alternate days or at even greater intervals. Furthermore, there is no convincing evidence that constipation causes 'poisoning of the system' or leads to disease in any other way.

Management of this group of patients is difficult and requires re-education of the patient to break the purgative habit, reassurance, advice to take as much exercise as possible, a diet containing natural roughage such as fruit and vegetables, and a high fluid intake.

Organic cause. The other group of patients with constipation is those in whom there is some organic cause. Among the simpler of these are painful haemorrhoids, anal fissure, and pregnancy. Among the more serious are carcinoma of the colon, as referred to above, and external pressure on the intestine from other varieties of abdominal growths (e.g. a large ovarian carcinoma pressing on the pelvic colon). It is obvious that the essential step in the management of patients in this group is detection and correction of the underlying lesion.

Hernia

Hernia is an extremely common abdominal condition. The term means the protrusion or herniation of a portion of the bowel (or other abdominal viscus) through the abdominal wall. There are a large number of herniae described but the common varieties occur in the inguinal and femoral region. They are characterized by a swelling which has a cough impulse and can commonly be reduced. Apart from the discomfort they cause, the importance of hernia lies in the fact that the loops of bowel they contain may become strangulated (cut off from their blood supply) and thus become gangrenous. This is a serious condition and threatens life. The treatment of hernia is to reduce the contents into the abdominal wall and remove the hernial sac (herniotomy) and then to repair the defect in the abdominal wall (herniorrhaphy). In case of strangulation the devitalized bowel must be removed and the continuity of the gastrointestinal tract repaired by end-to-end anastomosis. The hernia is then repaired.

Haemorrhoids

This is an extremely common condition in the western world, the piles presenting either as bright-red bleeding per anus or as a prolapse at the anal verge. Occasionally piles may strangulate with severe pain. Treatment is by the avoidance of constipation, by injection in the submucosa of the anal canal in early cases but haemorrhoidectomy may be necessary.

Diverticular disease

This is an extremely common condition particularly in obese middle-aged women. It is especially common in the western world and is said to be associated with a lack of dietary fibre. Small pouches bulging from the colonic wall form mainly in the left side of the colon and in the sigmoid region especially.

The symptoms consist of aching pain in the left lower abdomen, often accompanied by constipation. Occasionally one of the diverticulae perforate causing a pericolic abscess or peritonitis. This is a dangerous condition which is frequently fatal. Very occasionally a diverticulum bleeds heavily and can lead to collapse and shock.

Diagnosis is by barium enema X-ray examination. In the late stages when fibrosis and scarring have occurred the differentiation from cancer can be difficult and sigmoidoscopy or colonoscopy is necessary.

Treatment is by adjustment to the diet and the consumption of a high fibre or bran diet is often beneficial. Occasionally surgical resection is needed for advanced cases and is always needed for the treatment of pericolic abscess or perforation.

Investigation of patients with bowel symptoms

In the clinical examination of the patient particular attention should be paid to the nutrition, temperature, the presence of anaemia, and the presence of masses in the abdomen. The spleen and the liver should be particularly sought for and enlargement noted. Digital examination of the lower part of the rectum must always be performed since it is common for a small rectal carcinoma to be detected even though the symptoms may not suggest such a lesion. Visual examination of the lower bowel by the use of proctoscope and sigmoidoscope and more recently examination of the entire colon through a flexible fibre-optic colonoscope are also necessary and biopsy specimens may be removed for histological examination.

The stool should be examined by the naked eye (the appearances may be practically diagnostic as in steatorrhoea) for blood and for pathogenic organisms if there is any suspicion of an infective aetiology.

Radiological examination of the bowel after a barium enema is an extremely useful way of detecting structural changes and if air is introduced into the colon along with the barium then a more clearly defined picture is obtained. The characteristic changes in cancer are those of an irregular filling defect. Diverticulae can be seen as referred to above, and in ulcerative colitis or Crohn's disease the bowel wall can be seen to be rigid and narrowed with loss of characteristic mucosal pattern.

INTESTINAL OBSTRUCTION

Obstruction of the gastrointestinal tract can occur at any level. Obstruction affecting the oesophagus and pyloric outlet of the stomach have already been described.

Obstruction of the small bowel is usually the result of impaction of small bowel within a hernial orifice, or due to twisting (volvulus) of the bowel upon itself or in relation to an intra-abdominal band or adhesions. If the blood supply to the bowel is also obstructed, gangrene of the affected length of the bowel wall results. Obstruction of the large bowel is usually due to tumours.

The cardinal features of intestinal obstruction are abdominal pain, vomiting and distension. The pain is colicky, often abrupt in onset, and becomes progressively more severe. In small bowel or proximal colon obstruction it is felt in the central abdomen whereas the pain of distal colonic obstruction is subumbilical. Vomiting occurs early in obstruction of the small bowel but is often a late feature in colonic obstruction. It tends to be particularly early, profuse, and frequent in proximal small bowel obstruction and leads to dehydration and loss of electrolytes. Abdominal distension occurs earlier and is much more marked in obstruction of the colon but may be less prominent in upper small bowel obstruction. Obstruction in the distal colon causes initial swelling and tenderness in the right iliac fossa but this is soon followed by small bowel distension once the pressure forces open the ileocaecal valve. Complete obstruction of the bowel is associated with absolute constipation (failure to pass flatus or faeces) although one or two small motions may be passed shortly after the onset of obstruction.

The features of intestinal obstruction may be accompanied by evidence suggesting the underlying cause, e.g. the presence of a tender, nonreducible hernia indicating probable small bowel involvement, a history of change in bowel habit and perhaps the passage of blood and mucus per rectum suggesting a colonic neoplasm, or the patient may be known to be suffering already from a disorder such as Crohn's disease which predisposes to small bowel obstruction.

The level of the obstruction may be confirmed by taking a straight X-ray of the abdomen in the erect and supine positions. Fluid levels are seen within the distended bowel and the pattern of the gas shadows and their distribution may be helpful in reaching a diagnosis.

The principles of treatment are the early relief of pain, the passage of a nasogastric tube to alleviate vomiting and allow aspiration of fluid from the stomach and small bowel, the correction of dehydration and electrolyte deficits, and surgical intervention to relieve the obstruction. The abdomen is opened and the small bowel, if entrapped, is relieved. Any gangrenous segments of bowel are excised and the continuity of the bowel is restored by anastomosis. In obstruction of the large bowel, a similar approach may be possible but very frequently it is necessary to decompress the bowel temporarily by means of a colostomy opening on to the body surface. Such a colostomy may be permanent if the obstruction has been caused by an inoperable distal tumour, but may be temporary, allowing the surgeon to return at a second operation for removal of a resectable cancer and reconstitution of the bowel.

ACUTE APPENDICITIS

This is another common cause of 'acute abdomen' and is the commonest reason for emergency abdominal surgery. The history is often characteristic. The pain is initially central and colicky due to muscular spasm in the appendix. Vomiting and fever are common. When the inflammation involves the peritoneal coat of the appendix the pain moves to the right lower quadrant of the abdomen (iliac fossa) where tenderness occurs on palpation. Unless prompt appendicectomy is performed, the appendix may rupture causing diffuse peritonitis and shock, or a pelvic abscess.

10

Disorders of the liver, gall-bladder, and pancreas

ANATOMICAL AND PHYSIOLOGICAL CONSIDERATIONS

The liver is a large organ which plays an essential part in many body functions. It is situated in the right upper abdomen under the dome of the diaphragm. Venous blood from the alimentary tract is carried to the liver by the portal vein and arterial blood via the hepatic artery from a branch of the abdominal aorta. Bile is drained from the liver by the common hepatic duct and passes to the gall-bladder where it is concentrated. From the gall-bladder the bile passes to the duodenum by means of the common bile duct which, in its terminal portion, traverses the head of the pancreas.

The main functions of the liver may be considered under the following headings.

1. *Protein metabolism.* The liver plays a vital role in the breakdown of protein to a form that is suitable for energy use. It also synthesizes albumin, globulin, fibrinogen and most other clotting factors.

2. *Carbohydrate metabolism.* Glycogen is stored in the liver and released into the blood to maintain blood glucose levels. It is derived partly from the carbohydrate of the food but, in addition, the liver is able to synthesize glycogen from protein and from fat.

3. *Fat metabolism.* The bile salts produced by the liver are essential for the emulsification and digestion of fat. Liver cells also play a part in lipid metabolism and fat oxidation.

4. *Detoxicating function.* Many toxic by-products of metabolism and also a great variety of drugs are disposed of by the liver, some by direct excretion in the bile, some by oxidation (e.g. alcohol), some by conjugation with other chemical substances, and some by destruction.

5. *Secretion of bile.* One of the main functions of the hepatic cells is the extraction of bilirubin from the blood carried to the liver from the spleen and other parts of the reticuloendothelial system and the active secretion of it into the bile passages where it forms bile pigment.

6. *Other functions.* The liver is an important storage organ for a variety of essential substances including vitamins A, D, K, B_{12}, iron, and water.

JAUNDICE

Jaundice, or icterus, is a yellowish discoloration of the skin due to an increase in the pigment bilirubin in the blood and tissue fluids (plasma level normally less than 20μmol/l). When the increase is slight it is detectable only by chemical analysis of the blood but as the concentration of bilirubin rises a yellow tint appears in the sclera and is followed by yellow coloration of the skin and mucous membranes. In mild cases the yellowness is discernible only by careful examination in good light. In severe cases the yellow colour is intense and may assume a green hue.

The increase in pigment always occurs as a result of a disturbance in the normal metabolism of bilirubin and to understand the causation of jaundice it is necessary to have a simple appreciation of normal bile metabolism.

Normal bilirubin metabolism

This may conveniently be considered to occur in the following stages (Fig. 10.1).

1. The red blood cells survive for about 100 days and are then broken down in the spleen and other

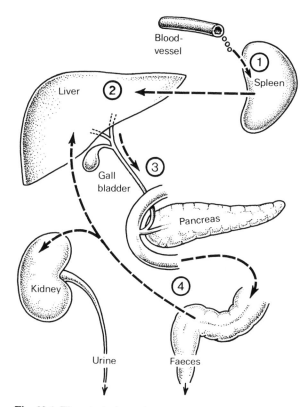

Fig. 10.1 The principal steps in normal bilirubin metabolism.

parts of the reticuloendothelial system. The haemoglobin from the cells is broken into haem and globin, and the haem is further divided into an iron-containing part, which is stored for further use, and an iron-free residue, which forms the bile pigment bilirubin.

2. Bilirubin is transported to the liver and in this prehepatic phase it is bound to plasma albumin and is said to be unconjugated. It is actively secreted by the hepatic cells into the tiny intrahepatic ducts of the biliary system and in its passage through the liver cells it becomes detached from albumin and conjugated with glucuronic acid. The unconjugated bilirubin is not soluble in water and cannot be filtered by the glomerulus of the kidney whereas the posthepatic or conjugated bilirubin can be filtered and hence can appear in the urine.

3. The biliary system drains the bile from the liver to the gall-bladder where it is concentrated by the absorption of water. The bile then passes down the common bile duct, which traverses the head of the pancreas on its way to the duodenum; as will be

seen later, this is a very important relationship. Bile pigment, altered to urobilinogen in the alimentary canal, is responsible for the normal colour of the faeces.

4. A small amount of urobilinogen is reabsorbed from the alimentary tract and some of it is excreted in the urine as urobilinogen. Normal urine does not contain bilirubin (bile).

Many classifications of jaundice have been proposed. The following is perhaps the simplest.

Haemolytic jaundice

This is due to excessive production of bilirubin resulting from abnormally rapid destruction of red blood cells. The liver secretes much of this bilirubin which is subsequently converted in the gut into urobilinogen. The stools therefore contain larger amounts of urobilinogen than normal and are consequently dark orange in colour. The urobilinogen content of the urine is also increased. In many patients, however, the liver is unable to deal with all the excess bilirubin which accumulates in the plasma and this results in jaundice. This excess bilirubin is unconjugated and cannot pass through the kidney and hence cannot appear in the urine.

A well-known example of this variety of icterus is congenital acholuric jaundice (congenital spherocytosis) which is discussed in the chapter on blood disorders. Other examples are the jaundice that accompanies diseases causing haemolysis of blood, such as malaria.

Obstructive (cholestatic) jaundice

Here there is no excessive production of bilirubin but there is an obstruction to the passage of bilirubin from the liver cells and it regurgitates into the bloodstream causing jaundice. The bilirubin is conjugated after its passage through the liver cells and is therefore water soluble and appears in the urine where it can be readily detected by simple tests. On account of the obstruction the bilirubin reaching the intestine is reduced in amount, or in complete obstruction is entirely absent. Consequently the urobilinogen is diminished or absent resulting in pale or even white 'clay coloured' stools.

Obstructive jaundice may be grouped into intrahepatic and extrahepatic disorders.

Intrahepatic cholestasis

Obstruction to the small biliary canaliculi can occur as a result of drug toxicity and in association with some diseases which damage the liver cells with disorganization of its structure. Thus severe intrahepatic cholestasis can occur following ingestion of the drug chlorpromazine and can also occur as part of the disease picture in infective hepatitis.

Extrahepatic cholestasis

Extrahepatic jaundice is due to obstruction to the flow of bile through the extrahepatic bile ducts system. The commonest cause for this is the presence of gallstones within the common bile duct but carcinoma of the common bile duct or head of the pancreas is also frequent. At first the obstruction is incomplete but progresses until no bile reaches the intestine at all and clay-coloured stools result.

Hepatocellular (hepatic) jaundice

A number of diseases directly damage the liver cells so that they are unable to metabolize the bilirubin that is delivered to them. In most of these conditions there is also an element of intrahepatic cholestasis so that the picture is intermediate between that of haemolysis and frank extrahepatic obstruction. Viral hepatitis (which includes hepatitis due to virus A, virus B, and non-A, non-B hepatitis) is the most common cause of jaundice due to hepatocellular damage in western countries. Other important causes include alcohol excess and drug-induced disease such as that occurring after overdosage with paracetamol.

Hepatitis A (infective hepatitis)

Aetiology

It is due to a virus (hepatitis A virus) spread by the faecal–oral route and has an incubation period of 2–6 weeks. Infective hepatitis has its maximal incidence in children and young adults; outbreaks are common in schools, institutions, and in the armed services. The infectivity is greatest for a week before to a week after the onset of jaundice; thereafter there is little danger of those in contact with the patient contracting the infection.

Clinical features

The common sequence of events is that for a few days the patient feels out-of-sorts, depressed, has a very poor appetite, and may vomit a few times. The diagnosis is made evident by the development of jaundice, first apparent in the eyes and later in the skin. The degree of jaundice varies from being very slight (perhaps detectable only by chemical analysis) to being very intense. The urine is darker than normal in colour and contains both bile and urobilinogen. The stools are usually only slightly pale in colour except in severe cases with gross intrahepatic obstruction. The liver is commonly slightly enlarged and tender. A haemorrhagic tendency, due to complex defects, is present in severe cases (see Ch. 12). The diagnosis is confirmed by high blood levels of bilirubin and enzymes (transaminases) released from necrotic hepatocytes, and by demonstration of hepatitis A antigen or antibody.

Course and prognosis

The majority of patients make a complete recovery after an illness lasting for a few weeks. In a small proportion the infection is so virulent that fatal hepatic necrosis is caused. Chronic liver disease does not occur.

Treatment

There is no specific treatment for infective hepatitis. The usual measures employed are rest, a diet low in fat but high in carbohydrate, and complete abstinence from alcohol during the period of jaundice and for several months thereafter.

Hepatitis B virus (serum hepatitis)

As discussed in Chapter 2, this virus is spread by percutaneous inoculation, either from mother to baby, by sexual intercourse, by injury with needles or other instruments, or by transfusion with contaminated blood or blood products. The incubation period is six weeks to six months. The clinical picture is similar to hepatitis A, but hepatitis B antigens and antibodies are detected in the blood; fatal hepatic necrosis is more common; and progression to chronic liver disease and/or hepatoma is common.

Non-A, non-B hepatitis

Non-A, non-B hepatitis is caused by one of several as yet unidentified viruses and is probably spread by direct contact as well as by percutaneous introduction. The incubation period may be as short as 10 days or up to 150 days. Our knowledge of the condition is still fragmentary since no viral markers are detectable in the blood. There are fluctuating increases in serum transaminases and a high risk of chronic liver disease.

Extrahepatic cholestasis

This variety of jaundice is often referred to as 'surgical' jaundice since it is amenable to cure or relief by surgical methods. It is important to realize that in operating for jaundice or (of importance to dentists) in the presence of jaundice, there is a haemorrhagic tendency (see Ch. 12) and prior to surgery injections of vitamin K must be given so that the prothrombin time is restored to normal within the blood.

In this variety of jaundice the pigmentation may be very marked and may assume a greenish hue but it is important to realize that the obstruction may be incomplete as occurs when a gallstone intermittently obstructs the common bile duct. The stools are usually pale as no bile pigment reaches the intestine and the urine contains large amounts of bile (bilirubin) and appears very concentrated and greenish-black in colour. In severe cases there may be bradycardia and pruritus due to the retention of bile salts.

Although clinical evidence of the cause of obstruction is usually present this is not always so and it is always important to think of obstruction as a cause of jaundice. In the case of gallstones there is frequently a typical history of attacks of colicky pain in the right upper abdomen associated with intermittent attacks of jaundice. By contrast in cancer, either of the pancreas or of the common bile duct, the classical picture is of progressive jaundice associated with loss of energy and loss of weight and usually without pain. There may be quite severe back pain in cancer of the pancreas. In extrahepatic

obstruction the diagnosis may be established before operation by radiological methods, e.g. ultrasound scanning which shows dilated bile ducts, and cholangiography which may show obstructing stone or carcinoma (Fig. 10.2). Exploratory operation with intraoperative radiology is only rarely necessary. Stones within the common bile duct are always associated with stones in the gall-bladder and treatment is by cholecystectomy and exploration of the common bile duct with removal of the stones. Occasionally a bypass operation between the common bile duct and the intestine is performed.

In cancer of the pancreas the prognosis is poor: most tumours are inoperable by the time the patient comes to surgery. All that is possible in these situations is to bypass the flow of bile to the intestine and so relieve the jaundice. Radiotherapy and

Fig. 10.2 Endoscopic retrograde cholangiogram showing a gallstone at the lower end of the bile duct (arrowed). The endoscope has been passed through the oesophagus and stomach to lie in the duodenum allowing the passage of a fine catheter into the bile duct from below.

chemotherapy may be employed but no great success has attended either. In the few patients in whom a small operable pancreatic or common bile duct tumour is found an extensive operation removing the entire head of pancreas and loop of the duodenum (pancreatico-duodenectomy) is possible. The risk of the procedure is high and reconstruction of the integrity of the gastrointestinal tract difficult.

There are a variety of rarer conditions which can cause extrahepatic obstruction and amongst these are carcinoma of the ampulla of Vater or duodenum, a number of congenital cysts of the extrahepatic bile duct system, benign stricture of the bile duct and chronic pancreatitis with fibrosis in the head of the pancreas.

Other hepatic disorders

Cirrhosis of the liver

Cirrhosis of the liver may be caused by chronic viral hepatitis (B or non-A, non-B), by autoimmune diseases, or most commonly by overindulgence in alcohol for many years especially if the diet has been neglected. In many cases, however, none of these factors is apparent and the cause is obscure.

The condition is characterized pathologically by a progressive replacement of liver cells by fibrous tissue and nodular regeneration of hepatocytes, causing disturbance of normal liver architecture. The fibrosis leads to deterioration in hepatic function with eventual liver failure and also to interference with the flow of blood through the liver resulting in portal hypertension.

The main clinical features of liver failure are a poor appetite, a tendency to morning dyspepsia, a sallow complexion with a trace of jaundice, ascites (excess fluid in the peritoneal cavity, causing abdominal swelling) and oedema. The liver is enlarged and firm in the early stages but later becomes small in size as the fibrous tissue contracts. Portal hypertension causes splenic enlargement and the development of oesophageal varices with the likelihood of recurrent alimentary haemorrhage. Small dilated blood vessels, descriptively termed spider naevi, may be seen on the face and on the upper part of the trunk. There may also be redness of the palms of the hands (palmar erythema) and finger clubbing. Cirrhosis is confirmed by isotope scanning and if necessary by needle liver biopsy. The course of the disorder is usually steadily progressive.

Surgical measures to reduce the portal hypertension by shunting portal blood to the low-pressure systemic system are sometimes feasible. In many circumstances it is preferable to rely on medical treatment, the main points being adequate nutrition and the avoidance of alcohol, the use of blood transfusion to deal with haematemesis, the control of ascites and oedema by diuretics, beta-adrenergic blocking drugs to reduce portal hypertension, and H_2 blockers to prevent peptic ulcers which are common.

Tumours of the liver

Primary tumour of the liver (hepatoma) is rare in Britain but it is a common malignant neoplasm in Africa and South-East Asia. It is usually caused by chronic hepatitis B infection (see Ch. 2). If the lesion is small, partial resection of the liver can be curative but this is rarely so. The results of palliative therapy are poor and there is usually a rapid progression to death.

On the other hand, secondary tumours involving the liver are a very common development following primary cancer of the stomach, bowel, lung, and breast. Here again the outlook is poor but effective palliative treatment can be afforded by the skilled use of chemotherapy and surgical resection has an occasional use for localized solitary lesions.

Hepatic failure

Acute hepatic necrosis, or acute yellow atrophy, is fortunately uncommon. There is massive death of hepatic cells due to overwhelming infection (severe cases of infective hepatitis or Weil's disease), gross nutritional deficiency, or chemical poisoning (e.g. paracetamol overdose). Hepatic failure also occurs in terminal cirrhosis. Patients develop deep jaundice, bleeding due to low clotting factor levels, and hypoglycaemia. Accumulation of gut bacterial toxins causes encephalopathy with drowsiness and coma. Patients are very sensitive to drugs and anaesthetics. In many cases there is an associated acute renal failure. Treatment involves correction of blood loss, hypoglycaemia and clotting factor defects, maintenance of fluid balance, and reduction of enterotoxins by laxatives and oral antibiotics (neomycin). The prognosis is poor.

Liver transplantation

Transplantation of the liver has been used in some patients for the treatment of liver failure and liver tumours.

DISEASES OF THE GALL-BLADDER

Cholecystitis

Inflammation of the gall-bladder may be acute or chronic. The condition occurs most often in middle-aged people and it is more common in women and more likely to develop in obese individuals. The disease is almost always accompanied by the presence of stones in the gall-bladder and the infecting organism is most frequently *Esch. coli*. The patient may suffer attacks of repeated inflammation which should be distinguished from the attacks of biliary colicky pain that occur in association with the presence of the gallstones.

In the acute stages of the disorder the patient has severe right sided upper abdominal pain which has a tendency to pass through to the right shoulder blade. The temperature is elevated, vomiting is common, there is tenderness over the gall-bladder, and a trace of jaundice is frequently present. In association with this the urine may be rather dark for a short period due to the presence of bile although the stools seldom become pale. In severe cases the acutely inflamed gall-bladder may become filled with pus (empyema of the gall-bladder) and in very severe cases gangrene and perforation of the gall-bladder may occur with consequent peritonitis. Acute cholecystitis usually settles following the use of an antibiotic and restriction to a fluid diet for a few days but the presence of a rising pulse rate, continued fever, and spreading abdominal tenderness are an indication for surgery. After subsidence of the acute attack, a low fat diet with a high carbohydrate content is prescribed but there is a considerable tendency for the infection to recur, with the subsequent development of chronic cholecystitis.

Chronic cholecystitis is characterized by a flatulent dyspepsia plus recurrent bouts of right sided upper abdominal pain due to acute exacerbations. Attacks are often precipitated by the taking of fatty foods. Mild cases may remain largely free from symptoms provided the patient adheres to a low fat diet but, if the attacks are recurring frequently and are severe, removal of the gall-bladder (cholecystectomy) is the treatment of choice. Indeed, provided the patient is otherwise well, many surgeons recommend cholecystectomy for chronic cholecystitis with associated gallstones because recurrence is so frequent and complications can be dangerous.

Gallstones

Gallstones arise because of the precipitation of cholesterol and calcium bilirubinate from the bile. This occurs in association with alterations in the constituents of the bile, with stasis in the gall-bladder with the presence of infection. Gallstones (cholelithiasis) are usually present in association with chronic cholecystitis. The attacks of pain are similar to those experienced by the patient with acute cholecystitis but fever and constitutional illness are not present. If a stone passes into, and becomes lodged within, the common bile duct obstructive jaundice results. This is a dangerous condition characterized by fever, rigor, and jaundice and may be complicated by infection passing into the bloodstream (bacteraemia). However, stones may remain within the common bile duct for many years and be quite symptom-free and revealed only by X-ray study. Very occasionally the gall-bladder may become adherent to the adjacent duodenum and a gallstone erodes into the small bowel. If such a stone is large enough it may obstruct the small bowel.

The treatment of gallstones is cholecystectomy, which should be performed if the general condition of the patient permits. The patient with stones within the common bile duct is seldom well and indeed the condition is sufficiently dangerous to warrant exploration of the common bile duct and removal of the stone. At operation for removal of the gall-bladder it is a good practice to X-ray the common bile duct at operation to ensure that stones within it are not missed.

PANCREATITIS

Inflammation of the pancreas may be acute, recurrent, or chronic. The disease is commonly associated either with the presence of gallstones or in association with a high alcohol intake.

In acute pancreatitis the patient is suddenly stricken with upper abdominal pain and repeated vomiting. There is considerable associated shock with a high pulse rate and low blood pressure and frequently the patient experiences respiratory difficulty and is cyanosed. The serum amylase is grossly elevated. Treatment is by conservative means including the use of intravenous fluids and pethidine for the relief of pain. The bowel is rested by means of nasogastric suction and oral fluids are prescribed. If gallstones are present they are removed and the patient is instructed to abstain from alcohol and to remain on a low fat diet.

In the presence of gallstones, particularly in the common bile duct, attacks may become recurrent and chronic pancreatitis is particularly likely to develop in those patients who consume much alcohol. Patients may develop malabsorption and steatorrhoea (see Ch. 9), which should be treated with oral preparations of pancreatic enzymes, or diabetes mellitus (see Ch. 15), treated with insulin. Chronic pancreatitis is an extremely difficult condition to treat. The patient must abstain from alcohol and any biliary pathology must be treated surgically. Occasionally, surgical removal of a portion of the pancreas (pancreatectomy) is effective. The fibrosis which occurs in the head of the pancreas with compression of the common bile duct and resulting in jaundice has been alluded to earlier.

11

Disorders of the renal system

PHYSIOLOGICAL CONSIDERATIONS

The kidneys, which measure about 12 cm in length, are situated retroperitoneally in the posterior part of the abdomen. Each is covered with a firm capsule. If the kidney is divided longitudinally the appearances are as shown diagrammatically in Figure 11.1. At the hilum, the pelvis of the ureter, the renal artery, and the renal vein are in close proximity. The blood supply is very abundant; the renal artery is short and arises directly from the abdominal aorta.

functional unit of the kidney; each kidney contains approximately one million nephrons. The glomerulus is a tuft of capillaries which invaginates Bowman's capsule, the expanded end of the renal tubule, as shown in Figure 11.2. The tubule comprises the proximal convoluted tubule, the loop of Henle, and the distal convoluted tubule. Collecting tubules carry the urine to the renal pelvis from where it passes to the ureters and the bladder.

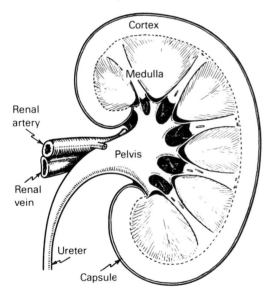

Fig. 11.1 The appearance of the kidney on longitudinal section.

The nephron

The nephron, comprising the glomerular tuft, Bowman's capsule, and the tubule, is the essential

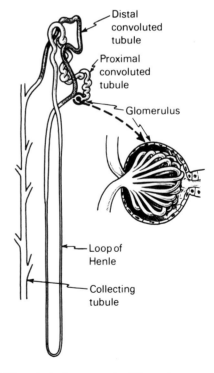

Fig. 11.2 The principal components of the nephron.

Formation of urine

The main steps in the formation of urine are as follows:

1. A large volume of filtrate, similar in composition to plasma except that it is free from protein and fat, is formed from blood flowing through the glomerular capillaries.
2. The filtrate is modified in its passage down the renal tubules in the following ways:
   a. The volume is greatly reduced by the absorption of water.
   b. Other substances which are of value to the body (e.g. glucose, electrolytes) are wholly or partly reabsorbed.
   c. Certain substances are excreted into the filtrate by the tubule cells (e.g. creatinine).
   d. The pH is adjusted according to the need to excrete excess acid or alkali.

Features of normal urine

The average 24-hour urinary volume in the healthy adult is 1500 ml. Normally the night volume is less than the day volume, a fact of considerable convenience.

Urine is a clear, straw-coloured fluid with a specific gravity which may vary from about 1.002–1.030 depending upon the concentration of solutes. It does not normally contain sugar or protein (albumin).

Functions of the kidney

The main functions of the kidneys are the elimination of waste products of metabolism and the control of fluid and electrolyte balance.

1. The kidney is the most important route for the elimination of the waste products of metabolism particularly the end-products of protein metabolism. A useful index of this function is the level of the blood urea (normal, 2.5–7.0 mmol per litre).
2. The kidney plays a vital role in regulating the fluid balance of the body. Thus if there is a high fluid intake the kidney compensates by excreting a large volume of dilute urine, while if there is a danger of dehydration (either from low fluid intake or from excess fluid loss by other channels as in diarrhoea and vomiting) the urinary volume is low.

3. Control of the pH of the blood within very narrow limits is essential for health, and the kidney is one of the main instruments by which this is achieved. If there is a tendency for an increase in the acid radicals in the blood (acidosis), the kidney excretes a more acid urine and, conversely, if there is an increase in the alkali radicals (alkalosis) an alkaline urine is formed. The lungs also play an important part in controlling acid–base balance.

4. Many drugs used therapeutically, or toxic substances taken accidentally or suicidally, are excreted by the kidney either in their original form or as breakdown products.

It is important to realize that the kidneys have a great reserve of function. This is amply illustrated by the fact that an individual can lead a perfectly healthy life should one kidney have to be removed (nephrectomy) because of traumatic damage or unilateral renal disease.

INVESTIGATION OF RENAL DISORDERS

In the investigation of renal disorders the customary practice of taking a full history and performing a full clinical examination is adhered to and is followed by examination of the urine, assessment of renal function, and, in certain cases, by radiological or visual examination of the renal tract or by renal biopsy.

History

The main points about which specific enquiry must be made are past history of sore throats, the presence of oedema, the occurrence of painful micturition (dysuria), or frequency of micturition, and any alterations in the appearance of the urine.

Clinical examination

Attention is directed particularly to the presence of oedema, the blood pressure, the size of the left ventricle, the appearance of the optic fundi, the presence of enlargement or tenderness of the kidneys, the bladder size, and, in males, the size of the prostate gland (this is assessed by digital rectal examination).

Examination of urine

This entails determination of certain physical characteristics (especially volume, specific gravity, colour, reaction), chemical examination for abnormal constituents (especially sugar and protein), microscopic examination (especially for blood and pus) and bacteriological examination. The more common urinary abnormalities are discussed below.

Assessment of renal function

A precise assessment of renal function is a complex matter but sufficient information may be gained in many cases by measuring the ability of the kidney to produce a concentrated urine and by determining the level of urea in the blood (normal, 2.5–7.0 mmol per litre).

After fluid restriction the normal kidney will produce a concentrated urine (specific gravity not less than 1.025) while after a copious fluid intake

the urine will be dilute (specific gravity around 1.004–1.002). In the presence of impaired renal function the specific gravity range becomes progressively less until finally the specific gravity becomes fixed at about 1.010.

Radiology and endoscopy

A straight X-ray of the abdomen may reveal the presence of opaque renal calculi or enlargement of the kidneys. Additional information is gained by radiology, either after the intravenous injection of a radio-opaque dye which is excreted by the kidney (intravenous pyelography, see Fig. 11.3) or after injection of the dye directly into the ureters following ureteric catheterization under direct vision through a cystoscope (retrograde pyelography). Cystoscopy also permits visual examination of the bladder mucosa and the taking of biopsy specimens. Ultrasonic or computerized tomographic (CT) scanning is also useful for non-invasive imaging of the kidneys.

COMMON ABNORMALITIES OF URINE

Polyuria

An increased volume of urine occurs physiologically after a high fluid intake, therapeutically after the administration of a diuretic, and pathologically in diabetes mellitus, diabetes insipidus, and chronic renal failure. When there is polyuria the specific gravity is low; the only exception to this is in diabetes mellitus, where, owing to the sugar present in the urine, the specific gravity is high.

Oliguria and anuria

A decreased volume of urine follows as a natural consequence of a low fluid intake. The more common disease states associated with oliguria are acute nephritis, cardiac failure, and excessive fluid loss from conditions producing diarrhoea and vomiting. Anuria, which is much less common than oliguria, means a complete cessation of urine formation.

Oliguria and anuria must always be differentiated from retention of urine caused by some obstruction to urinary outflow (a common example of this is prostatic gland enlargement).

Fig. 11.3 A normal intravenous pyelogram (IVP) showing kidneys, ureters and bladder.

Proteinuria

This is often referred to as albuminuria, but the term proteinuria is more accurate since globulin is also present. Protein in the urine may be detected by the appearance of a white coagulate on heating acidified urine; the reaction is the same as that which occurs on boiling an egg. A simpler test involving a colour change on a specially treated strip of paper which is dipped into the urine is now in general use.

The causes of proteinuria may be considered in three groups:

1. Due to kidney disease of which the most important are glomerulonephritis and diabetic nephropathy.

2. Associated with a disease process elsewhere, e.g. congestive cardiac failure or any febrile illness.

3. Orthostatic proteinuria which is seen in adolescents and young adults. It is believed that a postural defect (undue lordosis of the lumbar spine) leads to kinking of the veins concerned with venous return from the kidney when the individual is upright and that the consequent passive congestion causes proteinuria. Protein is present in the urine formed when the patient is ambulant but is absent from the urine formed during recumbency; there is no other urinary abnormality. There is no renal lesion and the prognosis is good. No treatment is required.

Haematuria

Copious blood in the urine produces a frankly blood-stained urine, lesser amounts lead to a smoky-brown appearance, while small quantities are detectable only by microscopy or by a test strip.

Haematuria may result from medical or surgical disorders of the renal tract (e.g. acute nephritis, tumour, renal calculus, trauma), from haemorrhagic disorders (e.g. acute leukaemia, purpura, haemophilia) or from subacute bacterial endocarditis.

Glycosuria

Sugar in the urine may be detected by a simple tablet test or the even simpler dip strip test.

The most important cause of glycosuria is diabetes mellitus. It is important to differentiate diabetes mellitus from the harmless condition of renal glycosuria which is due to a low renal threshold for glucose.

GLOMERULONEPHRITIS

The subject of glomerulonephritis is an extremely complex one but, from the dental student's viewpoint, it is sufficient to give a simplified account of the main clinical types of the disorder.

Acute glomerulonephritis

The condition is often akin to rheumatic fever in that it is caused by an immunological reaction to recent infection with haemolytic streptococci. It may also follow viral infections (especially hepatitis B), exposure to allergens (e.g. hair-dyes), or be part of a connective tissue disease (e.g. polyarteritis nodosa or systemic lupus erythematosus, see Ch. 17). The glomeruli of both kidneys show acute cellular proliferation which may be very marked. Immune complexes are deposited in the walls of glomerular capillaries, and may be shown in renal biopsy specimens by immunological techniques.

Clinical features

The condition is seen most commonly in young people. A history of sore throat about 10−14 days beforehand is frequently present. The onset is abrupt usually with headache and vomiting; there may be pain in the loins. There is a slight degree of generalized oedema which is most evident below the eyes in the morning, leading to a puffy appearance of the face (Fig. 11.4). The blood pressure is slightly or moderately elevated. The urine is reduced in amount and contains protein and blood. The blood urea is raised as a result of impaired renal function. Immune complexes may be detected in the blood or renal biopsy samples.

Course

The great majority of patients with acute glomerulonephritis completely recover after an illness lasting a few weeks. A small number die in the acute stage, from renal or cardiac failure, while others develop

Fig. 11.4 Facial oedema in glomerulonephritis.

chronic glomerulonephritis with progressive renal damage.

Treatment

No curative measures are available in most cases, the cause of the disorder being unaffected by the use of antibiotics or immunosuppressives. The intake of fluid, potassium, salt and protein require careful regulation as long as renal function is seriously impaired; dialysis may be needed. Careful follow-up is indicated and any further infections should be treated energetically. Corticosteroids or plasma exchange may be effective in some connective tissue disorders.

Nephrotic syndrome

This may be due to several types of glomerular disease, visible on renal biopsy. In children the most common is *minimal change glomerulonephritis*, which usually responds to treatment with corticosteroids or immunosuppressive drugs. In adults the most common causes are *membranous glomerulonephritis*, diabetes mellitus (see Ch. 15) or systemic lupus erythematosus (see Ch. 17).

Clinical features

The condition has an insidious onset and no history of previous sore throat is obtainable. The most striking clinical feature is oedema (Fig. 11.4). This may be extremely marked and, in addition to involving the limbs and the trunk, may produce ascites and pleural effusions. Pallor is usually prominent and may be out of keeping with the degree of anaemia that is usually present. The blood pressure is usually normal in the early stages of the disorder but may become elevated later.

The urine contains very large quantities of protein (more than 5 g/day) and this leads to a fall in the plasma proteins which results in a diminution in the colloid oncotic pressure of the plasma; this is the main factor in the pathogenesis of the oedema (Fig. 7.5). The blood urea may be normal in the early stages but later it becomes elevated.

Course

The prognosis is rather less favourable than in acute nephritis. Although some patients, especially children, recover spontaneously or on treatment, others may die from intercurrent infection to which these individuals are more prone, while others develop progressive renal failure and hypertension.

Treatment

It is customary to give a high protein diet in an attempt to replace the protein lost in the urine. The salt intake is restricted. The oedema can often be controlled by the use of a diuretic (a drug which acts on the renal tubules to increase the volume of urine). Corticosteroids or immunosuppressive drugs may be effective, especially in children.

Chronic glomerulonephritis

Chronic glomerulonephritis may follow a small proportion of cases of acute nephritis or it may develop in patients with the nephrotic syndrome who do not die from intercurrent infection. In some instances there is no definite history of previous renal disease. A similar clinical picture results from chronic pyelonephritis.

The kidneys are smaller than normal, scarred, and granular. Microscopic examination of a renal biopsy specimen reveals that many of the nephrons are replaced by fibrous tissue.

Clinical features

These are due to a combination of impaired renal function and hypertension. In the early stages of the disorder the kidney compensates for its inability to produce a concentrated urine by forming large quantities of more dilute urine and, in this way, the waste products of protein metabolism may be excreted. At this stage the main symptoms are polyuria and nocturia. The urine specific gravity is around 1.010 and there is little alteration from this figure following fluid restriction or increase. The urine contains protein, often in small amount, and a variable number of red cells and casts.

As the disease progresses, more and more nephrons go out of action and the kidney loses its ability to form a large volume of urine. When this occurs there is an inevitable retention in the body of the nitrogenous end-products of protein metabolism associated with electrolyte imbalance and acidosis. Anaemia develops and may be severe. The features of this stage of chronic glomerulonephritis are essentially those of uraemia which is described in the following section.

The blood pressure elevation leads to arteriosclerotic changes in the blood vessels and to left ventricular hypertrophy; breathlessness and headache are the most common symptoms. Cardiac failure may ensue. Changes in the optic fundi (narrowing of arteries, exudates, haemorrhages) are due to the hypertension.

Death may occur from uraemia, from cardiac failure, or from a cerebrovascular catastrophe.

Treatment

The hypertension is controlled with drugs and the diet is modified particularly in respect of the protein content which requires to be progressively reduced as the renal failure progresses.

A new lease of life can now be afforded to many patients with 'end-stage' chronic glomerulonephritis by regular dialysis therapy or by renal transplantation. The dentist should also be aware that some patients on regular dialysis may be receiving anticoagulants and also that renal transplant patients will be receiving steroid therapy to minimize the possibility of rejection of the graft.

URINARY INFECTION AND PYELONEPHRITIS (NON-TUBERCULOUS)

Infection of the lower urinary passages (cystitis) is a very common condition. In some cases the infection also involves the upper renal tract, causing pyelonephritis, and this is a much more serious disorder since it may lead to renal failure and to hypertension.

Aetiology

The majority of cases are due to Gram-negative organisms, especially *Esch. coli*. The organisms may reach the kidney via the bloodstream or from the lower urinary passages especially in females since the urethra is short and its orifice close to the anus.

Important predisposing factors, which interfere with urinary flow, are pregnancy, prostatic gland enlargement, renal stone, diabetes mellitus, hydronephrosis, congenital abnormalities, and disease of the nervous system (e.g. disseminated sclerosis). A further factor is catheterization; unless this is done with meticulous care, infection is likely to follow. Many cases of urinary infection, however, occur without any apparent predisposing factor.

Clinical features

The patient with acute urinary infection usually has frequency of micturition, pain on micturition (dysuria), and sometimes haematuria. If the infection is severe, the temperature will be elevated. Suprapubic discomfort is present if the bladder is inflamed (cystitis) and loin pain is present if there is acute pyelonephritis.

Many patients with chronic urinary infection affecting the lower urinary passages or with chronic pyelonephritis have relatively little or even no urinary symptoms. In these cases the condition may be detected on some routine examination of the urine, because the patient has an unexplained febrile illness or vague ill health, or, in the case of chronic pyelonephritis, because of the presence of renal failure or hypertension.

Diagnosis

The diagnosis is made in most cases by the

demonstration of bacteria and pus in the urine. In acute cases there may be some confusion with abdominal emergencies such as appendicitis. In chronic pyelonephritis characteristic structural changes occur in the pelvis and these may be detected by radiology.

Treatment

Acute infections usually respond promptly to treatment with an antibiotic to which the organism is sensitive, but recurrences are common. The infection tends to be more difficult to eradicate in cases of chronic infection and repeated courses of treatment may be required. In all cases it is important to consider and correct any underlying predisposing factor. If chronic pyelonephritis progresses to the stage of producing terminal renal failure, regular dialysis or transplantation may be undertaken as in chronic glomerulonephritis.

URAEMIA (RENAL FAILURE)

Uraemia, which literally means urine in the blood, is the term used to describe 'the metabolic disaster consequent upon renal failure'.

Aetiology

The causal factor may be primarily prerenal, renal, or postrenal; illustrative examples are given below.

Prerenal — severe hypotension leading to a fall in the filtration pressure in the glomerular capillaries (e.g. shock, heart failure).

Renal — acute or chronic glomerulonephritis or chronic pyelonephritis, diabetes mellitus, or long-term abuse of analgesic drugs.

Postrenal—chronic obstruction to urinary outflow by an enlarged prostate or stones.

Clinical features

Chronic renal failure leads to a characteristic clinical picture; the symptoms and signs are due to complex biochemical derangements, the chief being retention of nitrogenous end-products (e.g. urea, creatinine), accumulation of potassium, and acidosis. A chronic normocytic anaemia develops due to lack of erythropoietin.

Restlessness, apathy, mental confusion, and drowsiness are common *nervous* manifestations. Anorexia, nausea, and vomiting are common *alimentary* symptoms. The tongue is characteristically dry and covered with a dirty brown fur while the breath is foul and may smell of ammonia. Stomatitis may be present and the gums may bleed. There is a characteristic alteration in the *respiration*; the breathing is deeper and louder than normal (Kussmaul's respiration) due to stimulation of the respiratory centre by the retained acid products. Hiccough is a common and distressing symptom. Examination of the *cardiovascular* system usually reveals hypertension if the uraemia is of renal origin; pericarditis may occur terminally. Bleeding is common, especially from the gut, due to decreased platelet function (see Ch. 12).

Treatment

In cases of prerenal and postrenal uraemia there is good prospect of recovery if the patient can, by skilled correction of the biochemical derangements and dialysis in a renal unit, be tided over the renal failure until such time as there is a return of renal function or until a procedure such as prostatectomy may be performed. In end-stage renal uraemia the outlook has been transformed by the introduction of regular dialysis and transplantation.

When the serum urea rises to 30 mmol/l, dietary protein may be restricted to 40 g/day to decrease the protein load; the calorie intake is increased. The anaemia may respond to infusions of erythropoietin.

In chronic haemodialysis, an arteriovenous fistula is created surgically in the patient's arm, which can be connected by a large needle to an artificial kidney for two or three five-hour periods every week, either in hospital or at home. The patient is anticoagulated with heparin, and blood is pumped past a semipermeable membrane which separates it from sterile fluids into which the uraemic toxins diffuse down a concentration gradient. In chronic ambulatory peritoneal dialysis (CAPD), a sterile plastic catheter is inserted into the peritoneal cavity; the patient repeatedly connects bags of sterile fluid into which the uraemic toxins again diffuse across the peritoneal membrane. Chronic dialysis allows a relatively normal diet and reasonable health while a suitable transplant donor is found. However patients commonly have metabolic bone disease (see Ch. 17) and peripheral neuropathy (see Ch. 18).

The supply of kidneys for renal transplantation is sadly limited, since the usual source is 'brain-dead' persons after head injury or cerebral haemorrhage, who are mechanically ventilated. Many persons now carry consent cards for kidney donation in this event, and health care workers (including dentists) can play a valuable role in public education on the need for kidney (and other) transplants. After confirmation of brain death, the kidneys are removed prior to switching off the ventilator. This ensures a short time of 'warm ischaemia' which causes kidney cell damage. The kidneys are flushed and kept cool while matching for the most suitable recipient nationwide is performed. The kidney is usually implanted in an iliac fossa. To prevent rejection of the transplant, patients are given long-term corticosteroids and immunosuppressive drugs, which predispose to opportunistic infections.

When dealing with patients with chronic renal failure, dentists should be aware of several points:

1. There is a bleeding tendency and liaison is required to prevent bleeding after dental extractions (e.g. these should be performed after recent dialysis, but after the heparin effect has ended).

2. Immunosuppressive drugs in transplant recipients may cause opportunistic infections, which may be oral.

3. There was an increased risk of carriage of hepatitis B (see Ch. 2) in the past, although this is now uncommon.

4. There is increased susceptibility to drug toxicity due to diminished renal excretion, e.g. antibiotics.

OTHER RENAL DISORDERS

There are many other renal disorders and some of these are common and predominantly of surgical interest.

Hydronephrosis

The renal pelvis is dilated, often to a very considerable size. The condition follows chronic obstruction to the urinary outflow, e.g. by calculus, or by external pressure on the ureter or by an aberrant renal artery. In conditions of chronic obstruction to the outflow of urine from the bladder, back pressure may result in bilateral hydronephrosis. Infection is likely to supervene and the dilated pelvis becomes filled with pus (pyonephrosis).

If there is sufficient functioning renal substance remaining then an attempt to remove the obstructive lesion is worthwhile; the saccular dilated renal pelvis may be reconstructed by means of a plastic surgical operation. If there is very little renal substance remaining then the dilated sac, which is often filled with pus, should be removed by nephrectomy.

Renal calculus

Renal stones may be composed of phosphates, calcium oxalate, uric acid or urates, or rarely cystine. The phosphate variety is seen particularly as a complication of urinary infection, whereas the cystine variety is due to an uncommon metabolic error. The aetiology of other varieties is uncertain. The term *decubitus stone* is used for the calcium stone that forms in the kidneys of patients confined to bed for long periods particularly with skeletal disorders; there is decalcification of the skeleton and increased urinary excretion of calcium. Calcium stones are common in hyperparathyroidism (see Ch. 13).

Renal stones may cause a dull loin pain but, if the stone becomes lodged in the ureter, extremely severe pain associated with vomiting and collapse results (renal colic). There may be haematuria. Such stones are usually passed into the bladder and if small enough are voided in the urine; the patient is managed with analgesia until this occurs. However, it is important to make certain that the stone has been passed from the body since continued presence of the stone within the ureter is associated with subsidence of the pain and may be followed by the development of hydronephrosis. Stones that become impacted in the ureter must be removed (ureterolithotomy). Large stones within the renal pelvis can also be surgically removed. The pain caused by stones within the kidney or ureter must be distinguished from other causes of abdominal pain (e.g. gallstones).

Pyelonephritis is an important complication of renal stones, and surgical removal of the stones can be of great help in avoiding this problem.

Tumour

The most common symptom of a tumour in the renal tract is haematuria which is often painless, and in all such cases the renal tract must be thoroughly investigated. This includes the performance of intravenous pyelography and cystoscopy. Urinary tract tumours can present with other features such as hydronephrosis due to blockage of a ureter or by the presence of a secondary tumour.

The most important tumours of the renal tract are adenocarcinoma (hypernephroma) of the kidney which is particularly liable to cause secondary deposits in the bones and lungs, papillary adenocarcinoma of the renal pelvis, and papilloma or carcinoma of the bladder. These latter tumours are not nearly so likely to metastasize.

Hypernephroma is managed by surgical excision and even solitary secondary deposits may be excised with success in some cases. Tumours of the renal pelvis are usually also managed by a nephrectomy but papilloma of the bladder can be treated for long periods by endoscopic (transcystoscopic) fulguration. They are also sensitive to radiotherapy, and large tumours that have failed to respond to these means can be treated by cystectomy. In this instance the flow of urine must be diverted to a loop of bowel.

In men carcinoma of the prostate commonly presents with symptoms similar to those caused by simple hypertrophy of the prostate. Important differentiating features are hardness of the gland and biochemical (high serum acid phosphatase) and radiological evidence of metastases. Obstruction to flow of urine by a prostatic carcinoma can be managed by transurethral resection of tumour at the neck of the bladder. The tumour is hormone-dependent in many cases (see Ch. 6) and oestrogens (stilboestrol) can be used to manage the advanced disease and particularly to alleviate pain in bony metastases.

Prostatic hypertrophy

Enlargement of the prostate gland is very frequent in elderly men. There is progressive interference with urinary flow and, if not treated, renal damage results from back pressure and the development of bilateral hydronephrosis.

The treatment is surgical and the prostate may be removed either by open operation (transvesical or retropubic prostatecomy) or by the use of a diathermy cutting knife introduced with a special instrument through the urethra (transurethral resection).

Polycystic disease

Polycystic disease of the kidneys is a genetic disorder, one of the more common congenital abnormalities to affect the renal system. The kidneys are enlarged due to the presence of many cysts which, as they increase in size, cause progressive damage to the renal tissues. Renal failure and hypertension are common developments.

Renal artery stenosis

Very occasionally stenosis of the renal artery is associated with the development of hypertension. It is important to recognize this form of hypertension since it may be treated by surgical correction of the stenosed vessels.

Rupture of the kidney

The kidney is quite frequently damaged as a result of trauma. This may occur as a result of a direct blow (nonpenetrating injury) or from a penetrating wound such as that caused by a knife or bullet.

Non-penetrating injury is managed in the first instance by conservative means and cessation of bleeding usually occurs. If not then operation is necessary. Penetrating wounds frequently require operation and the kidney is often not the only organ damaged.

12

Disorders of the haemopoietic system

PHYSIOLOGICAL CONSIDERATIONS

The average healthy adult has a blood volume of approximately five and a half litres. If a sample of blood, to which an anticoagulant such as heparin has been added, is centrifuged or is allowed to stand in a tube, the cellular elements separate from the fluid plasma as depicted in Figure 12.1. The plasma contains the proteins albumin, globulin, and fibrinogen; fat, particularly as cholesterol; various electrolytes of which the most important are sodium, potassium, chloride, and bicarbonate; and minerals such as calcium and phosphate. The formed elements of the

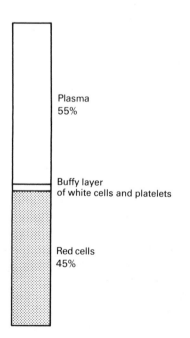

Fig. 12.1 The relationship between the formed elements of the blood and the plasma.

blood are the red cells, the white cells, and the platelets. The main steps in the formation of the red cells, white cells, and platelets are shown diagrammatically in Figure 12.2.

Red cells

The red blood cells, or erythrocytes, are non-nucleated biconcave discs with a transverse diameter of about 7 μ; they number approximately 4.5–5 $\times$ 10^{12}/l. They contain haemoglobin (composed of the iron-containing pigment haem and the protein globin) which has the ability to form a loose combination with oxygen and carbon dioxide. The red cells are thus enabled to transport oxygen as oxyhaemoglobin from the lungs to the tissues where oxygen is released, and to remove carbon dioxide from the tissues to the lungs where it is excreted. The average normal haemoglobin content is 14.8 g/dl.

Red cells are formed in the bone marrow from nucleated precursors called normoblasts. As the normoblast matures its cytoplasm becomes haemoglobinated and the nucleus becomes progressively smaller until it is extruded. For a period the very young red cell has a delicate structure of reticulum in the cytoplasm which may be demonstrated by a special staining technique; these young red cells, which are termed reticulocytes, are seen in the peripheral blood in cases of haemorrhage, haemolytic anaemia, and where an anaemia is actively responding to treatment, e.g. in pernicious anaemia following vitamin B$_{12}$ therapy. The average lifespan of a red cell is about 100 days and then the cells are broken down by the reticuloendothelial system, particularly in the spleen. The iron contained in the haemoglobin is conserved and used

The plasma labels in figure: Plasma 55%, Buffy layer of white cells and platelets, Red cells 45%.

PRECURSOR

ADULT FORM

Normoblast

Reticulocyte Erythrocyte

Neutrophil myelocyte

Neutrophil

Myeloblast

Basophil myelocyte

Basophil

Eosinophil

Eosinophil myelocyte

Lymphoblast

Lymphocytes

Monoblast

Monocyte

Megakaryocyte

Platelets

Fig. 12.2 The principal steps in the development of the red cells, white cells, and platelets.

for further haemoglobin formation; the non-iron containing residue goes to form the bile pigment bilirubin (see also Ch. 10).

The main substances known to be required for the formation of the red cells (erythropoiesis) are protein, iron, vitamin B_{12}, and folic acid. Vitamin C is also concerned with erythropoiesis but its precise role is less well understood.

White cells

The white blood cells, or leucocytes, number $4-11 \times 10^9/l$. In contrast to the red cells they all possess a nucleus. The granular white cells, or polymorphonuclears, have granules in the cytoplasm and a lobed nucleus; depending on the staining reaction of the granules they are classified as neutrophil, eosinophil, or basophil polymorphs. Lymphocytes have a round nucleus and a clear blue cytoplasm. Monocytes have a kidney-shaped nucleus and a foamy blue cytoplasm. In health, a differential white cell count reveals that about 70% of the white cells belong to the granular series, about 25% are lymphocytes, while the remaining 5% are monocytes.

The main function of the white cells is in dealing with infection and they usually increase in number (leucocytosis) in such circumstances. The polymorphonuclears are mainly increased in bacterial infections and the lymphocytes in viral infections. The polymorphs also deal with phagocytosis of necrotic or foreign material and also increase after injury or organ infarction (e.g. myocardial). The lymphocytes play an important part in antibody formation. The eosinophil polymorphonuclears are increased in certain allergic disorders such as hay fever, asthma, and urticaria (see Ch. 16), and in worm infestation.

The granular white cells are formed in the bone marrow and the lymphocytes in lymphoid tissue, particularly in the lymph nodes. The monocytes are also formed in the reticuloendothelial system but the exact details are uncertain. The primitive white cells are termed myeloblasts, lymphoblasts, and monoblasts respectively; the myelocyte is an intermediate stage in the development of the adult polymorphonuclear from the myeloblast. Primitive white cells do not occur in the peripheral blood in health and their presence is always suggestive of leukaemia. The white cells have a much shorter life than the red cells and the majority do not survive beyond a few days (the exception is lymphocytes which are long-lived and transfer between blood and tissues).

Platelets

The blood platelets, or thrombocytes, number $150-400 \times 10^9/l$. They are smaller than the red or white cells and have a varied shape. Platelets play an extremely important role in haemostasis. They are formed in the bone marrow from the cytoplasm of megakaryocytes.

INVESTIGATION OF BLOOD DISORDERS

History

Many of the symptoms associated with anaemia are common to all varieties of the condition; they result from an inadequate supply of oxygen to the tissues consequent upon the low haemoglobin level and they disappear when the anaemia is corrected. In general, the more rapid the onset of the anaemia, the more severe the symptoms. The most common symptoms are tiredness and breathlessness. Myocardial hypoxia may also produce palpitation, angina, and heart failure. Giddiness and mental confusion result from cerebral hypoxia.

After the history of the patient's immediate symptoms is elicited, enquiry is made regarding possible aetiological factors such as dietary deficiency (especially meat and vegetables), blood loss from the alimentary tract (haemorrhoids, peptic ulcer, oesophagitis, and carcinoma of stomach or colon), menstrual disturbances, obstetric history, drugs which might cause bone marrow damage (e.g. chloramphenicol), or alimentary blood loss (e.g. aspirin, anticoagulants). The family history is important in cases of haemolytic anaemia and haemorrhagic disorders. The ethnic background is important in haemolytic anaemia.

Clinical examination

Several clinical features of blood disorders are readily detected on general examination.

1. *Pallor* of the skin and mucous membranes is usually present in cases of anaemia but it is, at best, only a rough guide to the haemoglobin level; the colour of the conjunctivae is less misleading than the colour of the lips.

2. *Koilonychia*, a spoon-shaped depression of the fingernails, is diagnostic of iron deficiency anaemia (Fig. 12.3).

3. *Glossitis* is present in about 50% of cases of iron-deficiency anaemia and pernicious anaemia but it may occur also in certain vitamin B deficiency states (see Ch. 15) in the absence of anaemia.

4. *Jaundice*, which is most readily detected in the sclera, is seen in cases of haemolytic anaemia; slight traces of jaundice producing a lemon tint to the skin may be present in severe cases of pernicious anaemia.

5. *Petechial haemorrhages* are seen in platelet or vascular bleeding disorders, and extensive bruises in coagulation disorders.

6. *Lymph gland enlargement*, e.g. in the cervical region, should if local causes are excluded suggest

Fig. 12.3 Koilonychia.

the possibility of leukaemia, lymphoma, or infectious mononucleosis.

When the abdomen is examined, particular attention is paid to enlargement of the spleen or liver.

Laboratory investigations

Determination of haemoglobin level, red cell count, haematocrit or packed cell volume (HCT or PCV), mean cell volume (MCV), mean cell haemoglobin (MCH), mean cell haemoglobin concentration (MCHC), white cell count, and scrutiny of a stained blood film form the basis for the initial laboratory investigation. Apart from the blood film all of these measurements are now readily available from a single blood sample using a modern electronic counter. Further investigations which may be required include platelet count, differential white cell count, bone marrow examination, red cell fragility, and tests of blood coagulation and platelet function.

The *erythrocyte sedimentation rate* (ESR) may conveniently be described at this point although its application is greater in disorders other than those of the haemopoietic system. In the Westergren method a citrate anticoagulant solution is added to venous blood in a fixed proportion and the blood is drawn up into a long graduated tube which is allowed to stand vertically. The red cells sediment, leaving a top layer of clear plasma, at a relatively constant rate in normal individuals (not more than 20 mm/hour in young adults or 50 mm/hour in older adults). The principal factors that increase the

ESR are alterations in plasma proteins (increased globulins and decreased albumin) which occur in infections, other inflammatory processes such as rheumatic fever and rheumatoid arthritis, malignant growths, and other causes of tissue destruction such as fractures and surgical operations. The ESR also varies with the haematocrit, and is therefore not always reliable as an index of organic disease. Plasma viscosity and C-reactive protein are more reliable alternative tests, which are used increasingly. The ESR is useful as a screening test for organic illness and in assessing the activity of a disease process and its response to treatment (e.g. tuberculosis, rheumatoid arthritis).

ANAEMIA

Anaemia, which is a common disorder, is present when there is a reduction in the level of haemoglobin; in most instances this is associated with a fall in the number of the red blood cells. Anaemia is present when the haemoglobin concentration is less than 13 g/dl in men, 11.5 g/dl in women or children, or 10.5 g/dl in pregnant women.

Classification and causes

One classification is an aetiological one. In brief, anaemia may result from inadequate production of blood, from excess breakdown of blood, or from abnormal blood loss. The majority of cases of anaemia are due to iron deficiency, blood loss, or vitamin B_{12} or folate deficiency. Another classification is by cell size (MCV) into microcytic, normocytic, or macrocytic.

Disturbed production (dyshaemopoietic anaemia)

1. Deficiency of iron, resulting in inadequate haemoglobin formation, causes hypochromic microcytic anaemia.

2. Deficiency of vitamin B_{12} causes megaloblastic anaemia of which the main variety is pernicious anaemia. Megaloblastic anaemia may also be due to deficiency of folic acid, e.g. in pregnancy. These anaemias are macrocytic.

3. Aplasia or hypoplasia of the bone marrow which may be primary or secondary to certain drugs and industrial poisons or irradiation.

4. Anaemias of chronic disease. Disturbed production of blood is an important sequel of severe infections, especially if they are chronic, of malignant disease, and of certain metabolic derangements (e.g. uraemia, hypothyroidism).

5. Replacement of bone marrow by malignant disease, e.g. leukaemias, lymphomas, secondary carcinomas.

Excess breakdown (haemolytic anaemia)

1. Congenital acholuric jaundice (spherocytosis) which is due to increased fragility of the red cells.

2. Acquired haemolytic anaemia associated with certain infections (e.g. malaria), neoplasm, abnormal antibody formation, or drugs.

3. Haemolytic anaemia due to the inherited disorders of haemoglobin synthesis, haemoglobinopathies and thalassaemias.

Blood loss (posthaemorrhagic anaemia)

1. Acute blood loss due to trauma, bleeding peptic ulcer or obstetric complications (see Ch. 5).

2. Chronic blood loss, which may be occult, from the alimentary tract or, in women, from the uterus. This causes iron deficiency.

Iron deficiency anaemia

Iron is an essential constituent of haemoglobin and when the iron content of the diet is insufficient to meet the demands of new blood formation, hypochromic microcytic anaemia results; this is still the most common form of anaemia in Britain. It is most likely to occur where economic circumstances are poor because the iron-containing foods (meat, fish, vegetables) are the more expensive; in some cases ignorance of a proper diet is the causal factor. Hypochromic anaemia is much more common in women because their iron requirements are greater due to the demands of menstruation, pregnancy, and lactation; in many cases hypochromic anaemia becomes evident during or after pregnancy. In some instances malabsorption is a cause, e.g. after gastrectomy.

When hypochromic anaemia occurs in men, or in postmenopausal women, serious consideration must be given to the possibility of an underlying source of chronic blood loss in the alimentary tract (haemorrhoids, peptic ulcer, carcinoma of stomach or colon); in some, e.g. elderly widowers, it results from dietary deficiency.

Clinical features

Any or all of the symptoms of anaemia may be present. Pallor of the skin and mucous membranes is usually evident but the unreliability of pallor as a guide to anaemia has been stressed. Koilonychia (see Fig. 12.3) should always be looked for as its presence is a sure indication of iron deficiency. Glossitis occurs in about 50% of cases and in a small number is associated with dysphagia due to degenerative changes in the mucosa of the upper alimentary tract. The syndrome of hypochromic anaemia, glossitis and dysphagia, is termed the Plummer–Vinson or Kelly–Paterson syndrome or sideropenic dysphagia (see Ch. 9).

Investigations. The haemoglobin and the red cell count are both reduced, the MCV is low, and the MCHC is low. Blood film examination confirms that the red cells are smaller than normal (microcytosis) and stain poorly (hypochromia) due to their low haemoglobin content. The serum iron is low and the iron-binding capacity raised.

Treatment

The majority of cases respond satisfactorily to the

administration of an iron salt by mouth. A readily obtained, effective, and very cheap preparation is ferrous sulphate given in a dosage of one tablet (200 mg) three times daily. It should be taken after meals to minimize possible alimentary side-effects and the patient should be warned that the faeces will become black due to the fact that not all of the iron is absorbed. If a fluid preparation of iron (e.g. iron and ammonium citrate) is used it may be taken through a straw to prevent blackening of the teeth. Iron is also available for intramuscular injection in patients who are intolerant of, or refractory to, oral iron therapy; it is also useful where a rapid response is desired. It is common practice to administer iron tablets during pregnancy and lactation because of the increased requirements; folic acid is also given (see below).

In all instances consideration must be given to correction of any aetiological factors, e.g. haemorrhoids, or ignorance regarding the composition of a normal diet. Where the main factor is financial hardship it will probably be necessary to supplement the diet with periodic administration of iron tablets.

In severe cases of the Plummer–Vinson syndrome the oesophagus may have to be dilated by bougies.

Megaloblastic anaemia

Certain anaemias are characterized by an alteration in the red cell precursors in the bone marrow termed megaloblastic erythropoiesis. Our understanding of this group of anaemias was helped greatly by the work of Castle and his associates who put forward the hypothesis that the normal maturation of red cell precursors in the bone marrow required the presence of an anti-anaemic factor (formed by the interaction of an extrinsic factor, derived from the food, and an intrinsic factor secreted by the cells of the gastric mucosa) which was absorbed from the gut and stored in the liver until required by the bone marrow.

It is now known that vitamin B_{12} (cobalamin) is the so-called extrinsic factor, and that the role of the intrinsic or gastric factor is to promote the absorption of vitamin B_{12} from the alimentary tract. Vitamin B_{12} is present in protein foodstuffs and is formed by bacterial activity in the gut. The proper maturation of red cell precursors is also dependent upon the presence of folic acid, which is also a food constituent.

Pernicious anaemia

Pernicious anaemia is the most important variety of megaloblastic anaemia in Britain. It is due to a defect in gastric function (intrinsic factor deficiency) whereby vitamin B_{12} cannot be absorbed from the alimentary tract. The gastric defect may be the result of an autoimmune mechanism.

Clinical features

The disorder is seen particularly in middle age and in the later years of life. A family history is present in some instances. The onset is insidious and symptoms are often present for several months before medical advice is sought. Any of the symptoms of anaemia may be present; the most common are tiredness and breathlessness. In about half the cases there is soreness of the tongue due to glossitis. This may be limited to smoothness, due to papillary atrophy affecting perhaps only the sides of the tongue. In a smaller proportion of cases the tongue has a raw 'beefy' appearance. A sensation of pins and needles, or tingling, may be experienced in the hands and feet due to peripheral neuropathy. In severe cases the pallor has a yellowish or lemon tinge.

Investigations. The red cell level is low, often markedly so; the haemoglobin level is not reduced to quite the same degree. The MCV is increased. Blood film examination confirms that the red cells are larger than normal (macrocytosis), and they tend to be oval or pear-shaped (poikilocytosis) and are well filled with haemoglobin. The white cell count, platelet count, and serum B_{12} levels are reduced.

Bone marrow examination reveals that the red cell precursors are strikingly different from normal; the cells, which are termed megaloblasts, are larger and have a characteristic nuclear structure and other distinctive cytological features.

Examination of the gastric juice, obtained through a narrow tube known as a Ryle's tube, invariably shows that there is no hydrochloric acid present even after the cells of the gastric mucosa have been stimulated by an injection of histamine. This histamine-fast achlorhydria, unlike the bone marrow findings, persists after the anaemia has been treated. Decreased absorption of vitamin B_{12} can be demonstrated by the Schilling test.

Complications

Slight degrees of peripheral neuropathy are common in pernicious anaemia. A much more serious lesion of the nervous system, subacute combined degeneration of the spinal cord, may occur in cases of pernicious anaemia where treatment is inadequate or irregular, and is likely to produce permanent disability. There is muscle weakness due to involvement of the motor pathway or pyramidal tract, and sensory disturbance, particularly of posture, due to involvement of the posterior columns.

Treatment

This disease was formerly invariably fatal and therefore deserved the name 'pernicious'. Now, however, if properly treated the patient can be restored to health and afforded a normal expectation of life. The first effective step in the treatment of pernicious anaemia was the demonstration in 1926 of

the value of large quantities of raw or lightly cooked liver. At first these patients had to eat $\frac{1}{2}-1$ lb liver per day but soon oral liver extracts were available and these were followed by liver extracts suitable for intramuscular injection. The current treatment is to give frequent intramuscular injections of vitamin B_{12} (Fig. 12.4) until the blood levels have risen to normal and then to maintain normal blood levels with an injection every two months for the rest of the patient's life.

Other megaloblastic anaemias

The next most common form of megaloblastic anaemia in Britain occurs in the later stages of pregnancy. It is due to the combined effects of increased demands for folic acid and dietary deficiency. The therapeutic response to oral folic acid is excellent. Prophylactic folate and iron supplements are given during pregnancy.

Other varieties of megaloblastic anaemia include those due to severe nutritional deficiency of protein, resection of the stomach, and impaired absorption, e.g. folate deficiency in coeliac disease, B_{12} deficiency in Crohn's disease of the terminal ileum where B_{12} is absorbed. Folate deficiency may be due to anticonvulsant therapy (phenytoin).

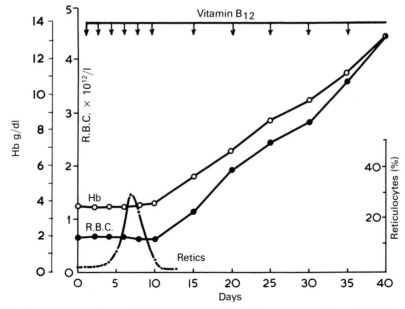

Fig. 12.4 Haematological response to vitamin B_{12} therapy in a case of pernicious anaemia. Note the initial reticulocytosis and the subsequent rise in haemoglobin and red cell levels.

Hypoplastic and aplastic anaemia

In this variety of anaemia the bone marrow becomes progressively less cellular and fails to produce an adequate number of red cells. The myeloid tissue and the megakaryocytes of the marrow are usually also involved so that low white cell and platelet levels are commonly associated (pancytopenia).

Aetiology

Some cases are secondary to bone marrow damage resulting from certain drugs and industrial poisons (e.g. cytotoxic drugs, chloramphenicol, phenylbutazone, benzene derivatives), from exposure to X-rays and to radioactive substances. In other cases, termed idiopathic or primary, no cause for the bone marrow depression can be detected.

Clinical features

The clinical features result from a combination of anaemia, leucopenia, and thrombocytopenia. The main symptoms resulting from anaemia are tiredness and breathlessness; leucopenia causes an increased liability to infection, while thrombocytopenia leads to bruising, bleeding from the gums, and purpura. The anaemia is normocytic and the bone marrow shows hypoplasia or aplasia of blood cell precursors.

Treatment

Careful enquiry must be made regarding any possible aetiological factor and, if still operative, this should be removed. Repeated blood and platelet transfusions are necessary to sustain life, and antibiotics may be required to control infection. With these measures life may be maintained for considerable periods even in the presence of irreversible bone marrow damage. In other cases a measure of bone marrow function returns. Steroid drugs occasionally are of benefit. Bone marrow transplantation may now be performed (see below).

Congenital acholuric jaundice (spherocytosis)

Congenital acholuric jaundice is the most important form of haemolytic anaemia in Britain. The basic abnormality is in the red cells which are spherocytic in shape and, in consequence, unduly fragile so that they are much more readily destroyed by the spleen. There is a compensatory hyperplasia of the bone marrow in its attempt to deal with the increased demands for new cells to replace those destroyed.

Clinical features

A family history of the disorder is readily obtained in most cases. The three main clinical features are anaemia, jaundice, and enlargement of the spleen.

The anaemia is variable in degree; for long periods the level of haemolysis appears to be more or less balanced by new red cell formation, but from time to time for reasons that are poorly understood, haemolytic crises occur during which the blood levels fall dramatically.

The degree of jaundice is closely related to the severity of the haemolytic process; between crises it is usually relatively slight. The condition is termed acholuric jaundice (i.e. without bile) because although the urine contains an excess of urobilinogen, which is derived from bilirubin, it does not contain bilirubin (Fig. 10.1).

Splenic enlargement is usually of moderate degree and readily detectable. The anaemia is normocytic and the reticulocyte count is increased.

Treatment

During haemolytic crises, blood transfusion is required. Once the crisis has settled, splenectomy should be performed. Although this does not alter the red cell abnormality it usually enables the individual to live a more or less normal life as the excessive haemolysis ceases.

Autoimmune haemolytic anaemias

These are due to antibodies in plasma or on the red cell surface, which destroy red cells. Causes include drugs, infections, and neoplasms, e.g. lymphomas, chronic lymphatic leukaemia. Treatment is with corticosteroids, and sometimes splenectomy.

POLYCYTHAEMIA

In polycythaemia there is an increased red blood

cell count, haematocrit, and level of haemoglobin. In the true (absolute) polycythaemias this reflects an increased red cell mass, confirmed by measurement of an injected radioisotope which labels red cells. The condition may either be primary or secondary.

Primary polycythaemia or polycythaemia vera

The aetiology is unknown. The red cell count and the haemoglobin level become very high (e.g. RBC $8–10 \times 10^{12}/l$, Hb 18–20 g/dl) and in consequence the skin and mucous membranes are redder than normal and the conjunctivae are suffused. There is often cyanosis present as the increased viscosity of the blood leads to slowing of the circulation permitting increased reduction of oxyhaemoglobin. The sluggish circulation also predisposes to venous and arterial thrombosis. The spleen is commonly enlarged. The white cell count and platelet count are often elevated and in some cases leukaemia develops. Bleeding is common due to decreased platelet function.

Treatment consists of venesections which may be followed by irradiation of the bone marrow with radioactive phosphorus (^{32}P).

Secondary polycythaemia

A compensatory secondary polycythaemia occurs where there is chronic oxygen deficiency. It is seen in high altitude dwellers (e.g. in the Andes), in cases of congenital heart disease associated with cyanosis, and in some cases of chronic lung disease or heavy smoking. The condition must always be differentiated from primary polycythaemia.

Relative polycythaemia

In this condition the high haematocrit is due to a low plasma volume. This occurs acutely in dehydration, or chronically in hypertension and cigarette smoking.

LEUKAEMIA

Leukaemia is a disease characterized pathologically by a purposeless proliferation of white cell tissue and clinically by a progressive course, often leading to death in a few months to a few years. The condition is perhaps most readily understood if it is thought of as a form of tumour of the tissues which form the white cells. The neoplastic cells replace the normal bone marrow cells, causing anaemia, thrombocytopenia, and reduced numbers of normal white cells.

Aetiology

It is now known that chromosomal abnormalities are present in leukaemia. The most consistent change is seen in chronic myeloid leukaemia in which chromosome 21 (the Philadelphia chromosome) is defective. Ionizing radiation causes chromosomal damage and is probably the mechanism of the increased incidence of leukaemia in survivors of the atom bomb explosions in Japan and in those children whose mothers had abdominal X-rays during pregnancy. Radiological studies during pregnancy are now strictly limited.

Classification

Leukaemia may be classified morphologically into myeloid, lymphatic, and monocytic leukaemia, or into acute and chronic forms depending on the rapidity of the disease; but, for practical purposes, it is sufficient to consider leukaemia under two headings.

1. Acute leukaemia — myeloid, lymphatic, or monocytic.
2. Chronic leukaemia—myeloid, lymphatic.

Acute leukaemia

Acute leukaemia is seen at any age, but particularly in children in whom it is usually lymphoblastic and the most common form of malignant tumour. In adults acute leukaemia is usually myeloid or monocytic and may develop from chronic leukaemia.

Clinical features

The condition has a rapid onset and within a few weeks pallor is evident and the patient is listless and obviously extremely ill. Bruising of the skin and purpuric spots are common and there is a great tendency to bleeding within the buccal cavity and from the nose. Hypertrophy of the gums may occur and is particularly a feature of monocytic leukaemia. Infection of the gums and of the throat is often present. Because of these changes in the buccal cavity, dental attention may be the initial help sought.

Examination usually reveals glandular enlargement but in many cases it is only slight or moderate. In the case of the cervical glands the enlargement may be partly due to the leukaemic process and partly to the associated infection in the mouth and throat. Enlargement of the spleen and liver may be found but again is not of great degree.

Laboratory features. The white cell count may be moderately elevated but may be reduced. Examination of the blood film shows that the great majority of the white cells are primitive 'blast' cells and it is often impossible to state whether they are derived from myeloid, lymphoid, or monocytic precursors. This requires special staining or immunological techniques. The haemoglobin and red cell levels are markedly reduced and in addition the platelet count is low. Normal marrow tissue is largely replaced with the primitive cells.

Treatment

Patients should be transferred at once to a specialized leukaemia unit. The anaemia is corrected with red cell transfusions, bleeding with platelet transfusions, and infection with antibiotics which should be bactericidal and given intravenously, and sometimes granulocyte transfusion. Courses of cytotoxic drugs in combination are then given to kill the leukaemia cells.

In *childhood acute lymphoblastic leukaemia* 90% of patients achieve a remission. Relapses are common, especially in the central nervous system, hence prophylactic cranial irradiation and intrathecal cytotoxic drugs are given. After five years, 40% are still in remission and many of these are probably 'cured'.

In *adult acute myeloid leukaemia* the remission rate is 70% but relapses usually occur within a few months or years. The prognosis has been improved by bone marrow transplantation. The patient is given 'lethal' doses of radiation and cytotoxic drugs to kill all leukaemic cells and also all normal bone marrow cells. Bone marrow, usually from a sibling, is then infused and 'seeds' in the marrow cavities to restore normal marrow.

Chronic leukaemia

Chronic myeloid leukaemia has its maximum incidence in the middle years of life while the lymphatic variety tends to occur rather later.

Clinical features

The onset is insidious and the patient usually presents with a complaint of tiredness, a dragging sensation in the upper left abdomen due to splenic enlargement, or enlargement of lymph nodes. The splenic enlargement is often extremely great in chronic myeloid leukaemia and the spleen may come to fill the left side of the abdomen; it is less of a feature in chronic lymphatic leukaemia. Lymph node enlargement is usually prominent in the chronic lymphatic type of leukaemia and relatively slight in the myeloid variety.

Laboratory features. The white cell count is characteristically very high (e.g. $100-200 \times 10^9/l$). Examination of the stained blood film shows that the great majority of white cells present belong either to the granular series (myeloid leukaemia) or are lymphocytes (lymphatic leukaemia). Most are mature. A slight or moderate degree of anaemia is usually present while the platelet count is normal or may be increased.

Prognosis

In most cases life may be maintained for some two to five years after the diagnosis of chronic myeloid leukaemia has been made and often rather longer in the lymphatic form. Towards the end of the illness the leukaemia may take on many of the characteristics of the acute variety, severe anaemia and haemorrhagic tendencies being prominent.

Treatment

Treatment may be with radiotherapy directed to the bone marrow, spleen, and lymph nodes or, alternatively, with an alkylating agent. In chronic myeloid leukaemia the drug is busulphan (Myleran®) while in chronic lymphatic leukaemia chlorambucil (Leukeran®) is employed. Treatment of chronic lymphatic leukaemia is required only if the patient is symptomatic. Autoimmune haemolytic anaemia and thrombocytopenia are common in this disease and respond to corticosteroids.

AGRANULOCYTOSIS

In agranulocytosis there is a great reduction or complete absence of the granular cells of the blood.

Aetiology

The condition may be secondary to drug administration or X-ray irradiation in the same way as aplastic anaemia. It also occurs as an accompaniment of idiopathic aplastic anaemia. Neutropenia is common in HIV infection (see Ch. 2).

Clinical features

The essential clinical feature is a greatly increased liability to infection, particularly affecting the throat, the respiratory tract, and the skin. The total white cell count is low and differential white cell count shows that the granular series is virtually absent.

Treatment

Antibiotics are given to control infection (not chloramphenicol in view of the possible bone marrow damage which it may cause) and transfusions of fresh blood or granulocytes may sometimes be required. Any possibly harmful drug should, of course, be stopped.

LYMPHADENOPATHY

In this section a brief account is given of the main steps to be taken in reaching a diagnosis. Cervical lymphadenopathy is of much greater importance to the dentist than lymph node enlargement in other areas and is discussed in Chapter 14.

It is most important on finding enlarged lymph nodes in a patient to consider: (a) whether there is a local disease within the nodes themselves; (b) whether the nodes are involved as a result of disease within their area of drainage (thus, for example, enlarged inguinal nodes may be associated with a lesion of the foot); and (c) whether the enlargement of the nodes is part of a generalized disease (e.g. leukaemia).

Diagnosis of lymph node involvement is made by taking a detailed history and by examination including palpation of all the lymph node areas of the body, the spleen, and in particular the areas drained by the affected group of lymph nodes.

Bacterial examination of any local infected lesions may be necessary and special diagnostic tests such as the Mantoux reaction in suspected tuberculous lymph nodes and serology for syphilis (see Ch. 1), HIV infection (see Ch. 2) or glandular fevers (see Ch. 1). The blood picture is often important as, for example, in acute leukaemia. In very many cases of lymph node involvement a precise diagnosis is not possible by these means and *biopsy* of the node with histology is necessary to establish a diagnosis. A small portion of any node removed should also be sent for bacteriological examination.

In some cases involvement of a lymph node with cancer is the first sign of disease elsewhere and a search must be made for the primary lesion utilizing other procedures such as a chest X-ray, barium meal examination, and endoscopy.

LYMPHOMAS

These are tumour-like conditions affecting primarily the lymph nodes and other parts of the reticuloendothelial system. Histologically they can be divided into Hodgkin's disease and the non-Hodgkin's lymphomas.

Hodgkin's disease

Aetiology

Hodgkin's disease has the proliferative characteristics of a malignant tumour and little more is known of its aetiology than of the aetiology of tumour in general.

Pathology

The normal lymph node structure becomes progressively replaced by a mixed proliferation of lymphocytes and large reticulum cells which may be multinucleated (giant cells or Reed−Sternberg cells); eosinophils and plasma cells may also be present. Caseation (softening) does not occur. Similar histological changes occur in the spleen and liver. Spread to skin and bones may occur.

Clinical features

Hodgkin's disease is seen most commonly in young adults and it is more frequent in males. The onset is insidious and the individual usually presents with a history that for several weeks he has felt unduly tired and has then become aware of lymph node enlargement most often in the neck. Any of the superficial lymph nodes may be enlarged and, in addition, the glands in the mediastinum and abdomen are also commonly involved. The mediastinal enlargement may cause dyspnoea, cough, and cyanosis through pressure on the bronchi and great veins. The enlarged glands are firm and rubbery on palpation. They are usually discrete, are not painful, and there are no signs of inflammation associated; pus formation and sinus formation do not occur.

Enlargement of the spleen is a frequent occurrence and the liver may also be involved. Anaemia is usually slight at first but in the later stages of the disease may become very marked. The erythrocyte sedimentation rate is characteristically elevated. There is no characteristic alteration in the white cells although in a small proportion of cases there is an increase in the eosinophil level. Pyrexia is present in some cases and may have an intermittent nature, the temperature being elevated for a few days and then falling to normal for a period before becoming elevated again (Pel−Ebstein periodic pyrexia).

Diagnosis

The differential diagnosis of the various causes of lymph node enlargement is discussed in the preceding section. A definite diagnosis of Hodgkin's disease cannot be made until a gland is removed for histological examination.

Treatment

The method of treatment chosen depends on the extent of the disease. This is determined by chest X-ray, lymphangiography, and often by laparotomy involving splenectomy, liver biopsy and biopsy of the nodes along the abdominal aorta.

For localized disease treatment is by radiotherapy directed to the affected tissue but for more generalized disease chemotherapy with multiple cytotoxic drugs is the treatment of choice.

With localized disease, 80−90% of patients with Hodgkin's disease can be cured. With more generalized disease the five-year survival is about 50%.

Non-Hodgkin's lymphoma

The clinical features, diagnosis, and treatment are generally similar to Hodgkin's disesase but the histological features are different and very variable. Disease is often more widespread at presentation and the overall prognosis is poorer.

MYELOMA

This is a tumour of plasma cells in the bone marrow which may be local or generalized (multiple myeloma, myelomatosis). The cells produce an abnormal monoclonal immunoglobulin. The main clinical features are bone pains, especially in the spine, pathological fractures, recurrent infections, anaemia, and renal failure. The ESR and plasma viscosity are very high due to the immunoglobulin, and the urine may contain immunoglobulin fragments (Bence−Jones protein). Radiology of the skeleton shows punched-out areas particularly in the skull, ribs and spine. Hypercalcaemia may occur. Bone marrow examination shows increased plasma cells. The prognosis is poor. Palliative treatment is with radiotherapy for bony lesions, corticosteroids, and the cytotoxic drug melphalan.

THE HAEMORRHAGIC DISORDERS

Those diseases which are characterized by an undue tendency to haemorrhage are of great importance to the dentist. An account will first be given of the way in which bleeding is normally controlled (haemostasis) and will be followed by a description of the main clinical disorders.

Haemostasis

Haemostasis, or the control of bleeding, depends on the close interaction of a number of processes. The subject is an extremely complicated one and the following is only a brief and simplified account. If a vascular tissue is incised or otherwise traumatized the first reaction to the injury is adhesion of platelets to subendothelial collagen fibres which in turn leads to the release of platelet adenosine diphosphate (ADP), thromboxane, and serotonin. These agents attract further platelets to the site of injury where they aggregate. A platelet plug is formed which occludes the transected vessel and this is the main factor in the primary haemostatic process. The release of serotonin and thromboxane also causes contraction of small blood vessels and this secondary vascular response augments the primary response. The third phase is the formation of fibrin due to activation of the contact mechanism of the blood, which is stimulated by exposure of blood to damaged tissue and by release of platelet phospholipid. The sequence of events leading to the production of fibrin is very complex and involves the interaction of many coagulation factors which have an agreed international nomenclature. Figure 12.5 gives a simplified version of the coagulation process following a dental procedure.

Fig. 12.5 A simplified version of the modern concept of the coagulation mechanism.

Tests of the haemostatic system

Platelet function is tested by the skin bleeding time. Using a sterile disposable device, a small incision is made in the skin of the forearm and the duration of bleeding is timed with a stopwatch. The normal time is less than 8 minutes; longer times are seen in thrombocytopenia or platelet function defects. Platelet function defects are diagnosed by platelet aggregation studies in which agents such as collagen and ADP are added to platelet-rich plasma and the extent of aggregation recorded.

Blood coagulation is initially tested by clotting time tests performed on platelet-poor plasma. The intrinsic system is screened by the activated partial thromboplastin time (APTT) in which a surface agent, phospholipid, and calcium are added and the clotting time recorded. The APTT is prolonged by defects in any clotting factor apart from factors VII and XIII. The extrinsic system is screened by the prothrombin time (PT) in which a tissue extract and calcium are added and the clotting time recorded. It is prolonged by defects in factors I, II, V, VII and X. Patients with haemophilia (factor VIII deficiency) or Christmas disease (factor IX deficiency) therefore have a prolonged APTT but a normal PT. In contrast, acquired defects (anticoagulant therapy, liver disease) usually have a prolonged PT. Specific assays of individual clotting factors can be performed after the coagulation system has been screened by clotting time tests.

Fibrin removal

After the clot has served its purpose the fibrin is removed by a complex fibrinolytic system which maintains the patency of the vascular tree. In health there may be a dynamic equilibrium between the fibrinolytic enzyme system and the coagulation system. Plasma plasminogen is activated to plasmin which digests fibrin. This can be stimulated by streptokinase, which is used for thrombolytic therapy in acute myocardial infarction (see Ch. 7), and can be inhibited by tranexamic acid (Cyclokapron®) to prevent postdental extraction bleeding in bleeding disorders such as haemophilia. The oral tissues and saliva are rich in plasminogen activators which may promote postextraction bleeding in such patients.

Classification of haemorrhagic states

A simple classification of the haemorrhagic states with an indication of the nature of the defect is given below. The term purpura is a purely descriptive one for any condition characterized by haemorrhages into the skin and mucous membranes. The haemorrhages may be very small (punctate, pin-point, purpuric spots) in platelet and vessel wall disorders. In coagulation disorders, skin bleeding is confluent so that large bruises, or ecchymoses, are formed.

1. Deficiencies of clotting factors
   a. Genetic defects
      (i) Haemophilia — deficiency of antihaemophilic factor (AHF or factor VIII).
      (ii) Christmas disease — deficiency of Christmas factor (factor IX).
      (iii) Von Willebrand's disease — deficiency of von Willebrand factor (carrier protein for factor VIII and co-factor in platelet adhesion).
   b. Acquired defects
      (i) Anticoagulant therapy.
      (ii) Liver disease — complex defect with deficiency of factors II, VII, IX, X.
2. Defects of platelets
   a. Thrombocytopenia — either primary or secondary.
   b. Impaired platelet function — von Willebrand's disease, uraemia, aspirin.
3. Defects in vessel wall
   a. Anaphylactoid purpura—vasculitis.
   b. Hereditary telangiectasia — focal capillary defect.
   c. Senile purpura, steroid purpura, scurvy — defect of supporting tissues.
   d. Septicaemia.

HAEMOPHILIA

Haemophilia is the most important of the hereditary haemorrhagic disorders. It is due to a defect in the production of an intrinsic system factor (factor VIII) which is synthesized abnormally. The condition is moderately common (about 4000 patients in Britain).

Family history

The condition is transmitted as a sex-linked recessive trait. The gene responsible is contained in the X-chromosome of the reproductive cells. The inheritance of haemophilia can be understood by a study of Figure 12.6 which shows a typical family tree. The main points regarding the inheritance of the disorder which should be remembered are:

1. If a haemophilic male marries a normal female none of his sons will have the disorder but all his daughters will be carriers of the disease.

2. If a normal male marries a carrier female there is a 50% chance of the sons being affected with the disease and a 50% chance of the daughters being carriers.

In clinical practice about one-third of individuals with haemophilia have no knowledge of a family history of the disorder. This is probably due to the passage down through several generations of female carriers without occurrence of the disease in males, or possibly due to gene mutation.

Some female carriers of haemophilia have a moderately reduced factor VIII level, and like mildly haemophiliac males have increased bleeding after surgery including dental extractions. Many carriers can now be definitively diagnosed by factor VIII assays and gene probe studies; they can be offered

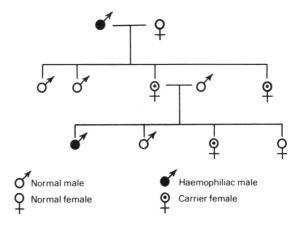

Fig. 12.6 A haemophiliac family tree.

antenatal diagnosis of affected male fetuses with the option of selective termination of such pregnancies.

Clinical features

These correlate with the plasma level of factor VIII (normal range 40–200 iu/dl). In *severe haemophilia* (factor VIII less than 2 iu/dl) the bleeding tendency usually presents between 6 and 18 months of age with 'spontaneous' bleeding and bruising after minor injuries of everyday life. Bleeding into the joints (haemarthrosis) is particularly common, the main joints involved being the knees, elbows, and ankles. The affected joint becomes swollen and very painful and the individual may be incapacitated for considerable periods. Permanent joint damage with chronic arthritis and flexion contractures is likely to occur following repeated haemarthrosis, and may be severe. Haematomata commonly occur in the subcutaneous tissues and in the muscles and, apart from causing bruising and pain, they may produce serious damage from pressure on vital structures such as nerves.

In *mild to moderate haemophilia* (Factor VIII 2–40 iu/dl) spontaneous bleeds into joints or muscles are uncommon, but excessive bleeding occurs after injury or surgery. Such patients are commonly first diagnosed when this occurs after surgery, including dental extractions. Following injury or any surgical procedure there is persistent bleeding which may be so prolonged as to endanger life. Thus after a dental extraction both mild and severe haemophiliacs may bleed from the tooth socket for days or even weeks and may, over this period, lose from a very small area many pints of blood.

Initially primary haemostasis is secured by the platelet plug, but after some hours or days bleeding recurs since there is a deficient fibrin plug. Large, offensive, greenish-purple clots build up in the mouth then break off with further bleeding from the socket. Patients may die from blood loss. Haematomas also occur after nerve block injections and may track down the neck causing tracheal compression and fatal asphyxia. Injuries (especially head injuries), surgery, and gastrointestinal bleeding may be fatal without proper treatment.

Investigations

The diagnostic finding in haemophilia is a deficiency in factor VIII which in severe cases may be manifest as prolongation of the APTT but in milder cases may be revealed only by specific factor VIII assay.

Management of haemophilia

The first essential is accurate diagnosis. All patients (male or female) with excessive bleeding after dentistry, injury, or surgery (current, previous, or in the family) must be referred to a haematologist before surgery for coagulation tests. All confirmed haemophiliacs (including female carriers with low factor VIII levels) should be registered and reviewed at least annually at the local haemophilia centre. They (and their general medical and dental practitioners) should be educated about the bleeding problems and asked to contact the centre in the event of injury (especially head injury), bleeding, or need for surgery including dental extraction or nerve block injection. They should be given a bleeding disorder card to carry, which gives details of their clotting factor defect and the name, address, and telephone number of their haemophilia centre. Patients are asked to show this card to any doctor or dentist whom they attend. They are advised to avoid aspirin which induces a platelet function defect and may precipitate bleeding (paracetamol or opiate drugs can be used instead for pain relief). Intramuscular injections should be avoided since they may cause large haematomata; intravenous and subcutaneous injections are safe (but not nerve block injections without cover).

Bleeding can be rapidly controlled (or prevented after injury or before surgery) by raising the low factor VIII level towards or into the normal range; the level and duration required vary with the site and severity of bleeding, injury, or surgery. In severe haemophilia (factor VIII less than 2 iu/dl) or moderate haemophilia (factor VIII 2–10 iu/dl), intravenous infusion of human factor VIII concentrate is required. (Unconcentrated plasma or whole blood does not contain sufficient factor VIII to raise the patient's factor VIII level adequately.) Patients with frequent bleeds are trained to give themselves this treatment at home to avoid delay in treatment and time off school or work.

Complications of factor VIII treatment include allergic reactions (see Ch. 16), the development of antibodies to factor VIII which greatly complicates treatment, and transmission of bloodborne virus infection (see Ch. 2). About one-quarter of haemophiliacs in Britain have positive HIV antibody tests and some have developed AIDS or other HIV-related disease; a smaller number are carriers of hepatitis B. A larger number have chronic non-A, non-B hepatitis (see Ch. 2 and Ch. 9). These viral infections may worsen the bleeding tendency, e.g. thrombocytopenia from HIV infection, extrinsic coagulation defects from cirrhosis (see later). The introduction of self-exclusion and screening of blood donors for HIV in 1985, plus the heat treatment of factor VIII concentrates, appears effective in preventing further exposure of haemophiliacs to HIV infection and in reducing further exposure to hepatitis B and non-A, non-B infections. In the future, production of factor VIII from microorganisms by genetic engineering will yield virus-free concentrates.

In mild haemophilia (factor VIII 10−40 iu/dl) which accounts for about half of registered haemophiliacs, and in those female carriers who have similarly low levels, the intravenous infusion of desmopressin (DDAVP®), a synthetic derivative of arginine vasopressin (AVP, antidiuretic hormone, see Ch. 13), raises the patient's own plasma level of factor VIII into the normal range by releasing its carrier protein (von Willebrand factor) from the vascular endothelium into the plasma. This treatment avoids the complications of blood product treatment. Side-effects include facial flushing, nausea, hypotension, and water retention. Because desmopressin also stimulates fibrinolysis (by releasing plasminogen activator from vascular endothelium), tranexamic acid is given to prevent excessive fibrinolysis that may increase bleeding. Desmopressin also increases platelet adhesion to vascular endothelium, partly by increasing von Willebrand factor levels and partly by a direct effect; it is therefore used to treat or prevent bleeding in von Willebrand's disease and other platelet function defects (see later).

Before dental extraction or other types of surgery, the patient's diagnosis and viral status are checked and plasma tested to exclude antibodies to factor VIII. The management plan is agreed between the haemophilia centre and the dentist (many centres liaise with their hospital dentist). The patient attends the centre to receive the first dose of tranexamic acid and also factor VIII concentrate (or desmopressin) to raise the factor VIII level to 50 iu/dl (lower normal range) one hour before the extraction. Extractions are performed with special care to the tooth sockets, which may be packed or stitched. Many patients can then be sent home with a ten-day course of tranexamic acid (1 g orally 8-hourly) and advice to contact the centre for further treatment if bleeding occurs. Some patients are kept in hospital for some days for observation (e.g. first extractions of adult teeth, difficult or multiple extractions, factor VIII antibodies, distance of home from haemophilia centre, etc.). The dentist or surgeon should take special care with haemophiliacs who are known or suspected cases or carriers of HIV or hepatitis B (see Ch. 2).

To minimize postextraction bleeding, all haemophiliacs should receive special, intensive education on dental hygiene and conservative dental care including fluoride treatment. This is especially important in children and young adults.

Christmas disease

Christmas disease is a haemorrhagic disorder which is clinically and genetically indistinguishable from haemophilia. The unusual name is derived from the surname of the first patient studied. The missing coagulation factor is termed the Christmas factor or factor IX. There are about 500 patients in Britain. The treatment is essentially as for haemophilia, except that concentrates of factor IX are used and not of factor VIII. Desmopressin is ineffectual, but fresh frozen plasma contains sufficient factor IX to treat mild Christmas disease. Antibodies to HIV are less common than with haemophilia, but occur in some patients, as does carriage of hepatitis B or non-A, non-B.

Von Willebrand's disease

In recent years there has been increasing recognition that von Willebrand's disease is the most common bleeding disorder, although at present probably only a minority of patients are registered at haemophilia centres. Unlike haemophilia and Christmas disease, its inheritance is autosomal dominant, hence women are affected as often as men and about half the family members are affected.

Von Willebrand factor is a high molecular weight protein which is released into plasma from vascular endothelium. It is composed of high and low molecular weight multimers, whose composition can be studied by electrophoresis of plasma. Von Willebrand factor has two functions: it acts as a carrier protein for factor VIII, and the higher molecular weight multimers also promote platelet adhesion to vascular endothelium.

The skin bleeding time is a useful *screening test* for von Willebrand's disease, in which it is prolonged despite a normal platelet count. The *diagnosis* is confirmed by measuring platelet aggregation in response to the antibiotic ristocetin, which is proportional to the plasma level of von Willebrand factor (normal range 40–200 iu/dl). In von Willebrand's disease the plasma level of von Willebrand factor as measured by this test is low. Study of electrophoresis of plasma multimers shows that there are several subtypes of the disease. The plasma factor VIII level may also be low.

Clinical features of von Willebrand's disease include easy bruising, nose bleeds, oral and gastrointestinal bleeding, and heavy periods in women which may cause iron deficiency anaemia. There is excessive bleeding after injury or surgery, including dental extraction, which may be fatal. Unlike haemophilia, the onset of bleeding is immediate rather than delayed, since primary haemostasis is defective.

Patients with von Willebrand's disease should be registered at haemophilia centres, educated, and given a bleeding disorders card as for haemophilia. Treatment is by infusion of desmopressin, which usually increases plasma levels of von Willebrand factor and factor VIII into the normal range. In some patients, factor VIII concentrate or cryoprecipitate (a cruder plasma concentrate which has a higher concentration of von Willebrand factor) is required. The regimens for dental extraction, block injections, or other types of surgery are similar to haemophilia. Antibodies to von Willebrand factor and HIV infection are less common than in haemophilia, but occur in some patients. Antenatal diagnosis is also possible.

Other platelet function defects

Congenital platelet function defects other than von Willebrand's disease are uncommon. The bleeding time is prolonged, von Willebrand factor is normal, and platelet aggregation to agents such as ADP and collagen is reduced. Platelet transfusion is required prior to dental extraction and other types of surgery. Patients with renal failure have long bleeding times and defective platelet function which is reversed by dialysis and/or desmopressin (see Ch. 11). Ingestion of a single tablet of aspirin decreases platelet aggregation (by blocking synthesis of prostaglandins and thromboxane within the platelet) and prolongs the bleeding time, but not sufficiently to cause postoperative bleeding unless the patient has another bleeding disorder: aspirin is contraindicated in all patients with bleeding disorders. Aspirin is, however, used after myocardial infarction, peripheral arterial disease, bypass grafting (see Ch. 7) and stroke (see Ch. 18) to prevent recurrent arterial thrombosis by its effect on platelet aggregation.

Thrombocytopenia

Thrombocytopenia, or reduction in the number of platelets, may be either primary or secondary. Haemorrhagic phenomena are likely to occur when the platelet count is $50 \times 10^9/l$ or less (the normal level is $150–400 \times 10^9/l$).

Idiopathic (immune) thrombocytopenic purpura

This disorder is seen particularly in young people. It is an autoimmune disease, due to formation of antiplatelet antibodies which cause increased platelet destruction by the reticuloendothelial system, especially the spleen. There is often a preceding infection. HIV infection (see Ch. 2) is an increasingly common cause. Some cases are due to drugs or neoplasms. Small haemorrhagic spots (petechiae) develop in the skin and mucous membranes and they may also occur in the internal organs, particularly the brain. The gums bleed unduly after brushing the teeth and nose bleeding is frequent. Dental extraction is a potential hazard because of haemorrhage although the problem is not of the same magnitude as that in haemophilia. Larger areas of bruising into the subcutaneous tissues are common after trivial injuries. Secondary anaemia commonly develops. Slight splenic enlargement may occur. The platelet count is very low and the bleeding time is prolonged.

The acute stage is treated by transfusion of platelets and by the administration of corticosteroid drugs or intravenous immunoglobulin. Splenectomy, which must be performed only after a remission, often leads to considerable improvement.

Secondary thrombocytopenia

Reduction in the platelet count, with resultant purpura, occurs in several diseases which reduce production of platelets from the bone marrow, of which the more important are acute leukaemia, primary aplastic anaemia, and bone marrow damage from drugs or irradiation. Increased pooling and destruction of platelets also occurs in patients with splenomegaly, e.g. in hepatic cirrhosis (see Ch. 10).

Liver disease

An undue tendency to haemorrhage is an important accompaniment of many forms of liver disease. In *obstructive jaundice* the absence of bile from the intestine leads to impaired absorption of the fat-soluble vitamin K and in consequence to low levels of factors II, VII, IX and X. This is an extrinsic coagulation defect with a prolonged prothrombin time. It is corrected by injections of vitamin K before surgery. A similar defect occurs in acute or chronic liver disease due to *hepatocyte failure*. It is not reversed by vitamin K, and requires intravenous infusion of fresh frozen plasma which contains the missing factors. This is required prior to surgery, including dental extractions and liver biopsies, to prevent excessive bleeding. Platelet transfusion may also be required for thrombocytopenia (see above).

Anticoagulant therapy

The dentist should have some knowledge of anticoagulant therapy as a number of people are receiving this form of treatment on a long-term basis, as a prophylactic measure in atrial fibrillation, in arterial or venous thrombosis, and in those with artificial heart valves or synthetic arterial grafts. The drug most commonly employed is warfarin which is a vitamin K antagonist and therefore reduces factors II, VII, IX and X. As with liver disease, this is an extrinsic defect with a prolonged prothrombin time. The dose of warfarin is adjusted according to the prothrombin time on regular visits to the anticoagulant clinic. All such patients are counselled about their increased risks of bleeding and carry a booklet to show any doctor or dentist whom they may attend.

If dental extraction is required in an individual receiving anticoagulant therapy, it should be performed only after consultation with the doctor in charge of the case. It may involve temporary correction of the clotting defect by either reducing the dose, injection of vitamin K, or infusion of fresh frozen plasma.

Hereditary haemorrhagic telangiectasia

This is an uncommon disorder in which there are areas of dilated blood vessels particularly on the mucous membranes of the lips, tongue, nose, and gastrointestinal tract. They may also be seen in the skin, especially of the face. A family history of the condition is usually obtained. The inheritance is autosomal dominant. Lesions appear in early adult life and become more frequent with age.

The most common complaint is of frequent epistaxis and gastrointestinal bleeding, and the chronic blood loss produces secondary anaemia. Undue haemorrhage after dental extraction may theoretically occur if there is telangiectasia in the operation field.

Senile purpura, steroid purpura, and scurvy

In elderly people there is decreased elasticity in the skin and subcutaneous tissues resulting in diminished support for the small blood vessels; these are more liable to rupture following minor injuries, and small purpuric areas result. These are seen particularly on the dorsum of the hands and forearms. The condition is not a serious one and there is no dental implication. Similar lesions are seen in patients receiving high doses of corticosteroids or with Cushing's syndrome (see Ch. 13), and in scurvy (vitamin C deficiency, see Ch. 15).

Henoch–Schönlein purpura

This is a vasculitis (inflammation of small blood vessels) which results in leakage of blood cells and a purpuric rash. The factor responsible is most frequently bacterial infection, especially streptococcal, and a history of a sore throat before the onset of the purpura is commonly obtained. In other instances an article of food is responsible while in some cases no cause can be detected.

The illness commonly starts with vomiting. Purpuric spots which are palpable as well as visible (in contrast to idiopathic thrombocytopenic purpura) occur on the skin, particularly of the legs, and may be very numerous. Joint effusions with pain may be present while in other instances bleeding from the alimentary tract is the main feature. Renal involvement, shown by proteinuria and haematuria, may also be present. The lesion is a vascular one and the platelet count is normal. The degree of blood loss is seldom great.

Corticosteroids may be given for the glomerulonephritis, but their benefit is not known.

Septicaemia

Septicaemia due to meningococcal (see Ch. 18) or Gram-negative bacterial infection (see Ch. 5) may damage small blood vessels causing an acute purpuric rash. The bacteria may be observed on skin biopsy.

13

Endocrine disorders

THE THYROID GLAND

The thyroid gland is situated at the front and sides of the lower part of the neck. It consists of two lateral lobes, each about four centimetres long, joined across the midline by a narrow isthmus. The gland is partly covered by the muscles of the neck in front. Posteriorly and medially the main relationships are to the trachea, the recurrent laryngeal nerve, and the oesophagus. The parathyroid glands lie along the posterior surface of the lobes. The thyroid gland has a fibrous sheath which is fixed to the larynx and trachea so that the gland moves with these structures on swallowing. The blood supply is derived from the external carotid artery (superior thyroid artery) and the subclavian artery (inferior thyroid artery).

The gland is composed of many follicles which are usually lined by a single layer of cubical epithelium; the follicles contain colloid. The size of the follicles, the colloid content, and the epithelial lining vary considerably in the different thyroid disorders.

The thyroid gland manufactures, stores, and secretes the two thyroid hormones, thyroxine (T_4) and triiodothyronine (T_3), of which iodine is an essential constituent. The synthesis of the hormones is regulated by the thyroid stimulating hormone (TSH) of the anterior lobe of the pituitary. The thyroid hormones stimulate the metabolic activities of the body generally, increase the heart rate, play a part in carbohydrate metabolism, and affect growth.

The first step on examination of the thyroid gland is a close inspection, in good light, of the lower neck, the patient's head being tilted slightly backwards; on swallowing the gland is seen to move upwards. Palpation is best carried out from behind, the patient's head being inclined slightly forward to relax the sterno-mastoid muscles; the swallowing test is repeated. If the vascularity of the gland is much increased there will be a systolic murmur, easily audible on auscultation, and it may be possible to feel a thrill.

Developmental anomalies

The isthmus and the medial parts of the lobes are formed from a central downgrowth from the floor of the primitive oropharynx; in adults the site of the downgrowth is represented by the foramen caecum. The downgrowth forms a hollow stalk called the thyroglossal duct, the lower end of which enlarges and forms thyroid tissue while the upper end atrophies and disappears. On either side of the central downgrowth, cells from the entoderm of the fourth arch proliferate to form the remainder of the lateral lobes.

The gland may not descend fully (lingual thyroid), may descend too far (retrosternal thyroid), may develop elsewhere, or the thyroglossal duct may persist in whole or part. None of these anomalies is common. The term *ectopic thyroid* refers to any portion of thyroid tissue which does not lie in the normal situation.

Lingual thyroid

This term is used where the thyroid does not descend as described above but develops in close proximity to the foramen caecum. The diagnosis is not usually made until after the gland enlarges at puberty. The gland may be completely buried in the root of the tongue or it may cause a rounded swelling on the posterior surface of that organ. If it is of considerable size it produces dysphagia and dyspnoea, and surgical excision is indicated; if there is no thyroid tissue elsewhere the patient will subsequently need to take sodium thyroxine.

Retrosternal thyroid

If the developing gland descends too far an intrathoracic, or retrosternal, thyroid is formed. Should the thyroid become enlarged in this situation, pressure symptoms (dyspnoea and dysphagia) are likely.

Other ectopic thyroids

Ectopic thyroid tissue may rarely be found in other sites, e.g. within the pharynx or laterally in the neck. In most cases thyroid tissue is also present in the normal thyroid situation.

Thyroglossal tract remnants

These are described under swellings of the neck (see Ch. 14).

GOITRE

The term goitre is used to describe enlargement of the thyroid gland. It may be a manifestation of several different disease processes which may be classified as follows:

1. Non-toxic, simple, or colloid goitre.
2. Toxic goitre, exophthalmic goitre, or thyrotoxicosis.
3. Thyroiditis.
4. Thyroid neoplasm.

Non-toxic goitre

Simple or non-toxic goitre is usually divided into endemic and sporadic categories according to whether many or few of the population are affected. The patient presents no other clinical evidence of disturbed thyroid function.

Deficiency of iodine is probably the principal factor in the production of endemic goitre. The deficiency is most commonly due to a low iodine content in water and locally produced foods. The cause of sporadic goitre is uncertain. In many in-

Fig. 13.1 Large simple goitre.

stances it is possible that a combination of factors is responsible, e.g. disordered synthesis of thyroid hormones due to genetically determined defects, and iodine deficiency either primary or conditioned by certain goitrogenic substances in the diet.

Whatever the basic cause of simple goitre it is generally believed that the enlargement is due to a compensatory thyroid hyperplasia initiated by inadequate circulating thyroid hormones. The hyperplasia is most likely to develop when metabolic demands are increased, particularly during the period of reproductive life in the female. Hence non-toxic goitre is much more common in females than in males.

The enlargement may be relatively slight or of such degree that the gland forms a large, disfiguring swelling causing pressure symptoms (Fig. 13.1). The surface of the gland may be smooth at first but it is likely to become increasingly nodular.

Prophylaxis by the addition of iodide to salt greatly diminishes the incidence of endemic goitre. In established cases of goitre the administration of sodium thyroxine may reduce the size of the gland but, if it is large and producing pressure symptoms, surgery is indicated.

Toxic goitre or thyrotoxicosis

Toxic goitre, thyrotoxicosis, or hyperthyroidism, is more common in women. Although it may occur at any age, it is seen most frequently in early adult life.

Fig. 13.3 Puffiness of the face in myxoedema.

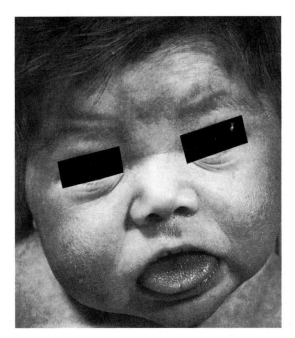

Fig. 13.4 Cretinism.

Diagnosis

The diagnosis is confirmed by finding a low serum T_4 level and high level of compensatory TSH.

Treatment

Substitution therapy is readily available in tablet form as sodium thyroxine. The initial dosage should be low and increases should be made gradually as cardiac function is often impaired.

Cretinism

Cretinism is the term used to describe hypothyroidism occurring in the early years of life (Fig. 13.4). There is physical and mental retardation and the child is slow to reach the usual stages of childhood development such as sitting, crawling, walking, talking, etc. The face is heavy and dull, the expression is vacant, the mouth is usually open, the tongue large and protruding, and the hair coarse and sparse. The abdomen is protuberant and umbilical hernia is common. Primary and secondary dentition is seriously delayed.

It is important that the diagnosis is made early otherwise there may be permanent mental and physical retardation. Screening of newborn babies is performed increasingly. Treatment consists of administration of sodium thyroxine.

THE PARATHYROID GLANDS

The four parathyroid glands are situated along the posterior surface of the thyroid, usually outside the capsule but occasionally just within the substance of the gland. The secretion of the glands, parathyroid hormone, controls the renal excretion of phosphorus, so disordered function of the parathyroids is associated with profound alterations in phosphorus and calcium metabolism.

Hyperparathyroidism

This is a relatively rare disease but the dentist should be aware of it as it produces important skeletal changes which may involve the jaws.

Primary hyperparathyroidism is usually due to an adenoma of one or more glands, or occasionally hyperplasia of all four glands. Secondary hyperparathyroidism occurs as a complication of severe chronic renal failure.

The excess parathyroid hormone causes increased urinary excretion of phosphorus and in consequence the serum phosphorus level falls. Phosphate, as calcium phosphate, is mobilized from the skeleton in an attempt to restore the blood level of phosphorus, and decalcification results. In a typical case the principal biochemical findings are a lowered serum phosphorus, an elevated serum calcium, and a high urinary calcium. The serum alkaline phosphatase level, which is an index of activity of bone breakdown and formation, is also raised.

Clinical and radiological features

The decalcification of the skeleton may show as a diffuse rarefaction or there may be multiple cysts present in addition (osteitis fibrosa cystica). The jaws are often decalcified but not the teeth. Compression of the vertebrae, pathological fractures, and deformities of the thorax and limbs may be present in severe cases. The bones and muscles may be aching and tender. Hypercalcaemia may cause thirst, polyuria, constipation, and mental changes. (Other causes of hypercalcaemia include tumours, e.g. bronchial carcinoma, myeloma.)

The excess calcium excretion by the kidney leads to the formation of renal calculi and progressive renal damage.

Treatment

Marked hypercalcaemia should be reduced by hydration, corticosteroids, or cytotoxic drugs. If a tumour of the parathyroids is present it should be excised while if a diffuse hyperplasia is found three of the four glands are removed.

Hypoparathyroidism

Hypoparathyroidism, which is uncommon, may be congenital, idiopathic, or may follow inadvertent removal of the glands during thyroidectomy. There is insufficient parathyroid hormone, the excretion of phosphorus decreases, the serum phosphorus rises, and the serum calcium falls. The lowered serum calcium results in tetany which is characterized by increased neuromuscular excitability.

Tetany

Tetany may be due to hypoparathyroidism or more commonly to a lowered serum calcium from other causes such as rickets, osteomalacia, and steatorrhoea. It may also occur in alkalosis probably as a result of lowering of the level of the ionized portion of the serum calcium. Alkalosis can be caused by abnormal losses of acid radicals as in severe vomiting, by a prolonged intake of readily absorbed alkalis such as sodium bicarbonate, or by overbreathing which causes increased carbon dioxide excretion. The latter may be seen in anxious individuals.

In severe cases there is spontaneous muscle twitching, convulsions, and in children a high-pitched cry due to spasm of the larynx (laryngismus stridulus). In less severe cases the neuromuscular excitability may be shown by twitching of the facial muscles after tapping over the facial nerve (Chvostek's sign) and by spasm of the hand after temporary partial occlusion of the blood supply of the upper arm (Trousseau's sign).

THE PITUITARY GLAND

The pituitary gland is situated in the sella turcica with the sphenoidal air sinuses below, the optic chiasma above, and the third, fourth and sixth cranial nerves, the cavernous sinus, and internal carotid artery on either side. The anterior lobe contains chromophobe, eosinophil, and basophil cells while the posterior lobe consists mainly of nerve cells and fibres. Although the pituitary gland is a tiny structure it exercises a dominating influence on development and through a variety of body function hormones:

1. Growth is controlled by the growth hormone secreted by the anterior lobe.

2. The activity of the adrenal glands is controlled by the adrenocorticotrophic hormone (ACTH) of the anterior lobe.

3. Thyroid function is controlled by the thyroid

stimulating hormone (TSH) of the anterior lobe.

4. The function of the ovaries and breasts are controlled by follicle stimulating hormone (FSH), luteinizing hormone (LH) and prolactin; and of the testes by FSH and LH. All these hormones are from the anterior lobe.

5. The antidiuretic hormone (ADH) of the posterior lobe promotes water reabsorption from the renal tubule and hence controls the volume of urine.

Clinical disorders of the pituitary gland are relatively rare and only a brief account is given of them, largely for general interest; only acromegaly is likely to be of direct interest to the dentist.

Prolactinoma

This is the most common pituitary tumour and is more common in women. It causes menstrual upset, infertility, and breast milk secretion (galactorrhoea). Treatment is with bromocriptine, surgery, or radiotherapy.

Gigantism

This is due to hypersecretion of the growth hormone of the pituitary gland occurring in childhood, i.e. before the epiphyses of the long bones have united. Heights of 7 or even 8 ft may be reached. These individuals are seldom strong and the majority die in early or middle age. Some gain their livelihood in circuses.

Dwarfism

Deficiency of the growth hormone in childhood produces pituitary dwarfism. The patient is usually well proportioned in contrast to the achrondoplastic individual in whom the head and trunk are normal in size but appear very large in contrast to the short limbs.

Dwarfism may also result from a general stunting of development caused by chronic severe illnesses occurring during childhood years (e.g. tuberculosis of the skeleton). It also occurs in cretinism.

Acromegaly

The term 'acromegaly' is derived from the Greek 'acros' meaning terminal and 'mega' meaning large, and thus is descriptive of the enlargement of the hands and feet which is a characteristic feature of the disorder. It is caused by hypersecretion of the growth hormone of the pituitary occurring in adult life, i.e. after the epiphyses have united. In most cases there is a tumour of the eosinophil cells.

The facial features (Fig. 13.5) become very coarse and heavy due to increase in the subcutaneous tissues, especially of the lips and nose. The mandible becomes enlarged to a much greater extent than the maxilla so that the lower jaw becomes very prominent. The frontal ridges and other bony prominences become enlarged. The hands and feet

Fig. 13.5 Acromegaly. Note heavy features, large jaw, large hands.

increase in size and the patient finds that larger gloves and shoes are required and rings no longer fit. Headache is a common complaint and later there is interference with vision because the pituitary tumour causes pressure on the optic chiasma.

No alteration takes place in the size of the teeth but they become well spaced because of the enlargement of the jaw. The lower teeth project beyond the upper, often to a considerable extent. If the patient has dentures they become progressively more ill-fitting as the lower jaw increases in size.

In the early stages of the disorder the diagnosis may often be made clear if comparison is made with a photograph of the patient taken some time before.

X-ray of the skull shows the enlarged lower jaw, prominent frontal ridges and enlarged air sinuses; in some cases enlargement and erosion of the pituitary fossa by the tumour is evident. Plasma growth hormone levels are high.

X-ray therapy directed to the pituitary gland is often successful in reducing the activity of the tumour. Surgical resection or cryosurgery (tissue destruction by extreme temperature reduction) are alternative forms of treatment.

Panhypopituitarism (Simmonds' disease)

Severe haemorrhage associated with child-bearing is the usual aetiological factor. For some ill-understood reason the shock leads to necrotic changes in the pituitary gland and thus to deficiency of several pituitary functions.

In the fully developed picture there is depressed thyroid function producing the features of hypothyroidism, depressed adrenal function, and depressed sexual function producing sterility and amenorrhoea. There is loss of body hair. Considerable improvement occurs following replacement hormonal treatment.

Cushing's disease

This is due to a basophil adenoma of the pituitary causing increased ACTH levels and hence increased cortisol levels. The main clinical features are obesity, muscle wasting, polycythaemia, hypertension, glycosuria and osteoporosis.

Fröhlich's syndrome

This syndrome is characterized by obesity, disturbances of the natural sleep rhythm, and sexual retardation. It has been suggested that the fat boy in *Pickwick Papers* may have been an example of this condition.

Diabetes insipidus

Deficiency of the antidiuretic hormone (ADH, arginine vasopressin, AVP), which controls the urinary volume, results in diabetes insipidus. The patient passes a very large volume of urine, possibly five or six times the normal amount, and in consequence suffers considerable inconvenience, loses sleep, and is constantly thirsty. The urine is of low specific gravity but does not contain any abnormal constituents. Diabetes insipidus can be controlled by supplying the antidiuretic hormone either by injection or as a snuff.

THE ADRENAL GLANDS

The adrenal, or suprarenal, glands are two in number, one lying on the upper pole of each kidney. The gland is composed of a medulla and cortex which have different embryological origins and different physiological activities.

The medulla

The hormones of the adrenal medulla are adrenaline and noradrenaline. Both substances cause constriction of blood vessels and elevation of the blood pressure. Adrenaline also has a powerful effect on carbohydrate metabolism causing mobilization of liver glycogen and a rise in blood sugar. Adrenaline may be used in the treatment of anaphylactic shock (see Ch. 16) since it relieves bronchospasm and results in vasoconstriction.

Disorders of the adrenal medulla are rarely encountered. *Phaeochromocytoma* is an actively secreting tumour which causes hypertension.

The cortex

A large number of steroid hormones secreted by the adrenal cortex have now been identified. The cortical hormones are secreted in response to stimulation by corticotrophin (ACTH) of the anterior pituitary. The steroid hormones play a vital role in many body functions and have a range of therapeutic usefulness which extends far beyond the replacement therapy of adrenal insufficiency. The principal actions of the steroid hormones may be grouped as follows:

1. *Carbohydrate metabolism.* The so-called glucocorticoids (especially cortisol or hydrocortisone) produce increased glucose formation from protein and possibly fat and decreased glucose utilization through an anti-insulin effect.

2. *Sodium metabolism.* The so-called mineralocorticoids (especially aldosterone) produce retention of sodium and increased excretion of potassium through effects on the renal tubule. There is a tendency to fluid retention and hypertension.

3. *Sex hormones.* The adrenal cortex produces male hormones (androgens) and female hormones (oestrogens) which are largely responsible for the development of the secondary sex characteristics.

Acute hypocorticalism

Acute adrenal insufficiency is a very serious condition which may occur as a rare complication of severe infections with septicaemia, or as an adrenal crisis in Addison's disease. The principal features are acute circulatory collapse, dehydration, hypoglycaemia, and vomiting. Intensive fluid, salt, glucose, and hydrocortisone replacement therapy is required.

Chronic hypocorticalism

The principal form of chronic adrenal insufficiency is Addison's disease which is of dental interest because of the buccal changes. It may be caused by tuberculosis of the adrenals or destruction by an autoimmune process.

The main clinical features are marked loss of energy, hypotension (e.g. a blood pressure of 90/50 mmHg), anorexia and vomiting, and pigmentation of the skin and mucous membranes. The skin pigmentation is more marked on exposed areas and may appear as a slaty-blue colour or, in some instances, like sunburn. Slaty-blue or dark-grey pigmentation frequently occurs in the buccal mucosa particularly along the line of closure of the teeth. It is practically pathognomonic of Addison's disease provided physiological pigmentation of racial origin is excluded. The deficiency of mineralocorticoids leads to excessive renal losses of salt and thus to characteristic alterations in the biochemical pattern of the urine and blood.

It is important for dentists to appreciate that patients with Addison's disease tolerate anaesthesia, surgical procedures, and illnesses such as infection very poorly. Injudicious surgery may precipitate an adrenal crisis which may prove fatal unless skilled replacement therapy is promptly instituted.

Patients should be given a card to carry and show any doctor or dentist whom they may attend. They should take hydrocortisone tablets twice daily and increase the dose in the event of intercurrent illness. Adrenal crisis is treated by intravenous fluids and hydrocortisone.

Hypercorticalism

Overactivity of the adrenal cortex, which may result from tumour or hyperplasia, is relatively uncommon. The clinical effects are largely determined by the steroid hormone that is preponderant. Excess secretion of the cortisol group (glucocorticoids) has features similar to those of Cushing's disease. Excess secretion of aldosterone (mineralocorticoid) produces sodium retention, potassium loss, and hypertension (Conn's syndrome). Excess secretion of androgens produces masculinization in the female (virilism) and excess of oestrogens produces feminization in the male.

Diagnosis is by laboratory estimations of the steroid hormones and by radiological studies of the adrenals. If a tumour is found it is removed. If hyperplasia is found bilateral adrenalectomy or subtotal removal of the adrenal mass is carried out.

Pharmacological steroid therapy

Long-term administration of supraphysiological doses of corticosteroids (e.g. prednisolone) may be given for asthma, rheumatoid arthritis and other connective tissue diseases, ulcerative colitis or Crohn's disease, autoimmune blood or skin diseases, or immunosuppression after organ transplantation. Such doses cause side-effects similar to Cushing's disease and also suppress adrenal function so that, as with Addison's disease, an adrenal crisis may follow anaesthesia, surgery, or intercurrent illness if treatment is interrupted. Patients should carry steroid cards to show any doctor or dentist whom they attend.

14

Swellings of the head and neck

It is important that the dentist has a clear appreciation of the various disorders that may be responsible for producing swellings in relation to the head or neck, and they are summarized in this chapter. Diseases of the salivary glands (see Ch. 9), of the thyroid gland (see Ch. 13), and certain disorders affecting the lymph nodes (see Ch. 12) have already been dealt with.

Physical examination of swellings of the head and neck

The precise anatomical situation of the swelling is important. It is particularly important to note whether the swelling is attached to surrounding tissue and to determine the plane in which it lies. Skin swellings are most likely to be sebaceous cysts or boils whereas lesions infiltrating the skin are much more likely to be cancerous in origin.

Thyroid swellings (see Ch. 13) occur below or on either side of the thyroid cartilage and move on swallowing. Thyroglossal cysts on the other hand lie in the midline but also move on swallowing or on protrusion of the tongue.

The common lateral swelling in the neck is due to lymph node enlargement but in the upper third of the neck anterior to the sterno-mastoid muscle branchial cyst must be considered.

Submandibular swellings characteristically appear just below the body of the mandible and swellings of the parotid gland behind the angle of the mandible and anterior to the mastoid process. If there is intermittent obstruction to a salivary duct, the relevant gland becomes tense and enlarged after a meal.

The *consistency* of the swelling is important, as is its *shape*. These may give a clue to its origin and to the cystic nature or otherwise of the swelling. Fluctuation can often be very difficult to elicit in the neck but tenderness usually indicates inflammation. The only neck swelling that transilluminates brilliantly is a cystic hygroma.

Branchial fistula and branchial cyst

These two conditions are congenital in origin and arise from the remnant of the second branchial cleft. The lowermost opening of the remnant of this cleft is at the anterior border of the sterno-mastoid muscle just behind and below the angle of the jaw. The track of the remnant then passes upwards between the internal and external carotid arteries and its inner opening is located in the region of the tonsil.

A branchial fistula stretching from the tonsillar fossa to the skin is most unusual. More commonly there is a sinus opening anteriorly, lined with squamous and occasionally columnar epithelium. The opening of the track may be tiny and only as the child grows and the track becomes infected does the orifice become evident, usually because of an intermittent discharge. Treatment is by excision of the entire track.

A branchial cyst is lined by squamous epithelium and the fluid contains cholesterol crystals. The cyst lies in the track of the second branchial cleft and presents in adult life protruding from the anterior border of the sterno-mastoid muscle. There may be a fibrous track passing upwards as in branchial fistula. Infection may occur particularly if attempts are made to aspirate the cyst. Treatment is again by complete excision.

Thyroglossal cyst

This is a cystic remnant in the length of the thyroglossal tract stretching from the junction of the anterior two-thirds with the posterior one-third of the tongue to the thyroid gland in the midline. The cyst lies anywhere in the midline above the thyroid cartilage and moves on swallowing or on protrusion of the tongue.

The track of the cyst runs anterior to and then curls up for a short distance behind the hyoid bone before descending to the thyroid gland. Excision of the cyst involves removal of the track; this often necessitating removal of the central portion of the hyoid bone.

Cystic hygroma. This is a multilocular cyst, often very large, and consists of a cavernous lymphangioma. The majority of cases present in early childhood or indeed may be evident at birth. Unlike many other swellings of the neck, a common site is in the posterior triangle or supraclavicular region. There are often deep extensions even reaching into the chest or axilla, and excision can be extremely difficult.

Skin lesions of the head and neck

Boils and carbuncles are extremely common, especially on the back of the neck, and the scalp is the most common site of the sebaceous cyst. This is a cystic swelling lying in the skin and lined by a squamous epithelium. The cyst arises from the sebaceous glands related to the hairs and may occur anywhere on hair-growing areas of the body. The cyst is filled with sebum and there is always a small orifice (punctum) visible on the surface. Sebaceous cysts commonly become infected and discharge intermittently. Treatment is by surgical excision.

Skin tumours have been dealt with elsewhere (see Ch. 6) but it should be remembered that nearly all varieties of the common skin tumours occur very frequently about the face.

Cervical lymphadenopathy

Swellings of the cervical lymph nodes are of great importance to the dentist. Some of these have already been referred to in discussing disorders of the haemopoietic system (see Ch. 12). The following

are common causes of lymph node enlargement in the neck.

Lymphadenitis

The cervical lymph nodes and in particular the submental, submandibular, and jugulodigastric glands are commonly infected from inflammatory lesions of the scalp and face, the tongue, oral cavity, nasal cavity, tonsils, and pharynx. The infected nodes are swollen, painful, and tender to touch, and as the inflammation progresses, they become adherent. Abscess formation may occur with the formation of fluctuant swellings and reddening of the skin, and the abscesses may discharge spontaneously.

Diagnosis is dependent on tracing the source of infection and this involves full examination of the head and neck, including a detailed examination of the teeth. Treatment consists of attention to the source of infection and appropriate antibiotic therapy. Abscess cavities in the neck may require incision and drainage. Long-continued chronic infected foci, as for instance a chronic periapical abscess, may result in chronically enlarged slightly tender cervical nodes which may resolve on appropriate treatment of the primary source of infection.

Tuberculous and syphilitic lymphadenitis (see Ch. 1) and lymphadenopathy due to HIV infection (see Ch. 2) have already been discussed.

Glandular fever

This is an important cause of lymph node enlargement, the main diagnostic points being the blood picture, the Paul–Bunnell test, and serology for the Epstein–Barr virus.

German measles or rubella

This may similarly be associated with enlargement of the glands in the upper part of the posterior chain of cervical lymph nodes.

Lymphoma and leukaemia

Cervical lymph node adenopathy is commonly seen in acute leukaemia, being due partly to the leukaemia per se and partly to the infection that occurs in the mouth and throat in these cases. The main diagnostic points are the presence of anaemia, bruising, and the characteristic blood and marrow findings. Cervical lymph node enlargement is common in chronic lymphatic leukaemia, and examination of the blood yields a diagnosis readily. Lymph node enlargement is much less common in other leukaemias.

The various forms of lymphoma may also lead to enlargement of the glands of the neck, and differentiation is on the basis of histological features.

Secondary carcinoma

The cervical lymph nodes are commonly enlarged as a result of a secondary spread from cancer anywhere in the upper alimentary or upper respiratory tracts. It is important to recognize that enlargement of the supraclavicular group of nodes, particularly on the left, can occur in cancer of the stomach or pancreas. Diagnosis involves appropriate investigation of the alimentary or respiratory tract, and excision biopsy with histology is often necessary.

Carotid body tumour

This is a tumour arising from the carotid body at the bifurcation of the common carotid artery. It is a slowly growing tumour and may occlude the carotid vessels.

The tumour does not move on swallowing and characteristically pulsates and is mobile in a horizontal but not in a vertical plane. Treatment is by surgical removal.

15

Disorders of nutrition and metabolism

It is important, for several reasons, that the dentist should have a clear understanding of what constitutes a well-balanced diet.

1. Proper nutrition throughout childhood is an essential factor in the development of sound primary and secondary teeth.

2. Dietary factors are of definite importance in regard to the causation and prevention of dental caries.

3. Several deficiency disorders have important manifestations in the buccal cavity.

4. Resistance to infection, including dental infection, is lowered in states of faulty nutrition and the powers of recovery from illness are impaired.

A sound diet may be defined as that which enables the body to develop to its full potentiality, yields sufficient energy for work and play, maintains the bodyweight at a proper level, and aids in keeping the individual in good health. The constituents of a well-balanced diet are protein, fat, carbohydrate, minerals, vitamins, water, and electrolytes.

CALORIE CONTENT

It is generally recommended that a young healthy adult male, of average weight, engaged in an occupation entailing moderate physical effort, should have an intake of about 3000 calories per day. The comparable figure for a young housewife is about 500 calories less. It should be appreciated that these are average figures and that there are considerable individual variations in energy expenditure among persons engaged in apparently similar occupations.

An increased calorie intake is required for those doing heavy manual work, during infection, during pregnancy and lactation, in hyperthyroidism, and in cold climates. Thus some heavy manual workers require about 5000 calories per day. The calorie requirements decrease with advancing years.

One may calculate the calorie content of the diet in a simple way by remembering the following approximate figures.

1 gram carbohydrate	yields 4 calories
1 gram protein	yields 4 calories
1 gram fat	yields 9 calories

Protein

Protein, which is composed of amino acids, is an essential constituent of all living cells. A certain intake is therefore necessary for growth, for the replacement of tissues, and also for the formation of some enzymes and hormones. Those amino acids which are termed 'essential' cannot be readily synthesized by the body from other sources whereas the 'nonessential' amino acids can be. The essential amino acids are eight in number — lysine, tryptophan, phenylalanine, leucine, isoleucine, threonine, methionine, and valine. Protein foodstuffs which supply all the essential amino acids are classified as first-class protein; those lacking some of the essential amino acids are referred to as second-class proteins.

For the average adult the protein intake probably should not be less than 60–70 g per day. A higher intake is required in pregnancy and lactation. In children the figure is relatively higher because of the demands of growth. The main animal sources of protein are meat, fish, milk and milk products, and eggs; peas, beans, lentils, oatmeal, and soya beans are good vegetable sources.

Kwashiorkor is a disease caused by gross protein deficiency in children. It is widespread in Africa. The main features are wasting, severe liver dysfunction, oedema, and failure to thrive.

FAT

Fat is important in the diet because it is a rich source of calories, it contains some fatty acids which are essential for health, and it contains the important fat-soluble vitamins A, D and K. The wide use of fat for cooking renders many foods more palatable. The amount of fat in the diet varies considerably according to individual taste, to racial customs, to the time of year, and to the climate. In Britain a daily intake of around 100 g per day is common. The intake is usually higher in cold countries.

Fat may be of animal origin such as meat and milk products, or vegetable origin such as margarine and many cooking fats. The possible role of a high animal fat intake in the pathogenesis of coronary artery disease has already been referred to (see Ch. 7).

CARBOHYDRATE

Carbohydrate is the main source of energy in the diet and the daily intake should depend largely on the required calorie expenditure. Obesity inevitably results if an excess is taken.

Given a protein and fat intake of 70–100 and 100–120 g per day respectively, this leaves approximately 1600 calories to be supplied by carbohydrate, i.e. an intake of about 400 g.

Carbohydrate foods are less expensive than either protein or fat and their proportion in the diet usually increases as the family income falls. Main sources of carbohydrates are potatoes, sugar, bread, other flour products such as buns, scones, biscuits, cakes, jams and other preserves.

MINERALS

Iron

Iron is an essential constituent of haemoglobin.

The daily requirement is about 12–15 mg. A considerably greater amount of iron is present in an average diet, but the body absorbs from the gut only what it needs. The principal dietary sources of iron are meat, fish, egg yolk, and green vegetables.

Deficiency of iron leads to hypochromic anaemia which is fully discussed in the chapter on blood diseases.

Calcium

Calcium is required for the formation of bone and teeth. It also regulates neuromuscular excitability and, if the level of calcium in the blood falls, tetany may be produced (see Ch. 13). In addition, calcium is one of the factors necessary for the coagulation of the blood.

The chief sources of calcium are milk, milk products such as butter and cheese, cereals, green vegetables, and eggs. The average adult requires about 0.75 g calcium per day and up to twice this amount in pregnancy and lactation.

About 25% of the calcium in the food is absorbed from the small intestine. Absorption is largely controlled by vitamin D and the parathyroid glands. Deficient absorption occurs if there is inadequate intake of vitamin D or if the hydroxylation of vitamin D in the kidney to its active metabolite is deficient as a consequence of chronic renal disease. Calcium absorption may also be impaired if there is defective absorption of fat (steatorrhoea) due to the fact that the inabsorbed fats combine with the dietary calcium to form insoluble soaps. It can be shown in experimental animals that phytic acid decreases calcium absorption although the significance of this in human dietetics is debated. Calcium carbonate is added to bread made from flour with a high phytic acid content, as a precautionary measure.

The blood level of calcium is normally 2.2–2.6 mmol per litre. The calcium level bears an inverse relationship with the serum phosphorus level so that the product Ca:P tends to remain a constant.

Iodine

Iodine is an essential constituent of thyroxine, the

hormone of the thyroid gland. The daily require-ment is about 0.25 mg. Normal sources of iodine are drinking water, fish, and vegetables. De-ficiency of dietary iodine is an important cause of simple goitre.

Phosphorus

Phosphorus, like calcium, is an essential constit-uent of bone and teeth. The diet should contain 1–2 g per day and the requirement is increased in pregnancy and lactation. Phosphorus is found in similar foodstuffs as calcium, and a diet adequate in the one mineral will be adequate in the other.

The normal serum inorganic phosphate level is 0.8–1.4 mmol per litre. Organic phosphate is to be found mainly within the cells where it is the principal anion. The organic intracellular phos-phates are connected with energy exchange and with the metabolism of fats and carbohydrate. The cells also contain phosphorus in the nucleopro-teins, phosphoproteins, and phospholipids.

Fluoride

Fluoride is a substance with a considerable dental interest. It is present in the bones and teeth, especially the dentine, in higher concentration than in other tissues of the body. The arguments for and against fluoridation of water supplies will be well known to the dental student and need not be repeated in this text.

WATER AND ELECTROLYTES

Water

It will be seen from a study of Figure 15.1 that water comprises more than half of the total bodyweight. The amount in the average adult is approximately 40 litres, of which 25 litres is within the cells and 15 litres is extracellular.

The water intake is derived from fluid drunk and from the water content of food. To this must be added the metabolic water derived from the oxidation of foodstuffs. The total water available from those sources is, on average, about $2\frac{1}{2}$ litres per day. This intake is balanced by insensible loss of water from the skin and lungs, by the urine, and by the faecal water.

In health, the body does its own regulating, largely through the medium of thirst and variation in urinary volume, but in diseases these mechan-isms may be deranged. It is of critical importance

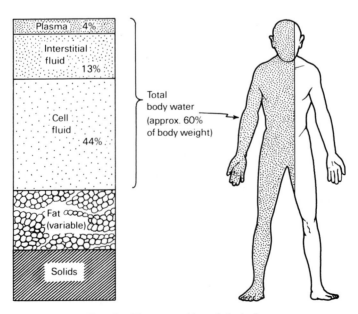

Fig. 15.1 The composition of the body.

to maintain a proper fluid balance in all who are ill.

Salt

Sodium and chloride are widely distributed through the body and, in health, their concentrations are kept within narrow limits. Sodium is the principal cation of the extracellular fluid and is one of the main agents responsible for controlling the acid–base balance of the body. Chloride is the main anion of the extracellular fluid.

The normal salt intake is about 5–15 g per day but there is considerable individual variation. The main route for salt excretion is the urine. Excess sweating may be an appreciable factor in very hot atmospheres and salt depletion is now known to be the cause of 'heat exhaustion'. Very large amounts of salt may be lost by diarrhoea and vomiting as in cholera and dysentery. The hormones of the adrenal cortex play an important part in regulating salt metabolism, and abnormal salt loss in the urine is a characteristic feature of Addison's disease.

Potassium

Potassium is the principal cation of the intracellular fluid. Hypokalaemia causes a form of muscle paralysis while hyperkalaemia leads to impaired cardiac function which may prove suddenly fatal.

THE VITAMINS

Historical

Probably the first clear-cut demonstration of the relationship between deficiency of foodstuffs and the development of a specific disease was the work of James Lind, the British naval surgeon. His *A Treatise of the Scurvy* published in 1753 showed clearly the value of fresh fruit in preventing scurvy among the crews of sailing ships and his work was responsible for the introduction of fruit juice in seamen's rations. The subsequent compulsory issue of lime juice in the British Merchant Service led to the use, by Americans, of the term 'limeys' for British seamen; it is still sometimes employed, often in a derogatory sense, for the English.

In the early years of this century, Hopkins and Funk published separate papers dealing with certain accessory food factors which were necessary for life. Funk coined the name 'vitamine' in the belief that the substances were amines; the 'e' was later dropped when it became apparent that this was not so. A tremendous amount of knowledge has now accumulated about the vitamins and they have been tried, often quite irrationally, as therapeutic agents, in practically every disease. Their use is indicated only where there is definite deficiency or at least a reasonable suspicion of deficiency.

Definition

Vitamins may be defined as organic substances that are essential for normal growth and the maintenance of health, are effective in very small amounts, do not yield energy directly, but are essential for the transformation of energy.

Classification of the vitamins

1. *Water-soluble vitamins*
   a. Vitamin B complex, the more important components being thiamine, riboflavine, nicotinic acid, vitamin B_{12}, and folic acid.
   b. Vitamin C or ascorbic acid.
2. *Fat-soluble vitamins*
   a. Vitamin A.
   b. Vitamin D.
   c. Vitamin K.

Normal requirements

The average daily requirements of vitamins are given in Table 15.1. These are increased in pregnancy, lactation, and childhood. The figures are internationally accepted and, owing to American influence, they are generous by the standards of many countries.

Causes of deficiency

Vitamin deficiency may result from one or more of the following causes:

1. *Inadequate intake.* This may be due to eco-

nomic factors, faulty cooking (especially vitamin C), food faddism, and alcoholism.

2. *Diminished absorption from the gut*. This may be caused by steatorrhoea, in which case the deficiency is multiple, or the absence of bile from the gut, in which case the deficiency is limited to the fat-soluble vitamins.

3. *Increased requirements*. There is an increased requirement for vitamins in infection, pregnancy, lactation, and hyperthyroidism.

4. *Impaired synthesis*. Antibiotic or sulphonamide therapy may lead to the destruction of the bacteria in the gut which normally synthesize vitamins of the B complex.

The vitamin B group

The vitamin B complex is now known to comprise at least 12 individual components, but only thiamine, riboflavine, and nicotinic acid are considered here. Vitamin B_{12} and folic acid are described in the chapter on blood diseases.

All the components of this group of vitamins are concerned with fundamental enzyme systems which control the later stages of energy production and cellular metabolism. Good plant sources of vitamin B are yeast, peas, beans, and grain, while satisfactory animal sources are egg yolk, liver, and milk. A simple and relatively inexpensive way to ensure a high intake of all the vitamin B group is to give three or four yeast tablets three times daily.

Thiamine (aneurine or vitamin B_1)

Deficiency of thiamine produces a disorder termed *beriberi* which is endemic in the Far East in people who live almost exclusively on highly polished rice. Beriberi has two main forms. The principal feature of wet beriberi is cardiac failure with oedema and dyspnoea. Dry beriberi is characterized by a severe polyneuritis with muscle wasting, paralysis, and limb pains; in severe cases mental confusion is present.

Riboflavine (vitamin B_2)

Riboflavine is especially concerned with the metabolism of the cells of the buccal cavity, cornea, and skin. Deficiency causes glossitis, the tongue often being magenta in colour, angular stomatitis, increased vascularity of the cornea producing photophobia and keratitis, and a scaly, greasy change in the skin around the nose, lips, and ears.

Nicotinic acid (niacin)

Deficiency of nicotinic acid produces a disorder termed *pellagra*; the word is derived from the Italian for rough skin 'pelle agra'. Pellagra is endemic in areas where maize, which may contain a toxic factor, is the staple item of diet. The main features are dermatitis, maximal in areas exposed to light, diarrhoea, and mental confusion progressing to complete dementia.

Occurrence of vitamin B deficiency

It is more common to see cases showing deficiency of several of the components of the B complex rather

Table 15.1 Recommended daily dietary allowance of vitamins

	Vitamin A i.u.	Thiamine mg	Riboflavine mg	Nicotinic acid mg	Ascorbic acid mg	Vitamin D i.u.
Moderately active man	5000	1.5	1.8	15	25	*
Moderately active woman	5000	1.2	1.5	12	25	*
Woman in pregnancy or lactation	6–8000	1.5	2.5–3.0	15	100–150	400
Child up to 12 years†	2–5000	.0.4–1.2	0.6–1.8	4–12	30–75	400
Child over 12 years	5000	1.3–1.7	1.8–2.5	12–17	80–100	400

* It is doubtful if the average adult requires to supplement from dietary sources the vitamin D derived from the skin.
† The requirements in childhood increase progressively with age.

than isolated deficiencies. Furthermore, there is often a deficiency of other substances, e.g. protein, iron, and minerals.

Vitamin B deficiency may occur as follows:

1. Endemic in certain areas of the world due to dietary inadequacy.

2. In special circumstances of deprivation such as Japanese POW camps in the 1940–45 war, famine, and drought.

3. Secondary to absorption defects such as steatorrhoea.

4. In chronic alcoholics in whom it is largely responsible for the mental symptoms of delirium tremens.

5. As a complication of antibiotic therapy.

Vitamin C

Sources

Vitamin C, or ascorbic acid, is present in good concentration in fresh fruits and in green vegetables. Although relatively small quantities are present in potatoes, we obtain a substantial proportion of our vitamin C requirements from this source because of the amount eaten. Vitamin C is destroyed by overcooking and by alkalis. The basic requirements are 25–30 mg per day.

Functions

Vitamin C is essential for the formation of intercellular substances in connective tissues, capillary walls, bone, and dentine. It plays a part in the development of red blood cells although its precise role is uncertain. Vitamin C is also concerned with the reactions of the body to infection and stress; in this connection it may be noted that it is present in high concentration in the adrenal glands.

Scurvy

Scurvy is caused by a deficiency of vitamin C. It used to be a very serious cause of disease among the crews of sailing vessels, and in the British Navy scurvy was probably responsible for more deaths than enemy action. In large towns such as Glasgow it is now seen particularly in elderly people, especially men, who are living in poor circumstances on a very limited diet often largely consisting of bread and tea. It may be seen occasionally in peptic ulcer patients adhering to a very rigid bland diet without proper supervision.

The main clinical features of scurvy are as follows:

1. Marked loss of energy.

2. Changes in the gums of those who still possess their own teeth. The gums become spongy, swollen, and bleed very readily, e.g. on brushing the teeth or after mastication. The changes are usually first evident in the interdental papillae. Infection of the gums is frequently superimposed leading to halitosis.

3. Bruises after trivial injuries. The bruises may be extensive and very painful. They are most often seen on the legs.

4. Small haemorrhages around the hair follicles especially on the thighs. Roughening of the skin at the base of the hair follicles also occurs (hyperkeratosis).

5. Delayed wound healing and a tendency for recently healed wounds to burst open.

6. A moderate degree of anaemia often largely due to an associated dietary deficiency of iron.

7. Subperiosteal haemorrhages, which may cause considerable pain, are a feature of severe scurvy in infants.

Scurvy responds to intensive treatment with oral vitamin C, e.g. 200 mg three times daily of the synthetic preparation. The essential step in prophylaxis is a liberal intake of properly cooked vegetables and of fresh fruit or fruit juices.

Vitamin A

Sources

Vitamin A is fat-soluble and is present in high concentration in fish liver oils, dairy products, and eggs. Carotene, which is converted to vitamin A in the body, is present in certain vegetables, especially carrots and tomatoes.

Functions

Vitamin A plays an important part in the regulation of the growth of epithelial tissue and is essential for the formation of visual purple.

Deficiency

If there is deficiency of vitamin A the main effect is shown on the epithelial tissues. The skin becomes hardened, scaly and roughened ('toad skin'), the cornea becomes dry (xerophthalmia) and in severe cases ulcerated, and there is impaired vision in the dark causing night blindness.

Vitamin D

Sources

Vitamin D is fat-soluble and, like vitamin A, is found in high concentration in fish liver oils, in dairy products, and in egg yolk. It is also formed in the skin from a precursor, 7-dehydrocholesterol, under the influence of ultraviolet light. It may be prepared synthetically from ergosterol by irradiation.

Functions

Vitamin D is essential for the proper absorption of calcium and phosphorus from the gut and for their subsequent utilization in bone formation. Deficiency leads to rickets in the child and osteomalacia (see Ch. 17) in the adult.

Rickets

Aetiology

Deficiency of vitamin D in the growing child is usually due to a faulty diet. Lack of sunlight often plays an important contributory role. Calcium absorption is impaired and in many cases an associated dietary inadequacy increases the deficiency of this mineral so that there is insufficient calcium for the body's needs. Calcium salts are not deposited in normal amounts in growing cartilage and newly formed bone which remains soft. These changes are particularly evident at sites of very active bone formation such as the ends of long bones and at costochondral junctions. The soft osteoid tissue is liable to be deformed according to external stresses. The lack of calcium also leads to loss of tone in the skeletal muscles and hyperexcitability of the nerves.

Clinical features

The main clinical features (Figs. 15.2 and 15.3) which may be found in florid cases can be grouped as follows:

1. *The limb bones.* The earliest change is thickening of the wrists and ankles due to enlargement of the epiphyses caused by the pull of muscles and tendons. As the child begins to crawl and walk, the softened long bones become curved and deformed.

2. *The pelvis.* The bones of the pelvis become deformed when weight-bearing occurs and in females this causes, in later years, serious mechanical obstruction to child-bearing.

3. *The skull.* Softening of the skull bones of the infant is one of the earliest skeletal changes in rickets. The change is usually most evident in the occipital and parietal regions where it may be relatively easy to depress the softened bone with

Fig. 15.2 Rachitic rosary.

Fig. 15.3 Thickening of wrist in rickets.

finger pressure. Delayed closure of the fontanelles is another important sign. Later there is abnormal thickening of the skull in the region of the frontal and parietal eminences so that the head may have a relatively square shape.

4. *The thorax.* Enlargement of the costochrondral junctions produces a line of swellings along the chest wall termed 'rachitic beading' or the 'rachitic rosary'. The sternum often projects unduly giving the chest a 'pigeon shape', and in severe cases the chest may be almost triangular on cross-section.

5. *The teeth.* Delayed dentition is invariable and the teeth when they appear are poorly calcified.

6. *Other points.* The nutrition may appear quite good owing to a high carbohydrate intake, but rachitic children are usually under-height for their age. The muscle hypotonia leads to a pot belly and weakness of the limbs.

Biochemical changes

The most consistent biochemical change in active rickets is elevation of the serum alkaline phosphatase level. There may be a fall in one or both of the calcium and phosphorus levels.

Radiological changes

The changes are most evident at the lower ends of the radius and ulna. The epiphyseal line becomes irregular or frayed, concave, and splayed out owing to the widening of the bone ends (Fig. 15.4). The bones are less dense than normal. The deformity of the long bones is confirmed. A thin white line develops in the epiphyseal area when healing occurs following treatment.

Prevention and treatment

Severe rickets is now uncommon in Britain due to the general adequacy of nutrition. Less severe rickets still occurs, however, and perhaps especially in immigrant children in whom the dietary intake of vitamin D is inadequate to compensate for the reduced amount derived from the skin in Britain's duller climate.

For the treatment of active rickets vitamin D is usually prescribed (as calciferol) to give a daily

Fig. 15.4 Rickets — irregular, concave, epiphyseal line with widened bone ends.

dose of about 2000 i.u. per day. A satisfactory calcium intake is also required.

Vitamin K

Sources

Vitamin K is fat-soluble. It is found in green plants, especially spinach, and it is formed in the large bowel by the normal bacterial flora.

Functions

Vitamin K is essential for the formation in the liver of coagulation factors II, VII, IX and X (see Ch. 12).

Deficiency

Deficiency of vitamin K often develops in obstructive jaundice because absence of bile from the gut causes impaired absorption of fat, including the fat-soluble vitamin K. Deficiency of factors II, VII, IX and X results and there is undue tendency to bleed with a long prothrombin time.

Uses

Vitamin K should be given by injection before any form of surgery in patients with jaundice. It is an efficient antidote to the oral anticoagulant drugs such as warfarin.

WEIGHT LOSS

The principal conditions which may produce marked loss of weight are listed below. A careful history and physical examination frequently yields a presumptive diagnosis but, in many cases, other investigations are required.

1. Inadequate food. Starvation is now rare in Britain but is a major problem in many areas of the world.
2. Diabetes mellitus.
3. Thyrotoxicosis.
4. Chronic infection, specially tuberculosis and HIV infection.
5. Malignant neoplasm of any site.
6. Obstructive lesions of the alimentary canal (e.g. pyloric stenosis) or impaired absorption (e.g. steatorrhoea).
7. Anorexia nervosa. This psychiatric disorder most often affects girls or young women. There is profound loss of appetite and weight loss.

SIMPLE OBESITY

The term simple obesity is used to describe an excess of fat unassociated with any apparent endocrine disorder. The condition, which is a common one, is more frequent in women and the incidence rises with age.

Aetiology

The basis of simple obesity is always a prolonged intake of calories in excess of the calories expended in energy, a state of affairs graphically described as a plethora of calories. Carbohydrate is the main source of the unnecessary calories.

Many individuals tend to put on weight as they get older because they do not decrease their food intake commensurate with the reduction in physical exercise that normally occurs in middle age and later. In other persons the appetite, for reasons that are not fully understood, is grossly excessive and even though the individual may remain quite active he (or more frequently she) becomes obese. Some consider that gluttony is often determined by psychological factors and that the pleasure derived from excessive eating is a substitute for some deep-seated unsatisfied desire.

Fat people commonly shelter behind the belief that they have some ill-defined glandular upset over which they have no control, but as far as is known at the present time there is no evidence that this is so in the vast majority of cases.

Prognosis

The obese may suffer little disability for many years, apart possibly from breathlessness on exertion and some limitation of physical activity. In middle age and in the later years of life, however, they are much more prone to develop coronary artery disease, gall-bladder disease, diabetes mellitus, cerebrovascular catastrophes, osteoarthritis, and varicose veins. Furthermore, the obese are greater risks for surgical operations and anaesthetics. It is not surprising, therefore, that the expectation of life is distinctly shorter for the obese. Life insurance societies are well aware of this fact and adjust their premiums accordingly.

Treatment

Treatment is extremely simple in principle but often difficult in practice. The calorie intake is reduced principally by cutting down on carbohydrates. A diet yielding about 1000 calories per day with a carbohydrate content not greater than 100 g is satisfactory in most cases until the body weight is near normal; it can then be carefully increased to a level that keeps the weight steady. Even lower calorie intakes may be used but, if so, careful supervision is necessary.

Difficulty arises because many fat people strongly deny that they eat excessively while others have a genuine problem in adhering to the diet. Firm handling of the patient is necessary together with frequent visits and remonstrations.

The use of the amphetamine group of drugs to depress appetite is undesirable; they have serious side-effects and may lead to addiction.

DIABETES MELLITUS

The term diabetes mellitus is derived from two of the cardinal features of the disorder, namely the passage of a large volume of urine which contains glucose. Patients with diabetes mellitus may be divided into three categories:

1. Those in whom the diabetes develops in early life (say up to 40 years), who lose weight, and who require insulin therapy (Type 1 or insulin-dependent diabetes).

2. Those in whom the diabetes develops in later life, who are often obese, and who do not require insulin therapy (Type 2 or non-insulin-dependent diabetes).

3. Diabetes secondary to other diseases, e.g. chronic pancreatitis (see Ch. 10) or Cushing's syndrome (see Ch. 13).

Insulin-dependent diabetes mellitus

Aetiology

The islets of Langerhans in the pancreas lose the ability to produce adequate amounts of insulin. The disorder may develop at any age. A family history is present in about 25% of cases.

As a consequence of insulin deficiency carbohydrate metabolism is seriously affected; the tissues cannot utilize glucose and the liver cannot store glucose as glycogen. The level of glucose in the blood increases (hyperglycaemia) and some of the excess is excreted in the urine. Protein and fat are utilized as sources of energy and wasting therefore occurs. Fat metabolism is also impaired and there is accumulation of ketone bodies which are excreted in the urine and breath.

Clinical features

Polyuria occurs due to the osmotic effect of the sugar present in the urine, and the increased fluid loss causes thirst. Pruritus, or itch, results from irritation of the urinary passages by the sugar.

There is loss of weight and loss of energy. The breath may have the characteristic fruity odour of acetone.

The urine is of high volume, pale, and contains glucose which gives it a high specific gravity. Ketonuria is a feature of severe, uncontrolled cases.

Diagnosis

The urinary findings plus a high blood glucose are usually sufficient to make a diagnosis, but a glucose tolerance test is necessary in doubtful cases. The fasting blood glucose is determined, the patient is given at least 50 g glucose in water to drink, and the blood glucose is estimated at half-hourly intervals for $2\frac{1}{2}$ hours. In the diabetic subject the fasting level is high, the curve rises out with the normal range, and does not return to normal (Fig. 15.5). The normal fasting blood glucose is 4.0–5.5 mmol per litre and the nonfasting range is 5.5–10 mmol per litre.

Complications

Diabetes mellitus, especially if it is poorly controlled, may be associated with complications affecting practically every system. There is a greatly increased liability to sepsis. This may show itself as boils and styes, while, from the dental point of view, infection and hypertrophy of the gingival tissues is important. Oral candidiasis may occur. There is an increased incidence of pulmonary tuberculosis and urinary infections. Atherosclerotic changes occur earlier and more severely in the diabetic, causing an increased tendency to coronary artery disease and peripheral arterial disease with gangrene. Peripheral neuritis is common while the eyes may be affected by cataract (loss of translucency of the lens) and by changes in the retina. Kidney function may be seriously impaired by a special variety of glomerular lesion. Autonomic neuropathy is common and may cause nocturnal diarrhoea, postural hypotension and, in men, impotence.

Prognosis

Despite the formidable list of complications that

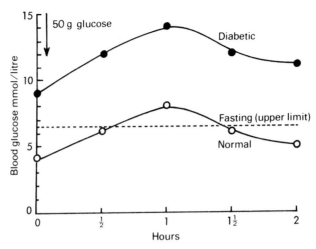

Fig. 15.5 Glucose tolerance curves in a diabetic subject and a normal person.

may afflict the severe and the poorly controlled diabetic, the student should remember that properly regulated insulin therapy now permits the majority of diabetics to live long and useful lives.

Treatment

The basic principle of diabetic treatment is to give a diet yielding sufficient calories for the patient's needs, and sufficient insulin to enable carbohydrate and fat metabolism to proceed normally.

The number of calories required varies with the age, sex, weight, occupation, and personal habits of the patient. The aim should be to keep the bodyweight at, or preferably just below, the ideal bodyweight as it has been found that 'a thin diabetic is healthier than a fat diabetic'. Consideration is given to a proper balance between carbohydrate, fat and protein, particular attention being paid to the carbohydrate content. In most cases, once stabilization has been achieved, it is sufficient for the patient to rely on simple measurements, e.g. an average slice of bread is equivalent to 15 g carbohydrate.

Insulin is given by subcutaneous injection in gradually increasing dosage until glycosuria is controlled. The diabetic must be instructed in the measurement of the dose and self-injection; the majority learn to do this very well. Short-acting insulin, the natural product, may be used for long-term treatment but as it has a short duration of action two or three injections per day are required to ensure diabetic control. A number of longer-acting modified insulins are available which have the advantage that they need be administered only once or twice daily. Insulin is available in different strengths and the patient must be fully aware of this, otherwise serious errors in dosage will occur.

The patient is taught to test the urine or blood for glucose regularly and to keep a careful weight record so that modifications in insulin dosage and diet may be made as required. Patients should attend the diabetic clinic regularly to review adequacy of control and to screen for complications.

Hypoglycaemia

A blood glucose below the lower limit of normal (4.0 mmol per litre) may occur in a diabetic in the following circumstances:

1. An overdose of insulin either through an error in measurement or an error in the strength of insulin.

2. Correct insulin dosage but insufficient food, e.g. due to being late for a meal.

3. Unexpected exercise or emotional upset leading to increased metabolism of glucose.

Symptoms are usually seen when the blood glucose falls below 2.0 mmol per litre.

The early stages of hypoglycaemia are characterized by mental confusion, slurred speech, headache, incoordination of movement, profuse sweating, and a full strong pulse. In some instances there may be confusion with drunkenness, a point of considerable legal importance. Unless corrected at this stage, unconsciousness will follow in all but mild cases. The urine is free from glucose and the blood glucose is low.

If seen and recognized in its early stages, hypoglycaemia responds quickly to the oral administration of carbohydrate, e.g. a glucose drink, sweetened tea, lump sugar, etc. If the patient is unconscious, glucose must be given by intravenous injection. An alternative treatment is to inject intramuscular glucagon, which may be useful in aggressive patients.

Diabetic ketosis or diabetic coma

This is a gross metabolic derangement which develops in diabetes mellitus when insulin dosage is inadequate. It used to be seen as the inevitable terminal event in pre-insulin days. When it occurs now it is usually associated with infection, which increases insulin requirements; in the presence of infection the diabetic should increase insulin dosage, but he may do the reverse because he is eating less due to poor appetite and vomiting.

The features of diabetic ketosis develop over many hours, or even a few days, and not suddenly as in hypoglycaemic coma. Nausea and sickness are prominent and drowsiness merging into coma occurs. The skin and tongue are very dry due to dehydration, the breathing deep due to acidosis, the blood pressure low, and the pulse weak; the breath has the fruity odour of acetone. The urine is loaded with sugar and acetone, and the blood glucose is high.

Diabetic ketosis calls for urgent treatment which is a skilled procedure requiring intravenous soluble insulin and intensive fluid and salt replacement.

Non-insulin-dependent diabetes mellitus

Aetiology

This usually occurs in men or women of middle age and over who have eaten excessively for many years and become progressively more obese. At first the excess carbohydrate is converted into fat and stored as such, but later this mechanism for disposing of unnecessary carbohydrate becomes overwhelmed and the blood glucose rises leading to glycosuria. There does not appear to be a primary deficiency of insulin; the pancreas is doing its best but it simply cannot deal with the prolonged excessive intake of carbohydrate. A family history is more common than in insulin-dependent diabetes.

Clinical features

Polyuria, thirst, and glycosuria are present but, in contrast to the other variety of diabetes, the patient is overweight. The complications mentioned above may occur, but they are usually less prominent.

Treatment

The essential step in treatment is to reduce the carbohydrate content of the diet and to ensure weight reduction, as described under simple obesity. In some patients an oral hypoglycaemic drug such as tolbutamide or glibenclamide may be required. There is a risk of hypoglycaemia with such drugs. As in insulin-dependent diabetes, patients should attend the diabetic clinic regularly for detection of complications and good control.

Surgery in diabetic patients

In patients treated by diet alone, the urine should be regularly tested for glucose in the postoperative period to detect hyperglycaemia. In patients taking insulin or hypoglycaemic drugs, the patient should be admitted to hospital 1–2 days before elective major surgery and the anaesthetist and diabetic physician informed. Control is achieved by multiple injections of short-acting insulins. The operation should be performed in the morning. On the day of surgery intravenous infusion of glucose and insulin is given, the dosage being adjusted according to regular blood glucose monitoring. When the patient is eating after surgery the normal regimen can be resumed.

Other causes of glycosuria

Renal glycosuria

In this disorder the kidneys have a low threshold for glucose, and glycosuria occurs even though the blood sugar level is perfectly normal. No symptoms are associated and the condition usually remains undetected until the individual has some routine medical examination, e.g. for the Armed Services or for insurance purposes. The diagnosis is confirmed by a glucose tolerance test (see Fig. 15.5).

Alimentary glycosuria

After short-circuit operations on the alimentary tract, such as gastroenterostomy, carbohydrate may be more quickly absorbed than normal leading to a transiently high blood glucose after meals. If the urine should be tested at this time it will be found to contain a trace of sugar. The condition is not important.

GOUT

Gout is a disorder of purine metabolism in which there is an accumulation of urates in the blood and the periodic deposition of urate salts in the tissues, especially of the joints. It is more common in men and there is often a family history. Alcohol and diuretic drugs are causal factors.

The individual experiences periodic attacks of acute pain and inflammation in the joints, especially the great toe, and after a time this produces chronic arthritis. Deposits of urates also occur in the subcutaneous tissues, particularly of the ears, causing small firm swellings, termed gouty tophi, which contain a chalky material. The blood uric acid is high. The diagnosis is confirmed by aspiration of the joint and examination for urate crystals.

An acute attack may be relieved by a variety of non-steroidal anti-inflammatory drugs. Further attacks can be prevented or minimized by the regular administration of drugs such as allopurinol which increase the urinary excretion of uric acid.

16

The allergic disorders

The term allergy describes an abnormal form of tissue reaction to a variety of agents (allergens) which in similar amounts are harmless to the majority of individuals. A family history is commonly present in those affected. The range of allergens is extremely wide and includes articles of the diet, microorganisms, drugs, topical applications, various chemicals, and pollens of grasses.

Types of hypersensitivity reaction

Type 1 (anaphylactic hypersensitivity). About 10% of the population produces excessive amounts of IgE antibodies in response to new antigens. In these 'atopic' persons the antibodies attach to mast cells and trigger histamine release which causes vasodilatation and bronchoconstriction. In the most severe form, massive systemic histamine release causes anaphylactic shock with circulatory collapse and severe bronchospasm.

Type 2 (autoimmune hypersensitivity). Antibodies are produced against antigens on the surface of the body's own cells. Complement is activated and the cells are destroyed. This type of reaction is seen in autoimmune haemolytic anaemia and immune thrombocytopenic purpura (see Ch. 12).

Type 3 (immune complex hypersensitivity). At certain ratios of circulating antibody to antigen, immune complexes are formed which deposit in small blood vessels, activate complement, and cause inflammation (vasculitis). This is seen in rheumatic fever, infective endocarditis (see Ch. 7), Henoch—Schönlein purpura (see Ch. 12), rheumatoid arthritis and other connective tissue diseases (see Ch. 17), and serum sickness.

Type 4 (delayed hypersensitivity). This is due to overactive T lymphocytes, and is classically seen in tuberculosis and graft rejection.

HAY FEVER

Hay fever is caused by a type 1 allergy to the windborne pollen of grasses and of some weeds and trees. It is seen especially in young people and it tends to lessen in severity with age. The maximum incidence of the attacks is in the early summer months.

The principal symptoms are a profuse, watery nasal discharge, paroxysms of sneezing, conjunctival irritation and lachrymation, headache and depression.

Those who are severely affected should try to avoid contact with the causative pollen. Specific desensitization by a series of injections of gradually increasing dosage of an extract of the pollen is often valuable. The injections should be started several weeks before the pollen season and may have to be repeated yearly. Beneficial drugs given locally as nasal sprays include sodium cromoglycate (which blocks the release of histamine from mast cells) and corticosteroids. Oral antihistamine drugs have a limited role since they cause drowsiness.

Allergic rhinitis may be due to causes other than hay fever. It is then termed vasomotor rhinitis. The allergens include bacteria and viruses, house dust, and locally applied drugs. The clinical features are essentially the same as in hay fever except that the disorder does not have a seasonal incidence. Nasal polyps (reactive outgrowths of nasal mucosa) can cause obstruction and may require surgical removal.

ASTHMA

Aetiology

In this condition there are recurrent and reversible attacks of acute breathlessness due to intense spasm of the smooth muscle in the walls of the bronchi, swelling of the bronchial mucosa, and an exudate of mucus. These three changes lead to marked interference with the flow of air during inspiration and expiration; expiration is affected to a greater degree since it is a less powerful action.

Many patients can be shown to be abnormally sensitive, or allergic, to various substances commonly inhaled, such as pollens, feathers, animal dander or house-dust mites, or ingested in the food. Both type 1 and type 3 mechanisms may operate. Emotional or psychological factors may also play an important aetiological role. In many instances the precipitating factor is an upper respiratory tract infection. Exercise, alcohol, and drugs such as aspirin may also provoke attacks.

There is frequently a family history of asthma or other allergic condition such as hay fever or urticaria. In late-onset asthma, allergy to external antigens is demonstrated less often.

Clinical features

The typical asthmatic attack is sudden in onset. The patient becomes intensely breathless and inspection shows that the main difficulty is in expiration. There is a short forceful inspiration, aided by the accessory muscles of respiration, followed by a longer, easily heard, wheezing expiration. Expiration is not successful, however, in deflating the chest which becomes distended and fixed in the position of full inspiration. The face is pallid, sweating and anxious while the lips, ears, nose and extremities may show cyanosis. The attack may last from half an hour or so up to several hours. Very prolonged attacks are termed *status asthmaticus*.

Sometimes the bronchospasm is not so severe and the individual is able to get about although he is limited somewhat in his activities because of breathlessness. The wheezing expiration may be readily audible. Asthma may present as recurrent cough rather than breathlessness and wheeze.

Course and prognosis

Childhood asthma sometimes becomes less severe in adult life and may even disappear. In other cases recurrent attacks of asthma occur throughout life and in those patients emphysema is likely to develop leading to severe incapacity.

Treatment

The treatment of asthma may be divided into the control of the acute attack and the general management of the patient.

Should a dentist be faced with the problem of dealing with a patient suffering from an *acute attack* of asthma he should first stop whatever dental procedure is going on, check that the airway is patent, loosen tight clothing around the neck, permit the patient to sit upright, and ensure that the atmosphere in the room is airy and cool. Many asthmatics carry an inhaler containing a bronchodilator drug (e.g. salbutamol, terbutaline) in metered doses. These are beta$_2$-adrenoceptor agonists which reverse bronchoconstriction. Patients should be encouraged to use their inhalers.

In severe or prolonged attacks other measures may have to be employed such as hospital admission, oxygen inhalations with nebulized bronchodilators, the intravenous injection of aminophylline, or a course of steroid drugs. An antibiotic is given if there is any suspicion that infection has precipitated the attack.

A careful history may reveal a substance to which the patient is allergic. He should try to avoid this substance, if possible, or an attempt may be made to desensitize him by the use of repeated injections of gradually increasing amounts of the substance, although the results of this procedure are often rather disappointing. Sodium cromoglycate, given regularly by an inhaler, prevents attacks by preventing histamine release from mast cells. It is useless in treatment of an acute attack. Inhalers of corticosteroids are also helpful in prophylaxis, and do not carry the risks of long-term oral steroids.

DRUG ALLERGY

Allergic reactions may occur to a large number of

drugs and, in some cases, may be serious and even fatal. The incidence is likely to be higher in those with a history of other allergic disorders such as asthma, and possibly in those receiving the drug for long periods of time. The reactions may develop after the first administration of the drug or, sometimes, only after the drug has been given on one or several prior occasions.

Important examples of common drugs that may produce allergic reactions are penicillin, barbiturates, aspirin, and local anaesthetics. Although the percentage of individuals reacting in this way is small, these drugs are used so frequently that the problem is a real one. Prior to their administration it is wise to ask if the patient has had any untoward drug reactions in the past.

Clinical features

Drug allergy may take any of the following forms singly or in combination:

1. *Serum sickness.* A type 3 mechanism causes systemic upset with sickness, fever, joint pains, and lymphadenopathy.

2. *Anaphylactic shock.* Following injection of a drug, massive systemic histamine release causes severe bronchospasm and circulatory collapse.

3. *Skin eruptions* ranging from transient reddening of the skin (erythema) or urticaria to severe exfoliative dermatitis.

4. *Haematological abnormalities* including agranulocytosis, aplastic anaemia, haemolytic anaemia, and thrombocytopenia.

5. *Angioneurotic oedema of the glottis* which may lead to asphyxia.

Treatment

If there is any suspicion that anaphylaxis is developing, the drug should be stopped immediately and an antihistamine preparation given (e.g. chlorpheniramine 10 mg) as well as a corticosteroid (e.g. hydrocortisone 100 mg), both intravenously. The subcutaneous injection of 0.5 – 1 ml of 1 in 1000 solution of adrenaline hydrochloride is a valuable emergency measure in severe cases. The management of cardiac arrest is described in Chapter 7. Prevention of further attacks by avoidance of the causal drug is important for the individual in the future. Allergic reactions should be noted in the patient's medical and dental records, and he should be advised to wear a warning bracelet.

URTICARIA

Aetiology

Urticaria is an allergic reaction of the skin to a variety of factors which include foods such as shellfish, nuts and fruits; drugs and blood products; bacterial infection; and infestation with intestinal parasites. Of dental interest is the view of some authorities that bacterial infection of the teeth and throat is an important cause of chronic urticaria.

Clinical features

Multiple, elevated wheals, which are intensely itchy, develop quickly on the skin. They last from an hour or two to a day or two. In severe cases a systemic upset shown by sickness and fever, and joint pain is associated.

Treatment

This is with antihistamine and, if severe, corticosteroid drugs. Calamine applied to the skin gives symptomatic relief. In chronic or recurrent cases consideration should be given to the possible role of bacterial infection in the mouth and throat.

Angioedema (angioneurotic oedema)

This may accompany urticaria, and the treatment is then identical; adrenaline may be required in severe cases. There is also an hereditary angioedema characterized by recurrent episodes of intense localized subepithelial oedema. The condition may affect many sites but is most serious when the soft tissues of the buccal cavity are affected as obstruction of the airway, with fatal outcome, may result. Physical trauma, which may be relatively minor or even trivial, is the most common precipitating factor and dental extractions, in those afflicted with the disorder, can cause life-threatening attacks. Other precipitating factors include extremes of temperature, infection, and emotional stress (hence the earlier term angioneurotic oedema). This disorder is now known to be due to an inherited defect in the functioning of the complement system and those affected have low serum levels of C_1 esterase inhibitor. The frequency of attacks may be lessened by the oral administration of an anti-fibrinolytic agent such as tranexamic acid or of an anabolic steroid such as danazol. Acute attacks do not respond to adrenaline, antihistamines, or corticosteroids, in contrast to allergic reactions to drugs, etc. (see above), but intravenous administration of freshly frozen plasma, which supplies the deficient complement factor, is beneficial.

CONTACT DERMATITIS

Aetiology

Contact dermatitis is an allergic reaction of the skin to contact with a wide variety of substances. The most important of these include soaps and detergents, antiseptics, local anaesthetics, sulphonamides or antibiotics applied topically, shampoos, cosmetics, hair dyes, dyes applied to fabrics, metals such as nickel and chromium, many chemicals used in manufacturing processes, and some plastics. The disorder is of great importance in industry, while some doctors, dentists, and nurses have the misfortune to react in this manner to substances they would customarily handle in their professional duties.

Clinical features

The initial reaction is swelling and redness of the skin followed by the development of small vesicles which rupture to produce a raw, oozing area. The lesion is itchy and secondary infection from scratching is common. The site of the lesion depends largely on the nature of the causal agent; the back of the hands and the face are common areas.

Treatment

Mild cases may settle once the cause is removed but serious cases require skilled treatment by a dermatologist. A barrier cream is often a helpful prophylactic measure.

STEVENS–JOHNSON SYNDROME

The Stevens–Johnson syndrome is usually considered to be a variant of a generalized allergic skin disorder known as erythema multiforme.

The principal features are the abrupt development, with fever, of ulcerative lesions of the buccal cavity and of the genital area, followed a day or two later by a generalized bullous eruption. The condition is treated by corticosteroids.

ERYTHEMA NODOSUM

Erythema nodosum is characterized by the development of red, tender swellings in the subcutaneous tissues, especially over the front of the lower legs. It is an allergic reaction to several processes including haemolytic streptococcal infection of the throat, tuberculosis, sarcoidosis, and some drugs.

17

Musculoskeletal and connective tissue disorders, including fractures

OSTEOMALACIA AND OSTEOPOROSIS

The first stage in bone formation is the laying down by the osteoblasts of an extracellular matrix, termed the osteoid, which is composed of nitrogenous substances. This is followed by the deposition in the osteoid of calcium salts, i.e. calcification.

Osteoporosis

Osteoporosis is characterized by a decrease in the bone matrix. There is no detectable abnormality of calcium or phosphorus metabolism and the blood levels of these substances, and of the alkaline phosphatase, are normal. Osteoporosis may occur in the following circumstances:

1. After disuse as in prolonged immobilization.

2. In old age probably as the result of androgen deficiency.

3. In many women after the menopause due to oestrogen deficiency.

4. In malnutrition due to deficiency of the nitrogenous components of the matrix.

5. In thyrotoxicosis due to increased metabolic demands.

6. Where there is an excess of certain steroid hormones of the adrenal cortex as in Cushing's syndrome or prolonged steroid therapy.

7. In fragilitas ossium, or osteogenesis imperfecta, which is a rare congenital disorder characterized by osteoporosis, multiple pathological fractures, hypermotility of the joints, deafness due to otosclerosis, and blue sclerae; dentine formation is usually defective and the teeth are malformed and prone to caries (dentinogenesis imperfecta).

The principal bones involved in osteoporosis are the vertebrae, the pelvis, and the long bones. Radio-logical studies show increased translucency, thining of the cortex and, in many cases, compression collapse of the vertebral bodies. Back pain and kyphosis due to collapse of thoracic vertebrae are common features. Fractures of the wrist or femoral neck are common, especially in older women. Characteristically the skull does not show radiological changes and the lamina dura around the teeth are not affected.

The main therapeutic aspects are correction of causal factors and the provision of a well-balanced diet with adequate calcium and protein (e.g. 500 ml milk per day). Women with premature menopause should be given replacement oestrogen therapy in physiological doses. No curative treatment is available for osteogenesis imperfecta.

Osteomalacia

Osteomalacia is due to defective deposition of calcium and phosphorus in the developing bone matrix of the adult. Rickets is the comparable condition in the child. The abnormality of calcium and phosphorus may be due to:

1. Dietary inadequacy of calcium and vitamin D combined with lack of exposure to sunlight (e.g. in Asian people living in Britain, in house-bound elderly people).

2. Defective absorption of calcium and vitamin D as in steatorrhoea.

3. Renal disorders which lead to chronic renal failure.

In most varieties of osteomalacia the serum calcium is low and the alkaline phosphatase high. The skeleton is much softer than normal and deformity of the weight-bearing bones commonly ensues. Bone pain and tenderness are usually present. The bones show increased translucency and, unlike in osteoporosis, this may be apparent in the skull where the lamina dura around the teeth may be absent. Muscle weakness causes a waddling gait.

Treatment varies to some extent with the cause but, in general, correction of any deficiency of calcium and provision of a vitamin D preparation which promotes calcium absorption are indicated.

PAGET'S DISEASE (OSTEITIS DEFORMANS)

Paget's disease is a chronic bone disorder, of unknown aetiology, which is common in elderly people. The long bones (Fig 17.1) the pelvis, the skull, and the spine are chiefly affected.

The initial process appears to be a patchy decalcification leading to areas of softening and this is followed by a rather disorderly recalcification. As a result of these two processes the affected bones are considerably thickened and deformed. In severe cases pathological fractures may occur.

The skull becomes enlarged and the face may become deformed by involvement of the maxillae and mandible. Rarely a 'leonine' appearance results. Changes in the bone around the roots of the teeth may cause their partial destruction. Bowing and deformity of the legs are commonly present. Involvement of the spine leads to kyphosis and a stooping posture. The only biochemical abnor-

Fig. 17.1 Advanced Paget's disease of the tibia showing a pathological fracture.

Fig. 17.2 Achondroplastic child with normal child of same age.

mality is an increased serum alkaline phosphatase. Radiological studies show areas of decalcification, areas of increased density, thickening of the cortex, and deformity. Osteosarcoma is a rare complication.

No generally effective treatment is available but calcitonin may produce some improvement in certain cases. Regular analgesics may be required to relieve the discomfort which many of these patients experience. If the jaws are markedly involved the teeth may have to be extracted, dentures refashioned, and excess bone removed.

ACHONDROPLASIA

Achondroplasia (Fig. 17.2) is an hereditary disorder of the skeleton due to defective cartilage growth and endochondral bone formation. The individual is dwarfed due to marked shortening of the limb bones. The gait is waddling. The limbs are often very powerful and muscular and the fingers short and thick. The trunk is relatively normal in size while the head is often rather enlarged.

The lips are thickened and the bridge of the nose sunken.

OSTEOARTHRITIS

In osteoarthritis, or degenerative arthritis, the cartilage which normally provides a smooth articular surface becomes thinned, irregular, and eventually worn away. The exposed bone becomes hardened and eburnated and bony outgrowths (osteophytes) tend to form at the articular margins producing 'lipping'. The weight-bearing joints, especially the hips, knees, and small joints of the spine, are mainly involved.

Aetiology

Minor osteoarthritic changes may be noted radiologically in a considerable proportion of elderly individuals and, to some extent, may be taken as a more or less inevitable accompaniment of ageing. More severe degrees of osteoarthritis are often largely caused by the abnormal strain which obesity throws on the weight-bearing joints. In

other instances faulty weight-bearing such as may occur after a badly aligned fracture or direct damage to the joint by a fracture extending into the joint and leaving residual distortion, are responsible. Malocclusion of the bite may cause osteoarthritis of the temporo-mandibular joint (see Ch. 18).

Clinical features

The dominant symptoms are stiffness and pain in the affected joints, and these are usually worse when movement occurs after a period of rest. In severe cases pain may be almost continuous. There are no signs of inflammation around the joint and no constitutional upset as shown by fever, anaemia, or elevation of the erythrocyte sedimentation rate. Small bony outgrowths, called Heberden's nodes, develop on the dorsal aspect of the terminal joints of the fingers in many cases (Fig. 17.3).

Fig. 17.3 Heberden's nodes.

Treatment

The main principles of treatment are correction of any aetiological factor such as obesity, the provision of a suitable analgesic drug such as aspirin, paracetamol or codeine, and the use of physiotherapy to improve joint function. In severe cases surgery may offer relief, particularly for osteoarthritis of the hip or knee joint. The joints are either realigned or in the case of hip the insertion of a prosthesis to form a new hip joint (replacement arthroplasty) is possible. Such developments are now feasible in the knee joint also. Occasionally, surgical fusion of the joint (arthrodesis) is necessary.

RHEUMATOID ARTHRITIS

Rheumatoid arthritis is a chronic disorder characterized by inflammatory changes in the synovial membrane, the capsule, and the surrounding soft tissues of the joints, leading to progressive destruction of the joint structures, deformity, and loss of function. The condition occurs at all ages and women are affected about three times more frequently than men. The aetiology is unknown.

Clinical features

The main joints involved are the small joints of the hand, wrists and feet, with the elbows and knees being next in order of incidence. In contrast to osteoarthritis there is local evidence of an inflammatory process revealed by tenderness and swelling of the affected joints. There is also evidence of a constitutional upset shown by pyrexia, elevation of the erythrocyte sedimentation rate, anaemia and loss of weight (Fig. 17.4). Morning stiffness is characteristic.

Movement of the joints is limited at first largely by pain and swelling, later by fibrous ankylosis, and still later by bony ankylosis. Progress of the condition is characterized by periods of activity, as shown by exacerbation of joint pain and constitutional disturbance, and periods of relative inactivity.

The appearance of the hands is often sufficiently characteristic to permit a diagnosis to be made at a glance (Fig. 17.5). The interphalangeal joints of the

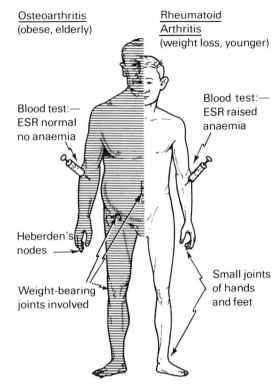

Fig. 17.4 Difference between osteoarthritis and rheumatoid arthritis.

fingers are enlarged and there is wasting of the intermediate soft tissues of the fingers leading to a spindle-shaped deformity. The finger joints are usually held slightly flexed, the patient is unable to close the fist properly, and the grip is weakened.

Fig. 17.5 Rheumatoid arthritis.

Fig. 17.6 Rheumatoid nodule in region of elbow.

Ulnar deviation of the hand at the wrist is commonly present.

Marked involvement of the knee joints may, in the absence of vigorous treatment, lead to the joints becoming fixed in a position of semi-flexion and the patient becomes bedridden; similar deformity may occur in the elbow joints. In some cases firm, painless nodules develop in the subcutaneous tissues, especially around the elbows (Fig. 17.6). Temporomandibular joint involvement is discussed in Chapter 18, and Sjögren's syndrome in Chapter 9.

Prognosis

Rheumatoid arthritis is a chronic disease which leads to serious disablement in a minority of cases. The disorder is particularly disabling should it affect those whose livelihood depends on use of the hands, e.g. dentists.

Treatment

No specific treatment exists for rheumatoid arthritis. Most authorities agree that the following measures are applicable to all cases and that their long-term use will help to control the disease and lessen disablement:

1. The use of *analgesics* to control the pain and stiffness of the joints (e.g. paracetamol, aspirin) and 'first-line' non-steroidal anti-inflammatory drugs (NSAIDs, e.g. aspirin, ibuprofen). NSAIDs act by inhibiting prostaglandin synthesis. Their main side-effect is gastric erosion and bleeding, which is common in older patients and can be prevented by use of an H_2-receptor blocking drug (see Ch. 9). NSAIDs do not affect the course of the disease.

2. The employment of *physiotherapy* to prevent deformity of the joints and to maintain as full a range of movement as possible. Heat and exercises are the main measures. Splinting may also be required.

3. The use of *rest* when the disease process is active, care being taken to avoid stiffness and loss of joint function from immobility.

4. Attention to the *general health* including the provision of a nutritious diet and the correction of anaemia.

Several 'second-line' drugs have been tried in the hope that they might have a specific effect on the disease process but none is curative. Examples are gold, which is given in a course of intramuscular injections; penicillamine; immunosuppressive drugs (e.g. azathioprine); and corticosteroids. Corticosteroids should be used only if the disease is actively progressing despite the use of the other measures referred to. If any of these drugs is employed, the patient should be under careful medical supervision by a rheumatologist as there are important toxic effects.

Surgical removal of the inflamed synovial membrane in the early stages of the disorder (synovectomy) is producing encouraging results in some cases, while surgical correction of established joint deformities can be of considerable value in long-standing severe cases. Joint replacement, even of the finger joints, is frequently performed.

Psoriatic arthropathy

An arthritis of the hands similar to that of rheumatoid arthritis occurs in patients with the common skin disorder, psoriasis. The distal joints are often affected and the fingernails pitted.

Ankylosing spondylitis

Ankylosing spondylitis is a disorder of unknown aetiology which has its maximum incidence in young men. It is strongly associated with the human leucocyte antigen type B27.

The small joints of the spine, especially in the lumbosacral region, and the sacro-iliac joints become affected by pathological changes similar to those of rheumatoid arthritis. In addition, there is a tendency for calcification to develop in the intervertebral ligaments leading to characteristic radiological appearances of the spine (bamboo spine).

The main symptoms are pain and progressive stiffness of the back. The normal thoracic curvature of spine becomes exaggerated and the patient develops an increasingly bent-forward posture. Eventually the spine may become entirely rigid. Treatment is with NSAIDs and physiotherapy.

Other forms of arthritis

Several other forms of arthritis are merely local expressions of some systemic disorder or infection which is described elsewhere.

1. Arthritis due to infection, e.g. tuberculosis, gonorrhoea, *Staph. aureus. Reiter's syndrome* is an immune reaction following infections such as non-gonococcal urethritis or Shigella dysentery (see Ch. 1). Like ankylosing spondylitis it commonly involves persons with human leucocyte antigen type B27. It consists in arthritis (usually of leg joints), conjunctivitis, and urethritis; mouth ulcers and pustules on the soles of the feet may occur. Treatment is with tetracycline and NSAIDs.

2. Arthritis associated with rheumatic fever (see Ch. 7).

3. Arthritis due to a metabolic disorder such as gout (see Ch. 15).

4. Arthritis due to recurrent bleeding into joints as in haemophilia (see Ch. 12).

5. Arthritis due to neurological conditions that cause loss of sensation in the joint structures, e.g. the Charcot joints of tabes dorsalis (see Ch. 1).

SOFT TISSUE RHEUMATISM

Fibrositis, or soft tissue rheumatism, is a very common disorder. Exposure to draughts, a sudden chilling or wetting, chronic muscular strain, and upper respiratory infections are all well-known predisposing factors, but the nature of the soft tissue changes is obscure.

The principal clinical features are aching pain, stiffness, and tenderness in the muscles and related soft tissues. Any of the fibromuscular tissues may be affected but the more common sites are the lumbar area (lumbago), the shoulder, and the neck.

The main aspects of treatment are the provision of rest, warmth, and analgesics. Injection of local anaesthetic and/or corticosteroids into the affected area may give valuable symptomatic relief.

COLLAGEN DISORDERS

The connective tissue of the body, which provides a framework of considerable stability, is composed of fibres largely formed of protein, set in a polysaccharide ground substance. Collagen is one of the main protein constituents of connective tissue representing about 30% of the total body protein.

The collagen disorders are characterized by extensive fibrinoid degeneration of collagen. The clinical manifestations are varied and usually involve many organs, as might be expected from the widespread distribution of connective tissue in the body, but certain features tend to be common to all: a more or less profound constitutional upset, elevation of the plasma globulin level, and marked acceleration of the erythrocyte sedimentation rate. Corticosteroid drugs are of value in treatment but are not curative.

Examples of collagen disorders are systemic lupus erythematosus, in which there is often a red rash on the cheeks, polyarteritis nodosa, in which there are widespread lesions of the small arteries, scleroderma, in which the skin becomes thickened and indurated, and polymyositis (see Ch. 18). Raynaud's syndrome is often seen in these diseases (see Ch. 7).

FRACTURES

A fracture (Fig. 17.7) is a break in a bone. It may be *simple*, in which case the skin overlying the bone is not breached, or *compound* where there is disruption of overlying skin. This carries the risk of infection, and compound fractures are therefore much more serious.

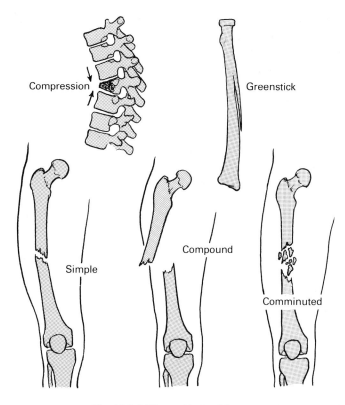

Fig. 17.7 Different kinds of fractures.

A fracture may be incomplete, the bone breaking along one border but remaining intact on the opposite side. Such fractures are prone to occur in young children and are known as *greenstick fractures*. More usually, however, the bone is completely broken; if many fragments are produced the fracture is known as *comminuted*. Occasionally, compression causes the bone to shatter and impact (this is a particularly common form of fracture in the vertebral column and in the calcaneum of the heel).

Healing of bone

Following a fracture in the bone bleeding occurs and a *haematoma* forms. The blood lost into this haematoma can be considerable. For example, in a fracture of the femur, as much as 2–3 litres may be involved. As in healing of wounds (see Ch. 4) the haematoma is organized from the periphery and from the broken bone ends by ingrowth of new blood vessels and connective tissue cells which fol-

low closely the macrophages that absorb the haematoma. The *granulation tissue* in this instance, however, contains many osteoblasts which begin to lay down immature (woven) bone. This mass uniting the bone ends is known as *callus*, which matures, the woven bone being gradually replaced by mature bone. The callus is remodelled by osteoclastic and further osteoblastic activity. The time for healing to occur varies in different bones.

Factors affecting the healing of bone are similar to those affecting wound healing. However, there are special circumstances in osseous tissue. Firstly, good reduction of the fracture with alignment of the bone so that there is not a large gap between the free ends is important. Secondly, movement tends to disrupt the forming callus so that immobility is crucial, and thirdly, infection is of particular importance in this instance since it is extremely likely to be followed by delayed or non-union healing. In addition, some bones have a peculiar blood supply such that the fracture produces avascular necrosis of a segment of the bone. This makes healing impossible.

Well-known examples are fracture of the neck of the femur, which may be followed by necrosis of the head of the femur, and fracture of the scaphoid bone of the wrist which can be similarly complicated.

Clinical features

A history is always useful since it may help in the diagnosis of fracture and be of value in the assessment of associated injuries. Furthermore, a good description of the force and direction of the blow that produced the fracture is of value. Thus a fall on the chin can produce a bilateral fracture of the neck of the mandible.

The patient complains of pain and swelling and on clinical examination the affected bone may show obvious deformity. This is not always present but local tenderness overlying the fracture is an invariable sign. There may be swelling and bruising of the surrounding structures and in compound fractures laceration of the skin through which a fragment of bone may protrude. Movement of the bone causes pain and may be accompanied by a grating sound (crepitus). Fracture of major bones (e.g. femur, pelvis) may produce sufficient haemorrhage to cause hypovolaemic shock.

It is extremely important to assess damage to adjacent structures caused by the fracture. Examples of nerve damage associated with bone fractures are damage to the radial nerve in fracture of the humerus, damage to the inferior dental nerve in fracture of the mandible, and damage to the lateral popliteal nerve in fractures of the neck of the fibula. Failure of the surgeon to detect such palsies before treatment are serious since the residual paralysis may well be attributed by the patient (and by his legal advisers) to the result of therapy. Major blood vessels may be damaged by fractures and assessment of the circulation of the limb distal to a fracture is essential. The fractured bones may also penetrate body cavities and damage underlying viscera such as the brain, lungs, liver, spleen or bladder.

Treatment

The object of treatment is to produce a good functional end-result. The management of a fracture can be considered under three headings.

1. *Emergency treatment.* The object is to lessen pain, prevent blood loss, treat shock, and prevent infection in compound fractures. This is achieved by the administration of analgesia and by a temporary splinting of the fracture (this not only relieves pain but slows blood loss). Blood is taken for grouping and cross-matching and blood transfusion used as required. Any wounds are covered with sterile dressing for later excision (see Ch. 4) in the operating theatre. Tetanus toxoid and penicillin are given for tetanus and gas gangrene prophylaxis as outlined previously. An assessment is then made of peripheral nerve and vascular function and of visceral damage. In particular the need to maintain an airway is important and the passage of an endotracheal tube may be necessary in the severely injured. Assessment of associated injuries to the brain, contents of the chest, or of the abdomen is made. If such injury is suspected the appropriate specialists are immediately consulted and management of severe thoracic, abdominal or cerebral injury takes precedence over definitive management of the fracture.

In facial fractures, particularly, the airway may be threatened and tracheal intubation and even tracheostomy may be necessary early in the course of management.

2. *Reduction.* When a bone is fractured the fragments may be severely displaced, not only by the fracturing force but also by the pull of muscles attached to the bone fragments. For example, in some fractures of the mandible, traction by the pterygoid muscles can produce quite marked displacement.

X-rays are taken to show the displacement and degree of comminution. It is important to take X-rays in two planes or the extent of the fracture may not be revealed; in addition, fractures on X-ray may show up not only as a break in the bone but also as a line of increased density if two fragments overlap.

Reduction of the fracture usually requires general anaesthesia, both to relieve pain and to relax muscle spasm. The fragments are reduced as much as possible but it is important to realize that good alignment is more important than perfect X-ray apposition. This ensures subsequent good function, particularly of related joints. Nevertheless, it is desirable to have the bones as closely approximated as possible without intervening muscle or other tissues. In the case of compound fractures excision is performed at this time and any small detached fragments of bone are removed, but such removal should be conservative since bony defects are difficult to close. In most instances of compound fracture the overlying wound is repaired as outlined previously but if gross infection is present the wound may be left open and dressed for subsequent management. Following reduction some means must be used to maintain the bones in correct position.

3. *Immobilization*. This may be affected by external splinting, by traction, or by internal fixation. *External splinting* is usually applied in the form of a plaster of Paris cast which should extend far enough beyond the lines of fracture to maintain the immobilization. However, as much function as possible should be allowed to surrounding joints so as not to unduly weaken the muscles in the area or to cause stiffness to develop in these joints. It is extremely important that plaster casts are accurately applied and checked frequently after the application since compression of the soft tissues with vascular impairment and subsequent gangrene can result. Splinting fractures of the jaw is performed by the application of cap splints or splints formed from dentures (Gunning's splints) to the fractured segments of bone. The fractured mandible or maxilla may also be fixed by penetrating struts and splinted by these to a skull appliance. This is a form of external splinting.

Traction is used to effect relative immobilization in fractures where muscle spasm is a major factor in the production of the initial deformity. The outstanding example is in fracture of the femur where the powerful thigh muscles tend to produce overriding of the fragments. Traction to the legs and the application of an external splint (Thomas' splint to the thigh) is usually sufficient. *Internal fixation* can be effected by wiring the fragments of bone together or by plating them with metal plates screwed to the opposing fragments or by insertion of a metal bar into the medullary cavity.

Rehabilitation following fracture is of great importance. A good functional result, not necessarily perfect alignment of bones, is the aim. To this end, appropriate exercises are commenced, sometimes during the period of fracture immobilization, and are continued in the phase following healing of the fracture. Thus, for example, in fracture of the femur, it is possible to achieve appropriate splintage and at the same time to allow exercise of the knee. This allows exercise of the great muscles of the thigh, which can be continued in the follow-up period. Function of the leg and its joints are preserved and recovery hastened. Rehabilitative exercises of this sort are particularly important in the hand where prolonged immobilization can lead to permanent damage and muscle contracture.

Facial fractures

Facial fractures are of considerable importance to the dentist and are covered in detail during the course of maxillofacial and oral surgery. As with other fractures, they may be compound and extend to communicate either with the external environment or with the mouth or nasal sinuses. They are often accompanied by head injury. The fractures may involve the zygomatic arch, the maxilla, the mandible, or all of the facial structures.

The immediate aspects of the management of facial fractures are occasionally the arrest of bleeding, the maintenance of a good airway, particularly in bilateral fractures of the mandible which allow the tongue to fall backwards and compromise respiration, and assessment of associated injuries, in particular cerebral injury.

Examination of the patient should include a careful history and an assessment of displacement of bone. This can be especially difficult once gross facial swelling has taken place. Assessment of the occlusion may give important clues, and abnormal mobility of segments of bone or of the alveolar arch may be detected. There may be areas of paraesthesia or anaesthesia due to entrapment of nerves by the fractured bone (e.g. an area of anaesthesia covering the upper lip and ala of the nose is not infrequent in fractured maxilla involving the infra-orbital nerve). There may be a disparity on examination of the eyes and the patient may complain of diplopia as a result of displacement of one or other of the orbital contents.

Special X-rays are taken to demonstrate the fractures and treatment is instituted as early as possible but may be delayed for a few days especially where other injuries take priority. However, if the condition of the patient is good, and especially if the fracture is compound, treatment should be instituted early.

The aims of treatment are to restore good function, good occlusion, and good appearance. In addition, if there are visual defects these must be corrected. If there are associated tears of the dura mater resulting in rhinorrhoea or otorrhoea, dural repair by a neurosurgeon is often necessary.

Fractures of the zygomatic arch are elevated by insertion of an appropriate instrument introduced through an incision in the hair-line and passed down deep to the temporalis fascia.

Fractures of the mandible and maxilla are reduced and are fixed either with wires, splints fixed to the teeth with external bars, by internal fixation by means of screwing bars to the fragments of bone, or by wiring methods. There is, of course, a necessity to treat associated soft tissue injuries and if there is skin loss extensive plastic surgical repairs may be necessary.

As with all fractures, a period of rehabilitation is necessary and any teeth damaged or lost at the time of injury must be adequately repaired or replaced by means of suitable prostheses.

Pathological fractures

Fractures following relatively minor injury occur when there is disease of the underlying bone, e.g. osteoporosis, osteomalacia, osteogenesis imperfecta, Paget's disease, myeloma, or secondary carcinoma. Metastatic bony deposits are common in carcinoma of the bronchus, breast, prostate, kidney, and thyroid, and may be the first presentation of the neoplasm.

18

Disorders of the nervous system, including head injury and management of the unconscious patient

ANATOMICAL AND PHYSIOLOGICAL CONSIDERATIONS

General structure

The principal parts of the central nervous system are the cerebrum, the cerebellum, the brainstem, and the spinal cord (Fig. 18.1). The peripheral nervous system consists of the cranial and peripheral nerves.

The cerebrum is divided into two hemispheres each comprising a frontal, parietal, temporal, and occipital lobe. The surface is mainly grey matter and within the substance of the hemispheres lie the basal ganglia, the third and lateral ventricles, the thalamus, and the internal capsule which contains many ascending and descending tracts (white matter), of which the most important is the pyramidal or motor pathway.

The cerebellum lies dorsal to the pons forming the roof of the fourth ventricle. The surface is composed of grey matter and the centre is mainly white matter containing three nuclei of grey substance. Tracts link the cerebellum with the spinal cord and other parts of the nervous system.

The brainstem is composed of the midbrain which lies uppermost, the pons which lies ventral

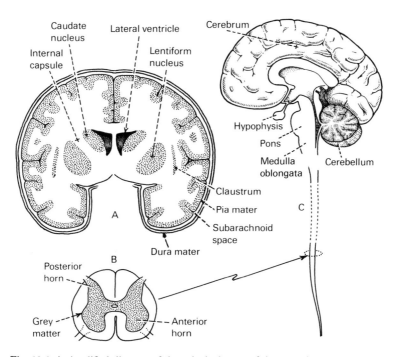

Fig. 18.1 A simplified diagram of the principal parts of the central nervous system.

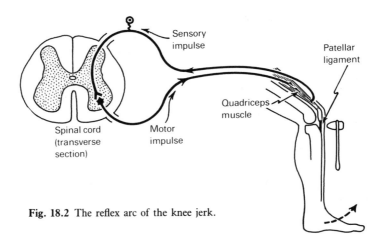

Fig. 18.2 The reflex arc of the knee jerk.

to the fourth ventricle and the cerebellum, and the medulla which is continuous with the spinal cord below. The brainstem contains ascending sensory and descending motor tracts and the cranial nerve nuclei from which the cranial nerves arise and emerge as shown in Figure 18.3. In the medulla the pyramidal fibres cross from the anterior aspect of the brainstem to the lateral part of the other side and descend in the cord.

The spinal cord occupies the bony vertebral canal between the foramen magnum and the first lumbar vertebra. Thirty pairs of nerves arise from the cord, each being made up of an anterior motor root and a posterior sensory root. The grey matter forms a central column, which is H-shaped on cross-section (see Fig. 18.2), throughout the length of the cord. The white matter is composed of ascending sensory tracts, ascending cerebellar tracts, and the descending pyramidal and extra-pyramidal tracts.

Reflex activity

A reflex occurs without conscious mental effort as an almost simultaneous response to a stimulus. There are many varieties of reflexes but in clinical neurology most use is made of the tendon reflexes, the plantar responses, and the reaction of the pupils to light.

The tendon reflexes, which include the knee, ankle, biceps and triceps jerks, are also termed deep or stretch reflexes. The reflex arc for the knee jerk, which is taken as an illustrative example, is shown in Figure 18.2. A tap on the patellar tendon below the kneecap causes a brisk forward movement of the lower leg due to contraction of the quadriceps muscle. Tendon reflexes are increased in pyramidal, or upper motor neurone lesions, and decreased or absent in lower motor neurone lesions.

The plantar response is a superficial reflex initiated by stroking the sole of the foot. In health there is plantar flexion of the great toe whereas in pyramidal tract lesions the toe dorsiflexes — the extensor or Babinski response.

The pupillary light reaction is a further superficial reflex. The pupil contracts in response to light. The light reflex is lost in many cases of neurosyphilis (Argyll Robertson pupil).

The motor system

The pyramidal pathway is composed of upper motor neurones and lower motor neurones.

Upper motor neurones commence in the motor area of the cortex, converge to pass through the internal capsule, traverse the brainstem giving connections to the cranial nerve nuclei of the opposite side, decussate in the medulla, and descend in the opposite side of the spinal cord, ending in synapses with the anterior horn cells.

Lower motor neurones are formed by the cranial nerve nuclei and the anterior horn cells of the cord, and run in the cranial and peripheral nerves respectively.

The difference between an upper and a lower motor neurone lesion is shown in Table 18.1.

Table 18.1 Comparison of the features of upper and lower motor neurone lesions

	Upper	Lower
Muscle power	decreased	decreased
Muscle tone	increased (spastic)	decreased (flaccid)
Tendon jerks	increased	absent
Plantar response	extensor	flexor
Muscle wasting	not present	present
Muscle fasciculation	never	sometimes

The extrapyramidal system is formed by the basal ganglia and certain nuclei in the brainstem from which tracts descend to end in relation to the anterior horn cells. Lesions of this system cause muscle rigidity and tremors but no paralysis.

Lesions of the cerebellar system cause incoordination of movement.

Sensory system

Sensory fibres pass in the sensory peripheral nerves to the cord via the posterior nerve roots, or via the sensory cranial nerves, and ascend to intermediate relay centres in the brainstem (deep sensation and position sense) and the thalamus (pain and temperature), from where fibres pass to the sensory areas of the cortex.

The cerebrospinal fluid

This is a clear, colourless fluid of similar composition to the plasma except that it contains very little protein. It is formed by the vascular choroid plexuses of the ventricles and the volume is about 120 ml. It circulates in the subarachnoid space providing a protective 'water-jacket' for the brain and spinal cord.

Cerebrospinal fluid may be obtained for diagnostic purposes by lumbar puncture in which a fine needle is passed, under local anaesthesia, between the spinous processes of the lower lumbar vertebrae (i.e. below the termination of the spinal cord) into the subarachnoid space.

PAINS ABOUT THE FACE AND HEAD

It is essential that the dentist should have a clear appreciation of the various disorders that may be associated with pain in the face and head. The symptom is a common one and, as with all forms of pain, it frequently leads the patient to seek advice. A simple classification of the causes is given in Table 18.2.

In patients with trigeminal neuralgia, and in many others with non-organic facial pain, a diagnosis may be made with reasonable accuracy on the basis of the history, provided the necessary time is taken to obtain a full description of the pain, its site, mode of onset, duration, precipitating factors, etc.; a careful clinical examination must never be omitted whether or not an organic basis is suspected and, in many instances, radiological studies and other special investigations are also required.

Trigeminal neuralgia or tic douloureux

This is a disorder that affects elderly people. The pain is usually experienced in the second and/or third division of the fifth cranial nerve and very rarely in the first. It is always confined to one side of the face. The pain occurs in paroxysms which last for a few seconds and it may be extremely

Table 18.2 Classification of pains about the face and head

No organic pathology	Secondary to		Associated with
Trigeminal neuralgia	Disorders of — teeth		Hypertension
Migraine	— sinuses		Toxic and febrile states
Migrainous neuralgia	— ears		Myocardial ischaemia
Postherpetic neuralgia	— eyes		
Anxiety	— temporo-mandibular joint		
Depression	Other bone and joint disorders		
Glossopharyngeal neuralgia	Temporal arteritis		
	Intracranial disorders		
	Disorders of mouth and tongue		

severe. It never radiates outside the distribution of the fifth nerve. A paroxysm may be triggered off by such simple factors as sitting in a cold draught, talking, swallowing, taking of hot or cold foods, washing the face, insertion of dentures, or by touching the side of the face. In trigeminal neuralgia there are no neurological signs and there is no numbness of the face.

Mild cases may be treated with analgesics or by the anticonvulsant drug carbamazepine (Tegretol®) but if the paroxysms are frequent and severe, more positive steps are required. The affected division or alternatively the Gasserian ganglion may be injected with alcohol or phenol, or destroyed by means of thermo-electrocoagulation and if this is not sufficient to produce long-lasting relief, surgical division of the preganglionic part of the nerve is indicated. Loss of corneal sensation may follow such procedures and secondary corneal ulceration results. This must be prevented by protective glasses.

Migraine

This disorder is believed to be due to recurrent spasm followed by dilatation of the intracranial arteries; the pain results from stretching of nerve endings in the arterial wall. A family history is frequently present. Migraine affects up to 10% of the population, usually in the first half of life. Attacks may be precipitated by stress, exercise, menstruation, foods such as chocolate, or red wine. In its classical form migraine shows the following characteristics:

1. A family history.
2. An onset in childhood or adolescence and a tendency for the attacks to lessen in severity after middle age.
3. Premonitory visual symptoms such as blurring or loss of vision, photophobia, or flashes of light in front of the eyes. These often affect one side only.
4. Headache, usually unilateral or mainly so (hemicrania = migraine), which may last for many hours and is often severe.
5. Vomiting, especially towards the end of an attack.

Most migrainous patients find some measure of relief by resting in a darkened room and by taking an analgesic such as aspirin or paracetamol, combined with an anti-emetic to aid absorption. Frequent attacks may be prevented by a beta-adrenergic blocker, or by the antihistamine, pizotifen.

Migrainous neuralgia

This is much rarer than migraine, and usually affects men. Attacks of pain usually occur in the first division of the trigeminal nerve and last for $\frac{1}{2}$–3 hours. They usually occur at night, in 'clusters' lasting several days or weeks, then remit for months or years. Lacrimation and rhinorrhoea occur during the attack. Treatment is with ergotamine which prevents vasodilatation.

Tension headache

This is the most common type of headache and is often associated with an anxiety state. A constant, dull discomfort is felt which may be frontal, occipital, or like a tight band around the head. It is attributed to muscle tension and there may be local tenderness. Diagnosis is by a typical history, evidence of an anxiety state (see Ch. 19), and examination to exclude other causes of headache. Treatment is by explanation, reassurance, and simple analgesics, e.g. aspirin or paracetamol.

Atypical headache or facial pain

This is often associated with depression (see Ch. 19). It is a constant, dull pain usually felt in a specific part of the head or face, often in middle-aged women. The patient may have delusions, e.g. of cancer or of worms eating away the bone. Examination and investigations show no evidence of organic disease. Patients should be referred to a psychiatrist for assessment and treatment with antidepressant drugs.

Postherpetic neuralgia

This follows herpes zoster infection of the trigeminal nerve (see Ch. 1). Elderly patients are more often affected. The pain may be relatively mild or very severe. It is experienced in the area in which the vesicles occurred and the presence of scars from the vesicles may give a clue to the origin of the disorder. Carbamazepine or antidepressant drugs may be helpful.

Dental causes

The various dental abnormalities that may cause facial pain will not be enumerated, but the following general remarks are not out of place:

1. Even a detailed clinical examination will not always reveal dental caries, especially at contact points, and small cavities below the gingival margin may be difficult to find. X-ray examination and particularly bite-wing films are necessary.

2. Pain of dental origin may be referred from the upper to the lower jaw and vice versa, but is never referred to the other side of the face. It may be referred to the temporal region on that side.

3. If a full clinical and radiological examination does not reveal any dental abnormality in a patient with facial pain, dental extractions should never be performed in the vague hope that this will produce a cure of the facial discomfort. It should always be remembered that just as dental pain may be referred elsewhere in the head and neck, so disorders elsewhere (such as maxillary sinusitis) may present as toothache.

Sinus disorders

Acute or chronic infection of the sinuses is a common complication of upper respiratory tract infection. Frontal sinusitis tends to cause pain in the first division of the trigeminal nerve and there is commonly tenderness on palpation over the affected sinus. Maxillary sinusitis is important to the dentist since it may produce pain in the teeth and indeed the upper teeth may be tender to percussion, the condition thus simulating peri-apical abscess. Sometimes the tenderness is confined to only one tooth. However, there is also pain on pressure in the infra-orbital region and above the apices of the upper premolar teeth intra-orally. The presence of pus within the sinus is easily demonstrated on X-ray since the affected sinus is opaque. Suppuration in the sphenoidal or eth-moidal sinuses may be impossible to diagnose with-out careful radiological study; severe headache may be caused, and some authorities have described anterior facial pain due to involvement of the sphenopalatine ganglion.

Treatment is by appropriate inhalations and postural drainage and the administration of anti-biotics, but surgical drainage may be necess-ary, most frequently in the maxillary sinus (Caldwell–Luc operation), since the normal opening of the sinus is high on its posterior and medial wall so that natural drainage is difficult.

Neoplasm of the sinuses is a serious cause of facial pain but is less common than simple infec-tion. Nevertheless, it is important to keep this possibility in mind. Facial swelling on the affected side, diplopia, unilateral nasal discharge, loosen-ing of the teeth, and perhaps the appearance of an ulcer in the mouth are all late signs. The diag-nosis is confirmed by biopsy and treatment is by surgical excision with appropriate reconstruction (this may need the provision of complicated dental prostheses) or by radiotherapy or by a combi-nation of the two.

Neoplasm of the sinuses is a serious cause of facial pain, but it is fortunately much less common than simple infection.

Aural disorders

Boils, acute otitis media, and mastoiditis cause local pain in the ear which may be intense. There is seldom any likelihood that these conditions will be confused with other causes of facial pain.

The geniculate ganglion of the facial nerve may be involved by herpes zoster or by chronic middle ear suppuration. Confusion may arise in these instances as the pain may be felt in the front of the ear and on the ipsilateral side of the tongue and hard palate, in addition to in the ear itself. Geniculate herpes is usually associated with facial paralysis through secondary involvement of the motor fibres of the nerve (Ramsay Hunt syn-drome).

Ocular causes

Errors of refraction are so well recognized as a cause of headache that testing of the visual acuity is often one of the earliest special investigations requested in patients with this complaint. Glau-coma, which is an eye disorder characterized by increased intra-ocular pressure, is a less common but very important cause of facial pain; the condition may be acute or chronic.

Temporo-mandibular joint disorders

Arthritis of the temporo-mandibular joint may occur in a relatively small number of cases of rheumatoid arthritis or as an uncommon meta-static complication of several infectious diseases, of which gonorrhoea is an example. However, pain arising from the temporo-mandibular joint is much more commonly caused by local factors that throw a strain on the joint structures and disturb the normal articular relationships. Osteoarthritis may result. This is termed the temporo-mandibular joint syndrome (or Costen's syndrome). It is usually associated with malocclusion of the teeth which may be of a relatively minor nature and follow loss of teeth with consequent drifting of others, unsatisfactory restorative procedures, improperly fitting appliances, and abnormal stresses after injury to the jaws. Overclosure of the jaws is also an important associated factor and may result from dentures which allow such over-closure. The pain is experienced in the side of the face and particularly on movement of the joint to the external auditory meatus, the auriculo-temporal nerve, and the middle ear structures. Common associated symptoms include discomfort in the ear, impairment of hearing, tinnitus, and temporal pain. Examination often reveals some tenderness over the affected joint and overclosure of the mandible, or deviation to one side on final closure may be evident.

It is very difficult to be precise about the frequency of the temporo-mandibular joint syndrome since the discovery of a dental abnor-mality can often be found in patients who do not have pain in the face or who have pain for some other reason. Many may suffer from a form of non-organic pain such as described earlier in this section. However, careful dental appraisal is important and the eradication of minor occlusive abnormalities is not difficult. Careful consider-ation must be given before embarking on major oral rehabilitation programmes. In very severe cases osteotomy of the ramus of the mandible produces relief.

Tumours as a cause of facial pain

Tumours of the nasal sinuses have already been referred to. However, there are a variety of dental tumours and tumours of the jaws which, although they usually present with swelling of the bone or pathological fracture, may occasionally present with facial pain. It is important to mention the rare tumours of the nasopharynx which are diffi-cult to diagnose and may present with pain in the face, sometimes associated with ear symptoms consequent upon blockage of the Eustachian tube. Secondary tumours also may present with facial pain and if associated with the jaws may cause loosening of the teeth.

Other bone and joint disorders

Involvement of the bones of the face and skull by Paget's disease, myeloma, or primary and secondary tumour (see Ch. 6) is likely to be associ-ated with headache and facial pain.

Osteoarthritis of the small joints of the cervical spine is a common disorder in elderly people. It may cause occipital headache and troublesome stiffness and pain in the back of the neck radiating into the shoulders and arms.

Temporal arteritis

This uncommon condition is a local manifestation of a collagen disorder (see Ch. 17). Other arteries of the head and neck may also be affected. The patient experiences severe temporal pain and headache. The diseased vessel may be palpable as a tender cord. Temporal arteritis is a serious disorder as it may cause blindness if untreated. The ESR is usually very high. Steroid therapy should be instituted without delay.

Intracranial disorders

The more important intracranial disorders that may be associated with headache are meningitis, cerebrovascular disorders, and cerebral tumour and abscess.

Hypertensive headache

Headache is often believed to be associated with

hypertension but in many instances the headache does not develop until the patient has been made aware of the presence of high blood pressure, or until the blood pressure is very high and damages the brain.

Toxic headaches

Headache may be experienced in a large variety of febrile and toxic states ranging from simple respiratory infections and 'hang-overs' to severe disorders of the liver and kidneys.

Myocardial ischaemia

Reference has already been made (see Ch. 7) to pain in the angle of the jaw resulting from myocardial ischaemia.

THE CRANIAL NERVES

The principal functions of the cranial nerves and their mode of emergence from the brainstem are shown diagrammatically in Figure 18.3.

First nerve

The olfactory nerve is of little clinical importance in disorders of the nervous system. Lesions of it give rise to loss of smell (*anosmia*) but this is also a feature of many local conditions of the nose due to mucosal changes.

Second nerve

The main steps on the visual pathway are the visual area of the cortex in the occipital lobe, the optic radiation which passes through the internal capsule, the optic tracts, the optic chiasma which is closely related to the pituitary gland, and the optic nerves. The medial fibres cross in the optic chiasma and, as a result, the lateral half of the retina derives its fibres from the ipsilateral visual area whereas the fibres on the medial side come from the opposite occipital lobe.

The effect of a pituitary tumour, e.g. as in acromegaly, is taken as an illustrative example of a lesion of the visual pathway. The central part of the chiasma is pressed upon, resulting in loss of vision in the lateral half of each visual field (bitemporal hemi-anopia). The term *papilloedema* describes the swollen ophthalmoscopic appearance of the optic disc which develops if the intracranial pressure is increased, e.g. in cerebral tumour or severe hypertension. A healthy disc has a distinct margin and a centrally depressed portion, or cup.

Third, fourth, and sixth nerves

The oculomotor nerves are collectively responsible for the nerve supply to the extrinsic ocular muscles. The nuclei lie in the brainstem and the nerves pass through the cavernous sinus on their way to the eye muscles. The fourth nerve supplies the superior oblique muscle, the sixth nerve the lateral rectus muscle, while the third nerve supplies the four remaining extrinsic muscles, i.e. the inferior rectus, superior rectus, internal rectus, and inferior oblique. The third nerve also supplies the voluntary part of the levator palpebrae superioris and the parasympathetic fibres to the muscles of accommodation, stimulation causing constriction of the pupil.

An isolated lesion of the fourth or sixth nerve on one side causes paralysis of one extrinsic muscle and this results in a squint, or *strabismus*. A third nerve palsy also causes a squint and, in addition, drooping of the eyelid (*ptosis*), and a dilated pupil which does not react to light or accommodation. Neurosyphilis produces a small, slightly irregular pupil which does not react to light.

Fifth nerve

The motor component is responsible for the muscles of mastication and the sensory component supplies sensation to the side of the face and head, including the cornea, and to the teeth and gums.

The principal disorders of the trigeminal nerve are trigeminal neuralgia and herpes zoster (see Fig. 1.1).

Seventh nerve

The facial nerve supplies the muscles of facial expression and also the taste fibres to the anterior

Fig. 18.3 The cranial nerves. An interrupted line (— — —) indicates a motor pathway and a continuous line (————) a sensory pathway. (After Frank H Netter, MD, The Ciba Collection of Medical Illustrations.)

two-thirds of the tongue. The nucleus is in the pons close beside that of the sixth nerve. The nerve passes across the posterior fossa of the skull in proximity to the eighth nerve, traverses the bony facial canal in the petrous portion of the temporal bone where it is related to the middle ear and the mastoid air cells, emerges from the skull through the stylo-mastoid foramen, and passes through the parotid gland before dividing up into

branches for distribution to the various facial muscles and to the mucosa of the tongue.

Paralysis of the facial nerve may be either supranuclear (upper motor neurone lesion) as in cerebral haemorrhage or infarction, or infranuclear (lower motor neurone lesion). The two varieties may be distinguished because in the lower motor variety the facial muscles around the eye are usually involved in the paralysis while they are spared in the upper motor variety as a result of their bilateral innervation.

Bell's palsy

This is the most common variety of facial palsy. The lesion is lower motor in type. The cause of Bell's palsy is not known with certainty, but it is generally believed that there is a localized inflammation of the nerve (neuritis) and that the resultant pressure on the swollen nerve at the stylo-mastoid foramen leads to paralysis. In a fully developed case the appearance is characteristic (Fig. 18.4). All the muscles of expression on one side of the face are paralysed. The patient cannot wrinkle the forehead, cannot close the eye properly, cannot purse the lips into the position for whistling, and when he attempts to show the teeth exposes less of them on the affected side. There is no sensory loss over the face, but if the fibres of the chorda tympani are involved, taste is lost over the anterior two-thirds of the tongue.

Fig. 18.4 Bell's palsy — patient attempting to show the teeth.

The majority of patients with Bell's palsy recover without any special treatment in a relatively short time. Corticosteroids are sometimes given with the aim of reducing the swelling of the nerve at the stylo-mastoid foramen. In severe cases it is desirable to fashion a simple splint which is hooked into the angle of the mouth and behind the ear to prevent stretching of the paralysed muscles. The paralysis is permanent in a few unfortunate individuals and they are left with disfiguring asymmetry of the face. Plastic surgery is often very valuable in such cases.

Surgical causes of facial palsy

Facial palsy is an uncommon complication of surgical procedures and most commonly occurs after operations on the parotid gland. Sometimes the mandibular branch of the facial nerve is damaged in excisions of the submandibular salivary gland. The facial nerve has also been reported damaged in operations involving the middle ear or the mastoid process, after an ill-directed injection of local anaesthetic and sometimes after prolonged forced instrumental opening of the mouth.

Eighth nerve

The eighth nerve has an auditory component and a vestibular component. The principal symptoms that may follow lesions of the eighth nerve are vertigo, tinnitus (noises in the ears) and deafness. These may occur singly or in combination.

Vertigo

The patient has an illusion of movement or of visible objects moving about him. If he is on his feet he staggers and may fall. Vomiting is often associated. Vertigo is caused by disordered function of the labyrinthine mechanism which is responsible for normal equilibrium. It is a much less common symptom than giddiness or light-headedness. *Ménière's syndrome* is a special form of paroxysmal vertigo, of obscure aetiology, associated with tinnitus and deafness. Labyrinthitis, of infective origin, is another important variety which may occur in small outbreaks.

Deafness

Impairment of hearing may be due to lesions of the eighth nerve (e.g. an acoustic neuroma) but more commonly it results from chronic suppuration in the middle ear, fusion of the bones of the middle ear (otosclerosis), or from primary nerve degeneration which is associated with increasing age, noise exposure, or increased blood viscosity.

Ninth, tenth, eleventh, and twelfth nerves

Isolated lesions of these nerves are rare. *Glossopharyngeal neuralgia*, which is much less common than trigeminal neuralgia, is characterized by paroxysms of pain in the throat and ear. In *bulbar palsy* there is a lower motor neurone paralysis, due to degenerative changes in the nuclei of the muscles supplied by the lower cranial nerves. The tongue becomes small, atrophic, shows muscle fasciculation, cannot be protruded, and, in consequence, there is great difficulty in eating, speaking, and swallowing. *Pseudobulbar palsy*, so-called because there is no wasting or fasciculation, is caused by a bilateral lesion, usually vascular, of the pyramidal fibres which supply the lower cranial nerve nuclei. *Unilateral hypoglossal paralysis* causes paralysis and atrophy of the muscles on the same side of the tongue. The tongue deviates to the paralysed side on protrusion (Fig. 18.5). Carcinoma of the tongue does not cause hypoglossal paralysis but fixes the tongue which protrudes to the side of the lesion.

Fig. 18.5 Appearance of the tongue in a left hypoglossal paralysis.

VASCULAR DISEASES

Disease of the cerebral blood vessels is one of the most common causes of disease of the nervous system.

Strokes

A stroke is an acute focal disturbance in the brain, usually due to cerebral infarction or cerebral haemorrhage. However, a small number of strokes are due to cerebral tumours, some arising acutely because of haemorrhage into the tumour. Stroke is the third most common cause of death (after myocardial infarction and cancer) and is the most common cause of hospital bed occupancy and of disability in the community. The incidence increases with age, and hypertension is the most important risk factor.

Cerebral ischaemia and infarction

80% of strokes are due to cerebral infarction. The usual cause of infarction is thrombosis occurring on a ruptured atherosclerotic plaque, commonly at the carotid bifurcation in the neck. The thrombus may fragment causing embolism in the distal cerebral arteries. Thromboembolism may also occur from the heart, e.g. from mural thrombus after acute myocardial infarction, atrial fibrillation especially in the presence of rheumatic valve disease, artificial heart valves, and infective endocarditis (see Ch. 7). Small emboli may cause *transient ischaemic attacks (TIAs)* whose duration is less than 24 hours, or *minor strokes*, whose duration is greater than 24 hours but from which patients recover with little or no disability.

Such patients should be treated with aspirin (300 mg daily) which reduces the risk of subsequent major strokes due to larger thromboemboli. Hypertension in such patients should also be treated, and anticoagulants considered in patients with proven cardiac lesions.

The *symptoms and signs* of transient ischaemic attacks and strokes due to cerebral infarction depend on the site of arterial occlusion. Occlusion of an internal carotid artery or its branches (the ophthalmic artery and anterior and middle cerebral arteries) is most common, and may result in ipsilateral monocular blindness (ophthalmic artery occlusion), contralateral hemi-anopia (visual tracts), contralateral hemiparesis (weakness of arm and leg) or monoparesis (weakness of only arm or leg) from motor cortex involvement, or contralateral hemi-anaesthesia (sensory cortex).

Involvement of the speech centres in the dominant hemisphere causes *dysphasia* — disability in understanding or using language (spoken or written). In right-handed people the left cerebral hemisphere is dominant, whereas in left-handed people either hemisphere may be dominant. Dysphasia must be distinguished from *dysarthria*, which is difficulty in speaking due to dysfunction of the ninth to twelfth cranial nerves (this may occur after stroke, e.g. pseudobulbar palsy) and which may be associated with difficulty in eating and swallowing.

Occlusion of the vertebral or basilar arteries or their branches may cause transient loss of consciousness, vertigo, or ataxia (infarction of the brainstem or cerebellum) or cortical blindness (infarction of the occipital lobe, supplied by the posterior cerebral arteries).

Intracranial haemorrhage

20% of strokes are due to intracranial haemorrhage, which is usually spontaneous. Post-traumatic intracranial haemorrhage is considered later in the section on head injury. 15% of all strokes are due to *intracerebral haemorrhage* from small aneurysms in the internal capsule (Fig. 18.6), cerebellum, or brainstem; these aneurysms are especially common in hypertension. 5% of all strokes are due to *subarachnoid haemorrhage* from aneurysms of the circle of Willis at the base of the brain. Such aneurysms are again associated with hypertension; prior to rupture they may press on adjacent cranial nerves (second to sixth) causing cranial nerve symptoms and signs.

Subarachnoid haemorrhage causes the abrupt onset of severe occipital headache, neck stiffness due to meningeal irritation by blood, and frequently transient or permanent loss of consciousness. Focal signs may be present, often due to cerebral arterial spasm. Suspected subarachnoid haemorrhage should be confirmed by computerized tomographic (CT) scanning; blood-

Fig. 18.6 The effect of a vascular lesion of the internal capsule. Note the decussation of the pyramidal fibres in the medulla.

stained cerebrospinal fluid is also seen at lumbar puncture but this should not be performed due to the risk of 'coning' of the brainstem through the foramen magnum, causing cardiorespiratory arrest and death. Cerebral angiography may show aneurysms which can be ligated by a neurosurgeon to reduce the risk of subsequent bleeding, which is high in the next few weeks and frequently fatal.

Progress and management of strokes

Strokes are usually sudden in onset; slowly progressive focal symptoms and signs are more suggestive of subdural haemorrhage, tumours, or degenerative diseases. In major strokes consciousness is often impaired or lost, with incontinence of urine and faeces. Loss of consciousness, headache, and vomiting due to raised intracranial pressure are common at the outset in intracranial haemorrhage, and occur after a day or two in major cerebral infarction due to cerebral oedema. Focal symptoms and signs depend on the site of the lesion. Contralateral hemiparesis, with or without hemi-anopia, hemi-anaesthesia or dysphasia, is the most common presentation of major strokes (see Fig. 18.6). An accurate diagnosis of the underlying cause cannot be made by the clinician, and requires CT scanning. Occasionally CT scanning reveals causes that are potentially treatable by a neurosurgeon (subarachnoid haemorrhage, subdural haemorrhage, tumour), but usually it shows untreatable pathology (intracerebral haemorrhage or cerebral infarction).

About one-third of patients with major stroke die, either in the acute stage from a large brain lesion, or in subsequent weeks of months from infection (bronchopneumonia, urinary tract infection, bedsores) or pulmonary thromboembolism. One-third recover but are dependent on others for their care. One-third recover to an independent existence but have an increased risk of subsequent cardiac or cerebral vascular events.

Treatment of major strokes is largely symptomatic, with nursing care and physiotherapy. Patients must be turned every two hours to prevent bedsores and pneumonia, and may require bladder catheterization. Care of the skin and mouth is important to prevent infection, and fluids are given by intravenous or nasogastric tubes to prevent dehydration since oral fluid intake is often poor because of impaired consciousness or swallowing.

Physiotherapy to the paralysed limbs initially involves passive movement to prevent contractures and maintain posture, and subsequently help to regain active movements and the ability to walk. The affected limbs are often stiff, with extension of the leg and flexion of the arm (see Fig. 18.6). The stiff leg aids return of walking, but arm function is often permanently lost. Dysphasia and dysarthria can be helped by speech therapy. Occupational therapists play an important role in adapting home circumstances to suit disability.

Medical treatment includes treatment of infections with antibiotics, and diagnosis of the small number of patients who may benefit from neurosurgery. No drugs are of proven benefit in cerebral infarction or cerebral haemorrhage. Patients with bleeding disorders (haemophilia, anticoagulant therapy, liver disease, thrombocytopenia) and intracranial haemorrhage must have their bleeding tendency reversed urgently by infusion of clotting factors or platelets.

After recovery from stroke, preventive measures against further strokes should be considered as for transient ischaemic attacks and minor strokes, i.e. aspirin in cerebral infarction, anticoagulants in cerebral infarction due to embolism from proven cardiac lesions, and hypotensive drugs for persistent hypertension. In younger patients with transient ischaemic attacks and strokes, ulcerated atherosclerotic plaques at the carotid bifurcation can be visualized by ultrasound scanning and arteriography, and may be removed surgically (carotid endarterectomy); however the value of this operation in preventing further strokes is controversial.

Multi-infarct dementia

Some patients suffer repeated cerebral infarcts which cause a dementia with step-wise progression, often with pseudobulbar palsy. This is much less common than senile dementia (see Ch. 19).

INFECTIONS OF THE NERVOUS SYSTEM

During the present century there has been a steady reduction in the incidence of infectious diseases of the nervous system. Poliomyelitis, neurosyphilis, and meningeal tuberculosis (see Ch. 1) are now rare in developed countries.

Herpes zoster is described in connection with chickenpox (see Ch. 1) since both diseases are caused by the same virus. HIV infection (see Ch. 2) is now becoming the most common neurological virus infection, causing encephalitis, peripheral neuritis, or dementia.

Poliomyelitis

Anterior poliomyelitis, or infantile paralysis, is due to a virus with an affinity for the anterior horn cells of the spinal cord and the cranial nerve nuclei. It has its maximum incidence in children and young adults, and the incubation period is about 12 days. The virus normally gains access to the body via the upper alimentary tract, including the oropharynx.

Clinical features

Not everyone who becomes infected with the virus develops a serious illness with widespread paralysis; many develop immunity without experiencing any symptoms while others have a short pyrexial illness without paralysis or a viral meningitis.

In the unfortunate minority who become paralysed the usual sequence of events is influenza-like symptoms followed by paralysis, usually asymmetrical and especially of the limbs (Fig. 18.7). The paralysed muscles are tender and the tendon jerks are absent. If the trunk is affected there is disturbance of respiration due to intercostal and diaphragmatic paralysis. Involvement of the cranial nerve nuclei causes difficulty in swallowing and further interference with respiration.

Prognosis

Mild paralytic cases may recover more or less completely, but if the paralysis is severe and extensive some permanent weakness is probable. The majority of adults whom one sees with a drop foot, or other evidence of limb paralysis, have suffered from poliomyelitis. In fatal cases death is usually due to respiratory paralysis.

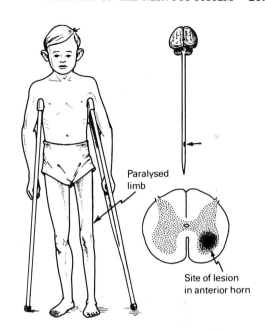

Paralysed limb

Site of lesion in anterior horn

Fig. 18.7 The lower motor neurone paralysis of poliomyelitis.

Treatment

The most important measure is prevention, and the incidence of poliomyelitis has been greatly reduced by the widespread immunization of children. Immunization boosters are recommended prior to visiting areas of high incidence.

Meningitis

Acute inflammation of the covering membranes of the brain and spinal cord may be due to many pathogenic organisms. Viral meningitis is common (e.g. measles, mumps, HIV, poliomyelitis). Of bacterial infections, *Haemophilus influenzae* is most common in young children, the meningococcus in older children and young adults, and the pneumococcus in older adults. Tuberculous meningitis should always be remembered.

The incubation period is short. The onset is abrupt and the main features of the illness are headache, fever, and stiffness of the neck due to meningeal irritation. A characteristic purpuric rash occurs with meningococcal infection (see Ch. 12). Lumbar puncture yields a purulent fluid containing the causal organism. The condition is a medical and bacteriological emergency, requiring high doses of the appropriate antibiotic given intravenously, to avoid death or brain damage. Antibiotic prophylaxis should be given to close contacts of meningococcal meningitis.

EPILEPSY

Epilepsy is due to recurrent paroxysmal bursts of uncontrolled cerebral electrical activity, and the nature of the attack depends on the area of brain involved and the intensity of the process. About 1 in 200 people are affected.

In the majority of cases the cause of the disorder is quite unknown. In some instances epilepsy follows local damage to the brain from tumour, trauma, or infection, and a cause such as this should always be considered when the disorder commences in middle age or over. Many people have only one seizure, often precipitated by obvious factors such as fever (especially young children), prolonged faints, or withdrawal of alcohol or drugs.

Clinical forms of epilepsy

In major epilepsy, or *grand mal*, the individual has recurrent convulsions. Sometimes there is a brief warning, or aura, but more frequently the seizure occurs without warning. Consciousness is suddenly lost and the patient may fall heavily to the ground and injure himself in so doing. For a few moments the limbs and trunk muscles are rigid and tense (the tonic phase) with cyanosis due to hypoxia. This is quickly followed by violent uncontrolled movements of the limbs. Frothing at the mouth is common and the tongue may be bitten. Incontinence of urine often occurs. Each attack may last from a few moments up to many hours; the term *status epilepticus* is used when seizures persist for hours. After the attack the patient is often drowsy and confused and may sleep deeply or be semiconscious for several hours.

Petit mal is characterized by a transient mental blank, but there is no convulsion. This form of epilepsy occurs only in children. The attacks occur without warning and last for a few seconds to a minute or so. The child is quite unresponsive during the attack and may be scolded by teachers or parents unless the diagnosis is known.

Other forms of epilepsy include *major nonconvulsive seizures* in which consciousness is lost but there is no motor activity, and *temporal lobe epilepsy* in which the patient does not lose consciousness but experiences peculiar complex sensory disturbances and may exhibit violent or other antisocial behaviour of which he has no recollection. In *Jacksonian epilepsy* the focus is in the motor or sensory cortex, causing unilateral convulsions or sensory disturbance.

Treatment

The most important step during a convulsive seizure is to prevent the patient injuring himself. He should be dragged away from anything dangerous such as a fire, machinery, or a cooking stove. He should be laid on his side and a clear airway maintained (beware the patient biting your fingers!). After the attack, the patient should be kept under supervision until he has returned to normal. Depending on the circumstances and duration of the attack, this may necessitate hospital admission. This is urgently required for status epilepticus to avoid hypoxic brain damage; intravenous anticonvulsants (e.g. diazepam) and/or general anaesthesia are given.

Management of the patient between seizures is very important. Patients should not drive unless free from seizures for two years, and cannot hold public service or heavy goods vehicle licences. They should avoid working at heights or with machinery. Special schooling may be necessary for epileptic children and, later, a suitable occupation should be chosen so that if seizures occur while at work the chance of injury to the patient and others is minimal.

The principal drugs employed to reduce frequency and severity of seizures are phenytoin (Epanutin®), sodium valproate (Epilim®) and carbamazepine (Tegretol®). These may be employed singly or in combination. The dentist should remember that hyperplasia of the gums (see Ch. 9) may follow prolonged use of phenytoin. In petit mal the principal drugs used are troxidone and ethosuximide (Emeside®, Zarontin®). Phenobarbitone is now little used in view of its sedative effects.

If dental treatment is required in a known epileptic the likelihood of seizures occurring will be lessened if attention is paid to the following points.

1. Ensure that prescribed anticonvulsant drugs are being taken regularly; liaise with the patient's doctor.

2. Use a local rather than a general anaesthetic since transient cerebral anoxia may occur with the latter and precipitate an attack. The anaesthetist should be aware of the patient's epilepsy and treatment.

MULTIPLE SCLEROSIS (DISSEMINATED SCLEROSIS)

Apart from the vascular disorders and HIV infection, multiple sclerosis is the most common serious disease affecting the central nervous system. The cause is unknown.

Pathologically the disorder is characterized by areas of demyelination scattered throughout the spinal cord, the cerebral hemisphere, and the cerebellum. Depending on the site of these lesions we may have a varied clinical picture but the most common sequence of events is as outlined in the following paragraph.

Multiple sclerosis usually starts in early adult life. The first expression of the disease is most often a transient weakness of a limb, sensory disturbance affecting a limb, or disturbed vision such as diplopia. Characteristically these first symptoms are of short duration but later the individual develops more areas of demyelination throughout the nervous system, and although there may be some temporary improvement after each episode there gradually builds up a background of permanent disability.

The fluctuating course of the disorder is of great diagnostic significance. In the fully developed case there is usually evidence of pyramidal tract involvement shown by weakness of the legs with increased tendon jerks and extensor plantar responses, loss of bladder control, slurring of the speech, and a tremor which is only apparent when the patient uses the hands. Euphoria, which is a sense of well-being or elation, or depression may occur.

No curative treatment is known for multiple sclerosis. Physiotherapy may help; sympathy and encouragement are essential. The duration and severity of acute episodes may be reduced by a course of adrenocorticotrophic hormone (ACTH). The disorder may be aggravated by anaesthetics or operations, even of a relatively minor degree, and this fact should influence the nature and extent of dental procedures in these patients.

PARKINSON'S DISEASE

Parkinson's disease may rarely follow a virus infection of the brain (encephalitis) in younger individuals, but usually occurs idiopathically in middle or later life. In both varieties the corpus striatum and related areas of the midbrain and cerebellum are depleted of dopamine. This leads to unbalanced cholinergic activity.

The clinical picture is characteristic and includes some or all of the following features:

1. Slowness and poverty of all movements but especially of facial movements so that the expression is mask-like.
2. Stiffness or rigidity of limbs.
3. Coarse tremors of the arms, head, and jaw.
4. A flexed posture of the trunk.
5. A shuffling gait.
6. Dysarthria.
7. Drooling of saliva, due to slow clearance.

The administration of levodopa (usually in combination with carbidopa as Sinemet®) benefits many patients with parkinsonism; it is converted into dopamine in the brain.

CEREBRAL TUMOURS AND ABSCESS

Primary tumours

The majority of cerebral tumours are malignant and they have the peculiarity that they never metastasize to other tissues.

The clinical features may be described conveniently in two groups:

1. Those due to increased intracranial pressure — headache, vomiting usually without nausea, visual upset due to papilloedema, and possibly bradycardia.
2. Those due to focal damage — muscle weakness,

sensory defects, personality changes, etc., depending on the position of the growth.

Further information regarding the site of the tumour may be obtained from CT scanning.

Treatment may be by radiotherapy or surgery. The prognosis is poor in the majority of cases. Symptoms of raised intracranial pressure are often helped by corticosteroids (e.g. dexamethasone) which reduce cerebral oedema.

Secondary tumours

The brain is a common site for secondary tumour, and bronchogenic carcinoma deserves mention in this connection since it often presents with cerebral symptoms.

Cerebral abscess

An important cause of cerebral abscess is chronic infection of the middle ear but abscess may also follow infection of the face, particularly of the lateral angle of the nose, or may be metastatic in nature, usually from the chest (lung abscess, empyema, bronchiectasis). The clinical features may be similar to those of cerebral tumour, though the cause of the illness is usually more acute, with fever. Precise diagnosis by CT scanning allows the surgeon to perform drainage which may be curative in combination with antibiotics.

PERIPHERAL NERVE DISORDERS

Mononeuritis

A neuritis involving a single nerve is usually due to some local pathological change in the tissues surrounding the nerve such as inflammation, tumour, and pressure. Examples are brachial neuritis due to pressure by a cervical rib, compression of the median nerve in the fascial tunnel at the wrist, and sciatica, which is described further.

Sciatica

This literally means pain in the distribution of the sciatic nerve. It is now appreciated that the majority of cases are due to pressure on the sciatic nerve by intervertebral disc protrusion (Fig. 18.8).

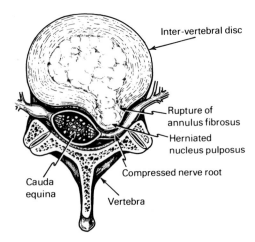

Fig. 18.8 Mechanism of production of sciatica by a prolapsed intervertebral disc.

This may follow some sudden muscular exertion such as lifting a heavy object. The patient experiences severe pain in the buttock and down the back of the leg. The pain is increased by attempting to raise the straight leg.

The majority of cases respond to rest on a firm mattress, analgesics, and spinal extension exercises. A plaster cast to hold the spine extended may be required in some instances. In refractory cases surgical removal of the offending disc (laminectomy) may be necessary before relief is obtained.

A few cases of sciatica are secondary to pressure from tumour deposits in the spine and this variety must always be carefully borne in mind.

Polyneuritis

This is a feature of many generalized toxic or metabolic disorders, and because of the diffuse nature of the cause many peripheral nerves are affected, usually symmetrically. It may occur in chronic lead poisoning, in poorly controlled diabetes mellitus, in chronic alcoholism, in deficiency states such as vitamin B_{12} deficiency or beriberi, while some acute cases are apparently due to a virus infection with a specific affinity for peripheral nerves. Plasma exchange is beneficial in treatment of this 'acute ascending polyneuritis', but ventilation may be required for respiratory paralysis.

The principal features are weakness of all limbs, wasting of muscles, loss of reflexes, sensory loss of all types over the distal parts of the limbs, and tenderness of the calves. Treatment is of the underlying cause.

Damage to peripheral nerves

Direct damage to peripheral nerves may occur as a result of involvement by tumour or their proximity to infected foci, but more usually is due to trauma. There is paralysis in the affected group of muscles with wasting and, in sensory nerves, associated sensory loss. Excision of the damaged ends with accurate suture can be followed by a remarkable degree of recovery. Dental examples of damage to peripheral nerves are the damage that may occur to the inferior dental nerve during extraction of teeth or to the lingual nerve during the removal of impacted lower molar teeth. The infra-orbital nerve may be damaged in fractures of the facial skeleton, as may the inferior dental nerve.

OTHER DISORDERS OF THE NERVOUS SYSTEM

Horner's syndrome

This results from paralysis of the ocular sympathetic fibres which arise from the lower part of the cervical cord, e.g. by pressure from an apical bronchial carcinoma. The syndrome consists of slight ptosis, a small pupil, and retraction of the eyeball (enophthalmos).

Syringomyelia

In this disorder cystic areas develop within the spinal cord, usually at the cervical level. They cause pressure damage to both motor and sensory pathways within the cord. The sensory loss is often 'dissociated' in that pain and temperature sensation is lost while deep sensation is not affected.

Subacute combined degeneration of the cord

This is a serious disorder of the nervous system caused by deficiency of vitamin B_{12} and characterized by degenerative changes in the pyramidal tract and the posterior sensory columns. Peripheral neuritis is usually associated. It is liable to develop in inadequately treated cases of pernicious anaemia (see Ch. 12), but in some patients the neurological lesions antedate the anaemia. Intensive vitamin B_{12} therapy is required.

Cervical spondylosis

In this disorder pressure damage to the cervical part of the spinal cord and the posterior nerve roots results from degenerative changes in the cervical intervertebral discs. The disorder may present because of pain in the back of the neck, shoulders and arms, or because of weakness and sensory disturbances in the legs.

Motor neurone disease

This is an uncommon disorder, of unknown aetiology, characterized by progressive degenerative changes in the anterior horn cells, the cranial nerve nuclei, and the pyramidal pathway. It causes severe disability. Bulbar palsy results from involvement of the lower cranial nerve nuclei.

Huntington's chorea

This rare form of chorea may be distinguished from chorea of rheumatic origin by a family history of the disorder and progressive dementia. The onset is in middle age. The involuntary movements are often extremely marked. The recent development of gene probes may allow antenatal diagnosis and selective termination of affected pregnancies.

Facial spasms

Involuntary spasms of the facial muscles may be due to either form of chorea, to habit spasms which are more common in children and are usually bilateral, and to clonic facial spasm. The latter disorder is usually unilateral and is more common in older people. It is believed to be due to an irritative lesion of the facial nerve; alcoholic injection of the nerve often gives prolonged relief.

MUSCLE DISORDERS

Muscular dystrophies

This is a group of genetic disorders of voluntary muscle which occur mainly in children and adolescents. A family history is often present. The affected muscles show progressive weakness and wasting. There are several different clinical varieties named according to the muscle groups involved. The facio-scapulo-humeral type is often recognizable by the fact that the zygomatic muscles are usually more markedly affected than the other facial muscles leading to weakness of retraction of the angles of the mouth and a characteristic 'transverse smile'. Treatment is symptomatic.

Myasthenia gravis

This is a disease in which the muscles show an abnormal fatiguability on exercise. It usually affects groups of muscles, especially those innervated by the cranial nerves, and common symptoms are double vision (diplopia), ptosis, and difficulty in chewing, swallowing or speaking. The symptoms are usually more prominent at the end of the day. The disease shows a tendency to remission and relapse. It usually affects younger women.

Myasthenia gravis is due to an autoimmune disorder of conduction at the myoneural junction which may be relieved by neostigmine or the closely related drug pyridostigmine.

Polymyositis

This is a connective tissue disease which affects older adults, with weakness and wasting of muscles, and often with a skin rash (dermatomyositis). Treatment is with corticosteroids. An underlying tumour may be present.

Metabolic myopathies

Muscle weakness may result from thyrotoxicosis, corticosteroid therapy, Cushing's syndrome, hypercalcaemia, hypokalaemia, or glycogen storage diseases.

HEAD INJURY AND CARE OF THE UNCONSCIOUS PATIENT

Head injuries

Head injuries are either closed, in that the brain and its meningeal coverings are not penetrated, or are open, in that there is direct penetration and exposure of the cerebral tissues and their coverings. The major problem both in diagnosis and management is the recognition and assessment of the extent of intracranial damage.

Head injuries, although they may be caused by a high velocity missile as in war-time, are most frequently caused by blunt impact from solid objects, and in civilian practice the large majority of these are related to car accidents. Indeed, more than 60% of all car accidents involve the head and in fatal accidents the percentage is over 70%. Lastly, if a patient is admitted unconscious after an accident, there is a high chance that he is suffering from intracranial haemorrhage and brain damage.

Local injury to the skull and underlying brain may give rise to haemorrhage and subsequent infection, but the effects are generally less than those that follow the more generalized injuries associated with sudden acceleration or deceleration. Such injury may deform the brain within the skull and cause injury at a point opposite to that of the direct impact (contre-coup injury). In addition, the force may be transmitted to the vital central tissues and brainstem structures.

Injury to the head may be limited to the scalp, but may also involve the skull, the brain, or all three.

Injuries to the scalp

The scalp is a layered structure consisting of the hair and skin, the underlying fat, the aponeurotic layer, and the subaponeurotic areolar tissue. Blunt injuries to the scalp thus tend to burst rather than crush the tissue and lacerations are common. The coarse nature of the skin and the underlying aponeurosis is important in consideration of head injuries since they tend to hold open blood vessels in the fatty layer between them and haemorrhage is often profuse. Once haemorrhage is controlled and the tissues sutured, healing occurs very readily.

Skull fractures

Skull fractures are either linear, depressed, with some compression of underlying brain tissue, or compound with exposure of the bone. A skull fracture indicates that there has been a severe blow to the head, but is not necessarily an index to underlying brain damage which may be severe even in the absence of fracture of the overlying bone.

A skull fracture that runs immediately across the middle meningeal artery or one of the venous sinuses may result in extradural or subdural haemorrhage and the patient must be carefully observed for signs that suggest the need for operation to relieve compression of the underlying brain.

Fractures of the base of the skull are not often seen on X-rays but depressed skull fractures are. It is important that X-rays be carefully examined, since palpation is often misleading due to overlying haematoma. Fractures that extend into the nasal sinuses or mastoid air cells are really compound in nature, since they are in communication with the external surfaces of the body and infection is likely.

Injuries to the brain

Injuries to the brain may be classified as concussion, contusion, or laceration. It is important to recognize that, although they may occur on their own, they are frequently seen in combination.

Concussion

Concussion is a clinical syndrome which is recognized by immediate and transient loss of consciousness due to a blow to the head. It is usually accompanied by a period of amnesia (loss of memory) to events immediately preceding the injury, and this is termed *retrograde amnesia*. In concussion there is usually no demonstrable permanent damage to the brain.

Contusion

This term implies a bruise within the brain. Contusions often occur along the base of the frontal lobe and posteriorly at the temporal lobe. There is underlying damage to the nerve tissues including the formation of local oedema and haematoma, and there may be ischaemia to brain tissue. If the injury is deep within the brain the results may involve a large mass of tissue.

Laceration

Severe injury to the head results in tearing of the brain tissue and this may occur at the point of application of a very considerable force to the head or at the directly opposite point (contre-coup).

Assessment and management

The assessment of a head injury is an emergency matter and early treatment important. Firstly, an adequate airway must be maintained and if necessary an endotracheal tube is passed. Secondly, it is important that there is a good blood supply to the brain. Although scalp lacerations may cause serious bleeding, shock is very rarely secondary to head injury alone and, if present, usually denotes haemorrhage within the thoracic cavity or the abdomen. Early control of bleeding and adequate blood transfusion is essential.

Diagnosis

Having obtained the history of a blow to the head, the cause of unconsciousness is usually readily evident, but it must be remembered that other conditions may be associated with the patient's state. Thus, a diabetic in coma may present with head injury. Similarly, patients in hepatic coma or drug-induced coma may have initially fallen and struck the head. The most important condition requiring differential diagnosis is that of alcoholic coma. The examining clinician should be wary of not attributing coma to one of these associated causes, but should be absolutely certain to exclude severe head injury. Usually a clear history taken from the patient's relatives or the ambulance driver, assessment of the clinical status, and appropriate special investigations provides the necessary information. The patient is then assessed.

Symptoms and signs of head injury

A quick examination of the nervous system is important in order to establish a base-line against which to measure subsequent events. The most important assessment is that of the level of consciousness.

Motor response. The patient's ability to move in response to command or stimulus is assessed and graded as to whether he responds to simple commands, shouted commands, localized painful stimulus, or whether the response is abnormal. There may be no response at all.

Verbal response. The patient's ability to speak and his speech is assessed. Does the patient simply make odd noises or give confused answers, or are his answers completely intelligible and appropriate?

Level of consciousness. This is a difficult matter of judgement and especially if the patient is intoxicated or under the influence of drugs prior to injury. The ability to open the eyes is an important assessment in this regard. It should be noted whether the patient opens his eyes in response to commands or stimulus, or whether he is aware and opens the eyes spontaneously. In addition to this, there should be a careful note made of any complaint the patient may make of headache, of the period of retrograde memory loss (amnesia), and of course of any scalp lacerations or cranial deformity. Traditionally, it is important to assess the eyes of the patient, especially if coma is evident. Pupillary size and their reaction to light is important and unequal size of the pupils, particularly unilateral dilatation of one pupil, is a sign of raised intracranial pressure.

Investigations

In severe head injury and with a rapidly deteriorating level of consciousness, there may be no time for investigation. In such cases, the skull should be opened by means of surgical burr holes in order to allow rapid diagnosis of extracerebral haemor-

rhage, and it may be necessary to proceed to craniotomy (elevation of a segment of the skull) in order to alleviate pressure by evacuation of haematoma.

Skull X-rays. Skull X-rays should be obtained as soon as possible. The major information to be obtained relates to the presence or absence of a fracture and whether this crosses the line of one of the major vascular structures or breaches one of the paranasal air sinuses. The pineal gland, which is calcified and radio-opaque in more than 70% of persons over the age of 20, may be detected and a shift of this gland to the right or the left on a good X-ray suggests an expanding intracranial haemorrhage.

Imaging of the brain. The brain may be imaged by means of CT scanning, which shows the presence and site of intracranial haemorrhage.

Haemorrhage within the skull

The brain, like the pulp of the tooth, is enclosed within a rigid cavity and is thus incapable of expansion. For this reason, haemorrhage, particularly if progressive, is associated with severe effects, the major one being compression of the cerebral tissue. A rising intracranial pressure forces the brain down through the foramen magnum and produces pressure on the brainstem.

Intracranial haemorrhage may occur within the extradural space, the subdural or subarachnoid space, or within the cerebral tissue itself.

Subarachnoid haemorrhage

Blood in the spinal fluid is a common finding with head injuries. The bleeding arises often from superficial cortical vessels draining the cerebral cortex, and quite large volumes of blood within the subarachnoid space may be relatively well tolerated. There may be headache, restlessness, and signs of cerebral irritation, but this in itself is not a sign for surgical intervention.

Extradural haemorrhage

The most common cause of extradural haematoma is laceration of a branch of the middle meningeal artery and this is usually associated with skull fracture. The injury is common since the artery lies in a groove in the inner table of the temporal bone. Extradural bleeding may also occur as a result from laceration of dural sinuses.

It is important to recognize that extradural haemorrhage may be produced by a relatively minor blow to the head and there may have been no period of amnesia. Indeed, an initially unconscious patient may have a lucid interval. That is to say, he may become alert and then subsequently relapse into coma. The haematoma enlarges and compresses the brain, producing a contralateral hemiparesis or hemiplegia. If allowed to continue, compression of the brain results in compression of the brainstem, and in irreversible damage resulting in death. It is important to realize that every patient with a history of even a minor blow to the head and unconsciousness for even a brief interval must have a thorough neurological examination and a skull X-ray. If the X-ray shows a fracture, careful monitoring of the level of consciousness (see above) and of vital signs is indicated. If the patient is admitted in coma with findings indicating unilateral cerebral compression (unilateral dilated pupils and hemiplegia), immediate burr holes are necessary in order to relieve the pressure.

Subdural haematoma

Although extensive injury may result in an acute presentation within 24 hours, the symptoms of this condition usually develop more slowly than those associated with extradural haematoma. The usual cause of subacute subdural haematoma is a tear to a small vein after relatively mild head injury, especially in infants, older people, alcoholics, and patients with coagulation defects (haemophilia, anticoagulant therapy, liver disease). A gradually enlarging subdural haematoma (due to continued oozing and the osmotic effects of breakdown of blood) may develop between one to three months after injury and an interval of up to six or seven weeks is quite common. The presentation is insidious and may develop after what has appeared to be a seemingly minor, perhaps forgotten, accident. The leading physical sign is one of progressive mental or personality change and there may be associated focal cerebral signs

and symptoms. There should be a high index of suspicion in middle-aged persons with any history of head injury who have shown a progressive deterioration in mental acuity associated with headache.

Intracerebral haemorrhage

Intracerebral haemorrhage results from injury to a vessel within the brain tissue itself. Accumulation of haematoma produces no particularly classical clinical picture but may present as a space-occupying intracranial lesion. Such lesions are often associated with laceration and contusion of the brain, and the patient's condition either becomes relatively stable or deteriorates progressively over days. A computerized tomographic scan is particularly valuable in diagnosis.

Cerebrospinal fluid leak

Leaks of cerebrospinal fluid through the nose (rhinorrhoea) or through the ear (otorrhoea) indicate a communication between the subarachnoid space or ventricular system (which contain the cerebrospinal fluid) and the nose and the ear. The particular hazard of such a fistulous opening is that it provides a pathway for the spread of infection leading to meningitis or brain abscess.

The leading clinical sign is a persistent clear, watery discharge from the ears or from the nose. Antibiotic prophylactic treatment is indicated and if the leak persists beyond ten days to two weeks then surgical repair of the torn dura is indicated.

Treatment of head injuries

1. Establish an adequate airway with tracheal intubation if necessary.

2. Provide respiratory assistance (by means of a respirator if necessary).

3. Control external haemorrhage and provide blood transfusion.

4. Assess the state of consciousness (see above).

5. If rapid deterioration is occurring, then carry out bilateral burr holes without further delay.

6. Counteract cerebral swelling by the administration of intravenous diuretic agents such as mannitol and corticosteroid injections.

7. Provide antibiotic prophylactic treatment in the event of cerebrospinal fluid leaks.

8. If the patient's condition deteriorates, this is an indication for CT scanning.

9. Compound fractures of the skull and penetrating wounds of the brain are clear indications for operation.

Prognosis

The prognosis and course of head injuries are related to the severity of intracerebral damage. The longer the period of unconsciousness and retrograde amnesia, the poorer the prognosis. Prognosis is very poor in an adult who presents with dilated fixed pupils and the signs of injury to the base of the brain.

The greatest improvement is likely to occur within the first two or three months but it should be noted that improvement following head injury can continue for nine months or more.

Late disability is one of the most important aspects of head injury and includes physical handicaps as a result of weakness, dysphasia, blindness or paralysis, or more mild forms of disability such as headache, difficulty in concentration, memory defect, dizziness, and fatigue. Some patients develop epileptic fits during the post-head-injury period. Indeed, the physical and psychosocial results of head injury are a major health problem.

The unconscious patient

A depressed state of consciousness may be due to a large number of causes and may occur suddenly, for instance following concussion (see above) or more gradually as might occur with the gradual accumulation of an intracranial haematoma (see above) or, for instance, as a result of the overdose of a drug. Repeated neurological examination will establish not only the level of consciousness but also its fluctuation. Depressed consciousness may be due to the following:

1. Trauma
2. Syncope as a result of transient cerebral ischaemia.
   a. Simple causes — vasovagal attack, postural hypotension.
   b. Serious causes — myocardial infarction, internal haemorrhage, Stokes–Adams attack.
3. A hypoglycaemic attack occurring in diabetes.
4. A non-convulsive epileptic seizure.
5. A stroke.

In addition to these causes, there are many others, e.g. diabetic ketosis, uraemia, poisoning of various kinds, and cerebral neoplasms.

The dentist will encounter but few of these in his practice, and for many of them complex investigations are necessary to establish a precise diagnosis. It is, however, important that the dental practitioner understands the care of the unconscious patient and the action to be taken should a patient suddenly become unconscious while undergoing treatment.

Management of the comatose patient

The maintenance of an airway and control of co-incident shock are the basic principles of the management of patients with a depressed level of consciousness.

Protection of the airway is perhaps the most fundamental procedure and attention to detail avoids many complications. A patient without a good cough reflex is unable to protect his own airway. Furthermore, the tongue tends to fall back and obstruct the oropharynx. Aspiration of vomit is a distinct risk.

The jaw should be pulled forward and the oropharynx cleared. An airway is maintained with an oropharyngeal tube, but it may be necessary to replace this with an endotracheal tube if there is no cough reflex. Tracheotomy may be necessary. Every effort must be made to reduce the likelihood of aspiration of gastric contents and to ensure unrestricted gas exchange at alveolar level.

A nasogastric tube should be passed in order to sample any ingested drugs and to remove gastric contents which might be aspirated into the lungs.

An intravenous line must be inserted in order to administer drugs and fluids to the patient. In prolonged unconscious states feeding may be carried out via a fine tube passed into the stomach. If gastric feeding is performed in this way, it should be always covered by an awareness on behalf of the staff of the dangers of aspiration.

An indwelling bladder catheter is used to prevent bedsores from soaked skin and to assist with the assessment of fluid balance, and the catheter must be carefully managed to prevent ascending infection.

The patient must be regularly turned and the skin cared for to limit the development of pressure sores, and passive movements must be performed by a physiotherapist. In addition, physiotherapeutic manoeuvres designed to keep the chest inflated and clear of secretions must be regularly carried out. The cause of coma must be diligently sought and treated.

Sudden loss of consciousness

If a dentist is faced with the problem of a patient who suddenly loses consciousness, the following are the most likely causes:

1. Syncope — usually as a result of a vasovagal attack, but sometimes due to a more severe cause.
2. An epileptic seizure.
3. Cardiac arrest (see Ch. 7).
4. Anaphylactic shock due to hypersensitivity to injected local anaesthetic or antibiotic (see Ch. 16).

In any event, the action to be taken is as follows:

1. The dental chair should be immediately lowered to allow the patient to lie flat; the patient should be rolled onto his side and, if possible, irrto a semiprone position. Dentures and all foreign bodies, including dental instruments and cotton-wool rolls, should be immediately removed from the mouth.

2. The mandible should be grasped and pulled forward so as to bring the tongue forward. The tongue is then grasped in a swab and also pulled forward, to maintain the airway.

3. The dental suction apparatus should be used to clear any mucus or secretions from the patient's mouth.

At this point, any constricting clothing about the patient's neck is immediately loosened. An immediate assessment is then made as to whether the patient is recovering from a simple syncopal attack or whether it is necessary to summon the help of a qualified medical practitioner.

It is perhaps important to mention that general anaesthesia should not be administered in the sitting position in a dental chair. Syncopal attacks can occur while under the influence of anaesthesia and serious brain damage may result consequent to cerebral hypoxia.

19

Psychological disorders

Psychological disorders, not all of which are of serious import, are so common that it is inevitable that some dental patients will be suffering from them. The recent tendency to discharge many previously long-stay psychiatric patients to their homes has increased this likelihood. In this chapter a very brief account is given of the more common psychiatric illnesses and also of some of the terms used when dealing with disordered function of the mind.

Disorders of the mind are traditionally classified into the psychoses, the neuroses, and mental retardation but it should be appreciated that the boundaries between some psychotic states and some neurotic illnesses and indeed between neurotic traits and normality are sometimes difficult to define with certainty. Lack of precise understanding of the aetiology of many psychiatric illnesses is a distinct hindrance to precise classification and although some psychiatric illnesses have a recognizable cause, such as organic brain damage, or are related to some 'toxic' factor, such as severe infection or drug abuse, in many instances of mental disorder there is no discernible organic pathological change in the brain or recognisable causal factor.

With this background mental disorders are considered under the following headings:

1. Mental disorders associated with organic brain disease.
2. Mental disorders secondary to organic disease elsewhere or to metabolic, hormonal, and deficiency states.
3. Alcoholism and drug abuse.
4. Functional psychoses.
5. Neurotic illnesses.
6. Personality disorders.
7. Mental subnormality.

MENTAL DISORDERS ASSOCIATED WITH ORGANIC BRAIN DISEASE

Senile dementia (Alzheimer's disease) is the most common organic brain disorder to result in mental abnormality. There is diffuse brain atrophy, shown on CT scanning. It is slowly progressive and usually occurs after the age of 65 years. *Multi-infarct dementia* (see Ch. 18) is less common and has a stepwise progression; CT scanning shows multiple infarcts. Other forms are cerebral tumours (primary or secondary), brain abscess, neurosyphilis (see Ch. 1), encephalitis (e.g. HIV infection), and cerebral trauma. Jacob–Creutzfeld disease is due to an infectious slow virus.

There are two principal clinical syndromes in this category of organic brain disorders — delirium and dementia. Delirium is characterized by acute onset, restlessness, irritability, marked anxiety, disturbed sleep or insomnia, and auditory or visual hallucinations which may be terrifying to the patient. In dementia there is a slowly progressive loss of the capacity of reasoning, inability to concentrate, inability to handle new information, loss of emotional control, narrowing of attention span, a poor grasp of the abstract, and an inability to separate the important from the unimportant.

Treatment involves detection and management of underlying disease; tranquillizing drugs (chlorpromazine, thioridazine); hospital admission for acute delirium; and supportive care in dementia, either from relatives at home, or in a home, sheltered housing, or psychiatric long-stay ward.

MENTAL DISORDERS SECONDARY TO ORGANIC DISEASE ELSEWHERE OR TO METABOLIC, HORMONAL, AND DEFICIENCY STATES

The functioning of the mind may be markedly compromised by a variety of processes which have their origin in organs other than the brain. The mental derangement may be acute and potentially reversible (e.g. severe febrile illnesses) but if the cause is either not recognized or is untreatable then the damage to the mental processes may be permanent. Acute processes tend to produce confusion that may progress to delirium; chronic processes may produce mental retardation in the child and progressive dementia in the adult.

Acute confusional states and delirium may be produced by severe infection (e.g. pneumonia or urinary tract infection), hypoxia (cardiac failure and respiratory disease), hypoglycaemia (e.g. due to inadvertent insulin overdosage), and other metabolic disorders such as hypocalcaemia, hepatic failure, and uraemia. Important deficiency states include hypothyroidism and vitamin B deficiency. Blood tests to exclude these treatable disorders should always be performed in organic brain disease. Drugs acting on the nervous system are common causes of delirium in older patients (e.g. tranquillizers, sedatives, antiparkinsonian drugs). Alcohol and drug abuse or withdrawal are common causes in younger patients.

ALCOHOLISM AND DRUG ABUSE

Alcoholism

The sense of relaxation and mild euphoria that follow consumption of a modest and socially acceptable amount of alcohol may not be unknown to the majority of students. Acute intake of larger amounts tends to lead to noisy and often aggressive behaviour and to a degree of disinhibition which is later regretted. Severe overdose can cause loss of consciousness during which serious complications such as pneumonia from inhalation of vomit or hypothermia may occur.

Chronic alcoholic dependence or addiction is a very common health problem. Perhaps as many as one million people in Britain have problems related to chronic excessive intake of alcohol, and the number is probably increasing. A common pattern is drinking that commences in adolescence or early adult life and gradually escalates in an insidious manner without the individual being aware that he is becoming dependent on alcohol. It represents a form of psychological dependence, usually with underlying emotional problems such as feelings of insecurity or inadequacy, lack of self-esteem, anxiety, or depression. At particular risk are those concerned in the manufacture and sale of alcohol, commercial travellers, company directors, journalists, entertainers, those in the merchant navy and the armed forces, dentists, doctors, and the increasing numbers of unemployed people. Dependence on alcohol may produce social problems, psychological problems, and physical problems. Detection in its early stages is obviously important, partly to prevent the development of complications and partly because at that stage management is rather more likely to be successful. The social problems may show as break-up of marriage after a period of time in which violence to the partner or children has occurred. The male's sexual impotence (a complication of alcoholism) aggravates his feeling of inadequacy and contributes to marital unhappiness. The alcoholic is liable to be off work more frequently and absences on a Monday after weekend alcoholic bouts are particularly characteristic. He is more prone to be involved in road traffic accidents whether as a driver or a pedestrian.

Psychological problems include depression, spells of amnesia during which he is unable to recollect recent events, delusions particularly of infidelity, and a gradual degeneration in moral standards with the result that many alcoholics become unreliable and untrustworthy. Acute alcoholic intoxication superimposed on chronic alcoholism can lead to delirium and in some cases a state of delirium, commonly termed *delirium tremens*, may develop following enforced abstinence from the usual daily intake of alcohol. The individual is extremely restless, commonly disoriented as to time and place, hallucinated often to a state of terror, and shows marked tremor, intense sweating, and may experience severe muscle cramps and intense nausea and retching. Seizures may occur.

Physical problems that may arise in the chronic alcoholic include peripheral neuropathy, cerebellar damage (dysarthria, tremor, ataxia), gastritis and peptic ulcer, pancreatitis, cirrhosis of the liver, cardiomyopathy and macrocytic anaemia.

Korsakoff's syndrome is specific impairment of short-term memory, with compensatory confabulation. *Wernicke's encephalopathy* causes delirium and oculomotor cranial nerve palsies.

Early detection along with insight into the problem by the patient and a determination to do without alcohol in the future are essential for success. He may require hospitalization in the initial stages and later may derive considerable support from membership of a body such as Alcoholics Anonymous or by firm adherence to a religious faith. Acute withdrawal symptoms such as delirium tremens require skilled hospital management involving adequate sedation with a drug such as chlorpromazine and correction of probable vitamin B deficiency by injection of thiamine and other B vitamins (Parentrovite®).

Heroin and morphine addiction

Addiction to opiates, once uncommon in Britain, is increasing. Even small doses of drugs can lead to dependence and the dependence is both physical and psychological. Tolerance is rapidly acquired and dependence increases as dosage increases. Most addicts tend to have been weak and rather inadequate and unhappy people before the addiction was acquired. Nevertheless it is a wise precaution to be extremely careful with administration of opiates in any individual who has a painful chronic disorder that is unlikely to progress to a fatal termination in a relatively short time.

Once addicted the addict will go to almost any lengths to acquire his necessary supply of drug. He becomes untrustworthy and may resort to crime. From the physical point of view he is prone to develop local infections due to lack of sterile precautions when injecting the drug, septicaemia and, of particular importance to the dentist, he is much more liable to acquire hepatitis virus B infection and HIV infection (see Ch. 2). Suspicion of addiction may be raised by tremors, restless movements, facial twitching, coryza, blood staining on the clothes from injections, injection marks particularly

over veins, or multiple superficial venous thromboses.

Barbiturate and benzodiazepine addiction

Barbiturates are effective sedatives and used to be extremely widely prescribed for use during the day and as hypnotics at night. In recent years it has been realized that addiction is easily acquired and that the chronic use of barbiturates can lead to confusion, defective judgment, and loss of emotional control. Addicted patients can show a picture similar to alcoholism, with dysarthria, tremor, ataxia, and seizures due to drug withdrawal. The use of barbiturates is now frowned on in Britain, their place being taken by benzodiazepine preparations such as diazepam and nitrazepam. However, addiction to benzodiazepines is now common, and also results in physical problems such as withdrawal seizures. They must be prescribed only in short courses for disabling symptoms.

FUNCTIONAL PSYCHOSES

In contrast to the organic psychoses, the functional psychoses are characterized by a pathological state of mind producing gross distortion of reality without any discernible physical abnormality in the brain or underlying abnormality in other systems of the body. The two most important forms are the depressive, manic or manic-depressive psychoses, and the schizophrenic psychoses.

Depressive and manic psychoses

These are characterized by a profound and morbid disorder of mood without intellectual impairment. They are often referred to as the affective psychoses. A family history is common.

The *depressive* variety is characterized by loss of enjoyment of life, inability to concentrate, tearfulness, remorseless self criticism, profound feelings of guilt and unworthiness, and by suicidal ideas which are sometimes translated into action. Associated with these morbid thoughts are symptoms which may be mistakenly interpreted as indicative of a physical disorder; indeed the patient frequently seeks medical advice for such symptoms rather than for the disorder of mood. The most common symptoms are loss of appetite, loss of weight, disturbance of sleep (difficulty in getting off to sleep and early morning awakening), constipation, atypical headache or facial pain (see Ch. 18), diminution in sexual desire, and amenorrhoea.

The *manic* variety of the affective psychoses is characterized by a markedly abnormal elevation of mood which makes the individual very restless, agitated and overactive, and leads him into a round of activities which he is unable to carry out efficiently and into which he has lack of insight. He may undertake financial or personal commitments he is later to regret or unable to meet and he is resentful of any advice that his actions are precipitate, ill-judged, and inappropriate.

Some patients, the manic depressives, may swing from one extreme of mood to the other or may display a mixed pattern of mood at the one time.

Management of the affective psychoses has been much improved by the psychotropic drugs which have powerful antidepressant or tranquillizing effects. The principal antidepressant drugs are tricyclic preparations (e.g. imipramine, amitryptiline) which tend to be more effective and to have fewer side-effects than the monoamine oxidase inhibitors. Electroconvulsive therapy (ECT) is now much less widely used for the treatment of severe depression but it is still employed where there has been an inadequate response to antidepressant drug therapy and particularly if a serious risk of suicide remains. The manic variety of the affective psychoses is often responsive to the tranquillizer drugs, particularly the phenothiazine group (e.g. chlorpromazine). Lithium salts are effective in long-term prevention of attacks of depression or mania. Careful monitoring of blood lithium levels at clinics is required.

The schizophrenic psychoses

The term schizophrenia, which literally means split mind, is a common and very serious functional psychotic disorder which affects 0.8% of the population. It usually commences between the ages of 15 and 25 years. Characteristic features include loss of initiative, withdrawal from social contacts, lack of emotional warmth, deterioration in intellectual capacity, and progressive disorder of thought processes. Hallucinations (especially threatening voices) are common; bizarre or paranoid delusions may be present; the individual may feel that he is under the control of external influences and that thoughts are being put into his mind. Phenothiazine drugs improve the symptoms in many patients, often quite dramatically, and they may be able to return to the community, hopefully to a sheltered pattern of life. Phenothiazine drugs are often given as intramuscular depot injections every 2–4 weeks. Relapses, often necessitating readmission to hospital, and with an increasing deterioration in personality, are a common pattern and some patients require long-term care in psychiatric hospitals. The patient with schizophrenia is particularly at risk of suicide, especially in the early acute stages.

A specific *paranoid psychosis* without other features of schizophrenia may develop in middle age, characterized by delusions of persecution, and resulting in inappropriate complaints and litigation.

NEUROTIC ILLNESSES

The neuroses are much more common than the psychoses and are less serious. Although the individual may develop quite disabling symptoms they tend to be an exaggerated form of many natural reactions (e.g. anxiety or fear of illness). Contact with the realities of everyday life is usually maintained and delusional ideas, hallucinations, or profound disturbances of thought processes are absent.

Anxiety neurosis

The major feature in this disorder is excessive anxiety which may express itself in recurrent bouts of panic, in intense fear of illness (hypochondriasis), of choking (globus hystericus), of being in enclosed spaces (claustrophobia), of being in open spaces (agoraphobia), of mixing with people, or of animals. The patient is usually tense, sweats excessively, sleeps poorly, may have a tremor, and commonly has tachycardia. Such patients frequently present to their doctors with insomnia, palpitations, atypical chest pains, or tension headaches (see Ch. 18). In managing such patients it is obviously important to exclude organic disease, including thyrotoxicosis, and to provide reassurance and support both medically and within the family. Sedation with a benzodiazepine preparation such as diazepam is commonly employed, but should not be continued for more than a few weeks, to avoid dependence.

Hysteria

The hysteric (from the Greek word for the womb, hystera, since this was considered the origin of the disorder) is usually an immature individual whose personality has not developed sufficiently to cope in a stable and constructive manner with the harsher realities, setbacks, and disappointments of life. When faced with problems hysterics tend to overreact, often in an extravagant and histrionic manner. They are often very suggestible and are easily hypnotized. Faced with difficulties they commonly indulge in childhood reactions such as denial or magical thinking and, like children, often look to others to solve their personal difficulties. At times of stress they may develop conversion symptoms (conversion hysteria) in which a physical illness is mimicked (e.g. paralysis of a limb, inability to speak, loss of sensation over part of the body), the apparent physical illness being quite unconsciously an honourable escape mechanism from an intolerable situation. Others may develop periods of amnesia as a reaction to unacceptable events (disassociation). As with anxiety states, it is important to demonstrate the absence of physical disease and to provide reassurance and support.

Obsessional or compulsive neuroses

An obsession is a fixed idea or delusion that the individual cannot dispel from the mind even though it is recognized that the idea is irrational if not absurd. A compulsion is an irresistible urge to perform a particular act even though the individual knows that it is pointless if not harmful. Obsessions may take the form of ideas or images which haunt the mind, or phobias, or of ruminations in which a problem or series of problems is turned over in the mind in an endless and senseless way. Compulsions can be very frightening and may involve acts of vi-

olence, or may be harmless although bizarre. Many individuals with milder forms of obsessional/compulsive states are able to lead reasonably normal lives although they tend to be preoccupied with detail, unimaginative, rigid in outlook, and conscientious to a fault. If obsessional ideas are severe the patient may become very distressed and agitated or may become quite severely depressed, and skilled psychiatric management will be essential.

PERSONALITY DISORDERS

The borderline between a normal personality and a personality disorder is almost always difficult to define and obviously may vary depending on the individual making the judgement. The adolescent punk rocker with strands of multicoloured hair and safety pins in his nostrils considers himself one of his peer group, and therefore normal, whereas he is likely to be classified as distinctly odd by the conformist majority. It is wise to reserve the term 'personality disorder' for someone who over a period of years has a pattern of maladjustment to society which exceeds that of the social misfit or eccentric. It is also important not to make dismissive value judgements bearing in mind that many very gifted individuals who could be classified as having had a personality disorder have made enormous contributions to our cultural life.

Within the framework of personality disorders will be included many chronic alcoholics, sexual deviants, drug addicts, and those with markedly antisocial traits who are considered to be psychopaths. A psychopath may conveniently be defined as someone who has a severe disorder of personality, emotional adjustment, or maturation which leads him to behave in an extreme and often violent manner and which renders him unable to develop and sustain a non-destructive and productive social and emotional relationship. Aggressive behaviour, lack of feeling, lack of remorse, inability to learn from mistakes, and lack of trust are common features. The condition is more likely to be seen in individuals who have had periods of emotional and social deprivation in childhood.

MENTAL SUBNORMALITY

The most common cause of mental retardation rendering the individual incapable of leading an independent existence is Down's syndrome or mongolism. This is due to trisomy of chromosome 21. Such children are mentally retarded and have stunted growth. The bridge of the nose is poorly developed, the eyes are slanting, the little finger is curved, the joints are hyperextensible, and the palms are broad. Children with Down's syndrome are more likely to be born to older mothers (over 35 years) probably because of faulty chromosome production by the ageing ovary. Antenatal diagnosis with the option of selective termination is now available for high-risk mothers.

People with Down's syndrome and other individuals who have severe mental retardation, frequently require to be cared for in institutions, and the dentist should always remember that in such institutions the incidence of infection with hepatitis B virus is increased. Special precautions are therefore required when carrying out dental treatment in any such individuals (see Ch. 2).

Index